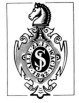

Arthritis of the Knee

Clinical Features and Surgical Management

Edited by M.A.R. Freeman

With Contributions of J.H. Aubriot, R.S. Bryan, J. Charnley
M.B. Coventry, H.L.F. Currey, R.A. Denham, M.A.R. Freeman
I.F. Goldie, N. Gschwend, J. Insall, P.G.J. Maquet, L.F.A. Peterson
J.M. Sheehan, S.A.V. Swanson, R.C. Todd

With 206 Figures

Springer-Verlag Berlin Heidelberg New York 1980

M.A.R. Freeman, M.D. F.R.C.S.
The London Hospital Medical College
University of London
Bone and Joint Research Unit
Arthritis and Rheumatism Council Building
25–29 Ashfield Street

London E1 2AD, Great Britain

ISBN 3-540-09699-X Springer-Verlag Berlin Heidelberg New York
ISBN 0-387-09699-X Springer-Verlag New York Heidelberg Berlin

Library of Congress Cataloging in Publication Data.
Main entry under title:
Arthritis of the knee.
Includes bibliographical references and index. 1. Knee-Diseases. 2. Arthritis. 3. Knee-Surgery. I. Aubriot, J.H. II. Freeman, Michael
Alexander Reykers. [DNLM: 1. Knee-Surgery. 2. Arthritis-Surgery. WE870 A786]
RC951.A74   616.7'22   79-27335
ISBN 3-540-09699-X
ISBN -387-09699-X

Typesetting, printing and bookbinding: Universitätsdruckerei H. Stürtz AG, Würzburg
2124/3140-543210

Preface

Early in its development, the subject matter of any field of surgery is too ill-defined and opinions are too fluid for the production of a book on the subject to be possible. Late in its development, controversy is at an end, and although it is still possible to produce a textbook, it is too late to produce a book that might stimulate discussion and crystallise ideas. This book has that objective, it being the Editor's view that the field of the surgical treatment of arthritis of the knee had reached an appropriate intermediate stage in 1978 when this text was written.

Three broad issues stand out as being in need of resolution before the optimum form of surgical treatment for a given knee can be defined more convincingly than is possible at present:

Firstly: What symptomatic and physical features of the knee are to be recorded pre- and post-operatively, upon the basis of which comparisons can be made between the results obtained by two different surgeons or with two different techniques. The resolution of this issue requires general agreement not only upon what features of the knee should be recorded but, crucially, upon how these features should subsequently be presented so as to characterise a particular group of knees.

Secondly: It has become clear that the success or failure of an osteotomy or arthroplasty is heavily dependent upon the surgeon's success in restoring the knee to its correct alignment under load. Clinical results presented without reference to this parameter (as have been most clinical results to date) are almost valueless. In view of the crucial importance of alignment, three questions must be answered: What is "correct" alignment? How can the alignment of a particular knee under load be measured accurately? How can the surgeon achieve the correct alignment with absolute reliability at operation? In the present author's view the answer to the third question is bound up with the design of appropriate instruments: in just the same way as it is difficult to draw a straight line by eye but easy with a ruler, it is difficult to put a leg straight by eye but easy to do so with instruments designed for the purpose.

Thirdly: If the malaligned knee is to be straightened surgically, it is essential for the surgeon to have a clear, accurate knowledge of the nature of the gross morbid anatomical events that are responsible for that malalignment. Only then can he reverse them. That a surgeon should have a good working knowledge of surgical pathology is axiomatic in most fields of surgery: oddly this area seems to have been neglected in arthritis, so that there is still controversy, for example, as to the extent to which medial bone destruction as against lateral soft-tissue elongation is responsible for varus instability and why such a malalignment should sometimes be fixed, sometimes passively correctable.

Turning to surgical treatment, the position, although still confused, is steadily becoming clearer. Thus arthrodesis is now used only as a salvage procedure. Soft-tissue operations, with the possible exception of meniscectomy, have nothing to offer in osteoarthritis (OA), and osteotomy has little or nothing to offer in rheumatoid arthritis (RA). Thus the early osteoarthrosic knee should be treated by conservative means, by osteotomy, or possibly by unicompartmental replacement – osteotomy being perhaps most appropriate for young adults with a varus knee without flexion deformity. Many surgeons and rheumatologists feel that early RA is now best treated conservatively, although some feel that synovectomy still has a place if disabling synovitis persists in spite of adequate conservative treatment. To understand this indication the surgeon must know what constitutes "adequate conservative treatment" and what it can achieve.

For all other knees some form of replacement is now thought to be appropriate. Although at first sight, there appears to be a bewilderingly wide range of implants with which the knee can be replaced, these devices in fact fall into a limited number of families, each of which is described in one of the chapters of this book.

Most implants replace all the articular surfaces of the tibio-femoral joint, but some can be used to replace only one compartment. The role of such unicompartmental procedures is unclear: some surgeons do not use an arthroplasty of this type at all, while others use it in early unicompartmental OA that might otherwise be treated by osteotomy.

If both compartments are to be replaced, the surgeon has a choice between retaining or sacrificing the cruciate ligaments. If they are retained, a two-component or a four-component prosthesis can be used. If they are sacrificed, the knee can then be replaced with a fully stabilised implant (i.e., a hinge), a semistabilized implant, or an implant having little or no inherent stability. Of these three categories, the first two require intramedullary stems for fixation to the skeleton, but the third can be confined to the surfaces of the bones. Counter-balancing this advantage for the minimally stabilised implants, however, is the fact that such surface prostheses, used after cruciate sacrifice, require special instruments for their insertion if the knee is to be correctly aligned and stabilised.

Finally, the necessity for and advantages of patello-femoral replacement are controversial: perhaps another 3–5 years will be required to resolve this issue. Should patello-femoral replacement turn out to be desirable, four-component implants retaining the cruciate ligaments will be at a disadvantage, since the addition of two further components to such a device would hardly be practicable.

These and other issues are dealt with in separate chapters of this book. The basic biomechanics of the natural and replaced knee is dealt with by Prof. S.A.V. SWANSON, Professor of Biomechanics at Imperial College London. The question of how best to record and present clinical data describing the knee is covered by Mr. R.C. TODD, who has been in charge of the Knee Clinic at The London Hospital for some years, and by Prof. N. GSCHWEND, Zürich, Switzerland. That these two surgeons have a shared view on the subject and that this view is so closely similar to that of the British Orthopaedic Association encourages the hope that agreement on this fundamental issue cannot be far away. Mr. R. DENHAM, a busy practising orthopaedic surgeon in Southampton, England, has spent some years investigating methods by which the alignment of the leg in relation to the line of action of the body weight can be determined in routine clinical practice. Since it is perhaps the English-speaking countries that have most particularly neglected the radiological assessment of knee alignment, it is appropriate to mark our conversion by placing this chapter in the hands of an Englishman. Finally, I have taken the liberty of setting down some of my own observations of the surgical pathology made at operation over the last 10 years. I have also contributed to some of the other chapters.

With regard to treatment, Prof. H.L.F. CURREY, Professor of Rheumatology at The London Hospital Medical College, describes the best that modern conservative management can offer in OA and RA. It is essential for the surgeon to understand the rheumatologists' capabilities, since only when these have been exhausted does surgery have a part to play. A Scandinavian surgeon, Prof. I. GOLDIE, writes on soft-tissue procedures, since synovectomy remains popular for RA in Sweden. Osteotomy is described by one of its most ardent protagonists, P.G.J. MAQUET. Arthrodesis has been described by Sir John CHARNLEY, whose contribution to this field is too well known to require further mention. Finally, there are five chapters describing the results to be achieved with one member of each of the families of replacement procedures described above. In each case the originator of one of the most widely used examples of each group has been asked to contribute, the choice of author being an invidious editorial task, arbitrarily discharged.

If this volume helps to clarify the issues and does nothing else, its production will have been justified.

London, March 1980   M.A.R. FREEMAN

Table of Contents

**Chapter 11. Tibio-femoral Replacement Using
a Totally Constrained Prosthesis and Cruciate
Resection. (The Guépar Prosthesis)**
(J.H. Aubriot)

**Chapter 12. Tibio-femoral Replacement Using
a Semi-stabilised Prosthesis and Cruciate Resection
(The Sheehan, GSB, Attenborough and
Spherocentric Prostheses)**
(J.M. Sheehan)

**Chapter 13. Tibio-femoral Replacement Using Two
Un-linked Components and Cruciate Resection.
(The ICLH and Total Condylar Prostheses)**
(M.A.R. Freeman and J. Insall)

List of Contributors

J.H. AUBRIOT, Professor
Centre Hospitalier Universitaire de Caen
Service de Chirurgie Orthopédique
Avenue George-Clemenceau,
Caën/France

R.S. BRYAN, M.D.
Department of Orthopaedic Surgery
Mayo Clinic and Mayo Foundation
Rochester, Minnesota 55901, USA

Sir JOHN CHARNLEY, Professor
Wrightington Hospital,
Wigan, Lancashire WN6 9EP
England

M.B. COVENTRY, M.D.
Department of Orthopaedic Surgery
Mayo Clinic and Mayo Foundation
Rochester, Minnesota 55901, USA

H.L.F. CURREY, Professor
The London Hospital
London E1 2AD, England

R.A. DENHAM, F.R.C.S.
The Royal Portsmouth Hospital
Commercial Road
Portsmouth, Hants, England

M.A.R. FREEMAN, F.R.C.S.
The London Hospital
London E1 2AD, England

I.F. GOLDIE, M.D. Associate Professor
Department of Orthopaedic Surgery
University of Göteborg, Sweden

N. GSCHWEND, Professor
Schulthess Stiftung
Neumünsterallee 3
CH-8032 Zürich

J. INSALL, M.D.
517 E 71st Street
New York
NY 10021/USA

P.G.J. MAQUET, Docteur
25, Thier Bosset
B-4070 Aywaille, Belgium

L.F.A. PETERSON, M.D.
Department of Orthopaedic Surgery
Mayo Clinic and Mayo Foundation
Rochester, Minnesota 55901, USA

J.M. SHEEHAN, F.R.C.S.I.
St. Vincents Hospital
Elm Park
Donnybrook
Dublin 4/Ireland

S.A.V. SWANSON, Professor
Biomechanics Unit, Department of Mechanical
Engineering
Imperial College
London SW 7 2 BX/England

R.C. TODD, F.R.C.S.
Essex County Hospital
Lexton Road
Colchester, Essex/England

Chapter 1

Biomechanics

S.A.V. SWANSON

Biomechanics Unit, Department of Mechanical Engineering, Imperial College, London SW7 2BX, England

Mechanics is the science of forces and movements. In most systems, the forces acting are related to the movements occurring, and a complete description must therefore include forces, movements, and their interactions. This is certainly true of any joint of the human skeleton when the activities of ordinary living are being performed; yet something can usefully be said about the forces and the movements separately. This Chapter will deal with the biomechanics of the knee by describing what is known of the movements and the forces, first with reference to the natural knee and secondly with reference to knee prostheses.

Movements of the Normal Knee

Movements Under Load and Under No Load

One special aspect of the interdependence of movements and forces is that the motion of the normal knee is indeterminate (within limits) unless load is applied. This is easily verified by direct observation; even in the fully extended (or slightly hyperextended) position, which is generally supposed to be the one position in which the joint is "locked" by a "screw-home" mechanism, laxity or elasticity of the ligaments allows a few degrees of ad- or abduction if the knee is not carrying a compressive load. In all other positions, the fact that force is needed to make the movements determinate is more obvious. In kinematic terminology, the knee joint is a "force-closed mechanism", whereas the normal hip joint, for example, is a "self-closed mechanism". The practical significance of this is that all descriptions, some of which have been elaborate, of the movements of the knee joint should be accompanied by a specification

of the force system acting when the movements were observed.

Three-dimensional Nature of Movement

The basic movement at the knee joint when it transmits compressive loads between the femur and the tibia is rotation about an axis which is not fixed relative to either the tibia or the femur. An axis that moves relative to the bodies concerned is known in kinematics as an instantaneous axis, because it occupies any one position for only an instant while the motion is taking place. To find the successive positions of an instantaneous axis that has a significantly three-dimensional movement is fairly complicated, but the principle can be described with reference to a simplified system in which the axis always remains parallel to one particular direction, i.e., it moves in space by translating sideways but not by tilting. In this case all motion takes place in planes perpendicular to the axis, and if one of the two bodies (e.g., the femur) is fixed, any one point fixed in the other body (the tibia) will move in a plane perpendicular to the axis. If this plane is made the plane of a diagram (Fig. 1), successive positions of the instantaneous axis will all be perpendicular to the plane of the diagram. In any movement small enough for the instantaneous axis not to move significantly, a point A in the tibia will describe a small arc of a circle; the line drawn as the perpendicular bisector of the chord of this arc must pass through the instantaneous axis. The same is true of any other point fixed in the tibia. Thus if the problem is to find the unknown positions of the instantaneous axis, the solution is now apparent: choose two points, say A and B, select a set of corresponding positions A_1B_1, A_2B_2, A_3B_3 etc., draw the chords A_1A_2, B_1B_2, A_2A_3, B_2B_3, etc., draw the perpendicular bisector of each chord, and the inter-

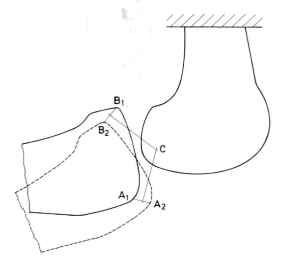

Fig. 1. Finding the instantaneous centre of the moving tibia relative to the fixed femur, assuming the motion to be only in the plane of the diagram. A and B are points fixed in the tibia; their positions at the beginning and end of a small movement are A_1, B_1 and A_2, B_2; the instantaneous centre C for that part of the motion is the point of intersection of the perpendicular bisectors of $A_1 A_2$ and $B_1 B_2$

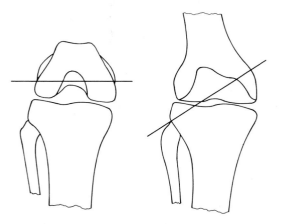

Fig. 2. The positions of the instantaneous axis of flexion-extension according to ELFTMAN (1954), with the knee flexed (*left*) and extended (*right*). In flexion, rotation about the long axis of the tibia is possible in addition to flexion-extension; the axis of this motion is not shown

sections of the corresponding perpendicular bisectors define the positions of the instantaneous axis. Thus in the diagram shown in Fig. 1, the intersection of the perpendicular bisectors of $A_1 A_2$ and $B_1 B_2$ defines, for that interval of the motion, the

point C at which the instantaneous axis intersects the plane of the diagram. Ideally the intervals chosen should be infinitesimally small for a truly instantaneous centre to be found; but in practice a few trials on a particular system will show how small the intervals need be to obtain the relevant degree of accuracy.

If the instantaneous axis really does not tilt, i.e., if the motion is truly two-dimensional, then any plane perpendicular to the axis could be chosen for the procedure described above. If the direction of the instantaneous axis is not known, or is variable, then the procedure for finding successive positions of the axis is considerably more complicated than that described above, though based on the same principles.

Treating the system as three-dimensional, ELFTMAN (1954) stated that the instantaneous axis occupied the positions shown in Fig. 2. According to this description, at or near full extension the axis is inclined at about 60° to the long axis of the femur, while in flexion it is roughly perpendicular to the shaft of the femur.

Extensive observation of the movements of the leg segments during level walking was an essential part of the "*Fundamental Study of Human Locomotion*" performed at the University of California in 1945–1947 (EBERHART et al., 1947). Some observations were made on subjects who had volunteered to have lightweight pylons screwed into the cortices of the iliac crest, a femoral condyle, and a tibial condyle under local anaesthesia, so that the relative movements of the bones themselves could be observed without errors due to the movement of skin relative to bone. Other observations were made in subjects walking with small visual targets or light sources attached to the skin close to each joint of the leg, multiple-exposure photography being used to record the position of these points in three dimensions. Figure 3 shows the rotation of the tibia relative to the femur during a walking step, as observed in three mutually perpendicular directions: from the side, from the front, and from above. The three components of rotatory movement thus described are not, of course, the three customarily described as flexion, abduction, and rotation, because only in special cases, and then only at a few instants, is the axis of the femur perpendicular to two of the viewing directions (from the side and from the front). Nevertheless, the existence of significant movement (a range of 17° in the subject chosen for Fig. 3) as seen from the front shows that the instantaneous axis cannot

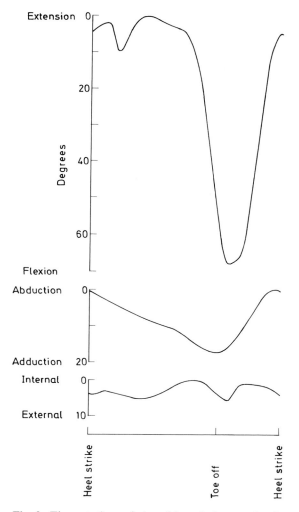

Fig. 3. The rotation of the tibia relative to the femur during level walking, as seen from the side (*top curve*), from the front (*middle curve*) and from above (*bottom curve*). From EBERHART et al. (1947): 19 year old male subject

Movements at the Knee and at Adjacent Joints

At first sight, the provision at the knee of a joint so much more complicated than a simple hinge might seem out of place for one of the chief uses of the leg: locomotion by level walking. It is therefore worth noting that the several joints of the normal leg collectively provide what is needed for an economical translation of the torso. The hip is, for all macroscopic purposes, a ball-and-socket joint with three rotational degrees of freedom. The knee, as has just been outlined, is a joint whose rotations about three axes are determinately related when under load. The tibio-talar joint is very nearly a uniaxial pivot with its axis almost horizontal and transverse. The subtalar complex is less simple than it may appear, but during walking it provides rotation about an axis that is roughly horizontal and parallel to the direction of walking. The path of the centre of gravity of the torso is not a straight line as seen from either the side or above; during the swing phase, the foot is obviously free to rotate about any axis relative to a fixed frame of reference, but it is not free to do so during the stance phase, unless friction between the shoe and the ground is unusually low. This is not the place for a full description of the kinematics of walking; these facts are mentioned partly to show that the complicated nature of the movements at the knee fits into the characteristics of the complete system, and partly as a reminder that even the most elaborate knee replacement implants are much less subtle than the natural joint.

Two-dimensional Simplifications

It is common to write of the "instantaneous centre" of the knee, which implies that the instantaneous axis is always perpendicular to a fixed plane, usually implicitly the sagittal plane. If this is so, the points at which the successive positions of the instantaneous axis intersect the chosen plane are called the instantaneous centres, and the curve joining the successive positions of the instantaneous centre, often called the centrode, characterises the motion. Since the two bodies (the femur and the tibia) move relative to each other, the path of the instantaneous centre relative to the femur will not be the same as that relative to the tibia, and it is important to specify which of the two is meant.

always be parallel to any given direction. During the swing phase of a walking step, the knee joint is under muscular loads only, and may then be thought to be "unloaded" in the conventional sense of weight-bearing; but it should be observed that during the stance phase, when the joint is certainly weight-bearing, the ranges of movement were 44°, 17°, and 4° as seen from the side, the front, and above, respectively, in the one subject for whom all three measurements were reported; other subjects showed larger ranges of movement as seen from above (see Table 1).

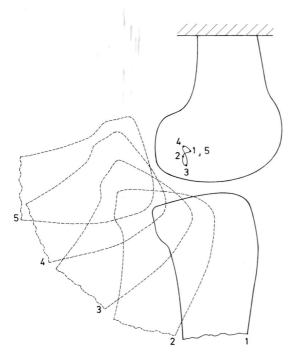

Fig. 4. Positions relative to the femur of the instantaneous centre of the tibio-femoral motion in extension and at four angles of flexion. Normal knee, 17 year old male (subjects aged up to 48 years showed similar patterns). Re-drawn from FRANKEL et al., 1971

This simplification was used by FRANKEL et al. (1971), who took lateral radiographs at intervals of 10°–20° from full extension to 90° of flexion with the knee not bearing weight; they discarded radiographs showing evidence of significant rotation about the long axis of the tibia, thereby making some attempt to stay within the restrictions implied by the assumption that the instantaneous axis does not tilt. The instantaneous centre was found to move; a representative set of positions is shown in Fig. 4 (this has been re-drawn to show the position relative to the femur instead of relative to the tibia as presented by the authors). It will be seen that the total movement of the instantaneous centre is only a few millimetres, either vertically or horizontally. Such movements may be important for the internal mechanics of the knee (and the main point of the paper by FRANKEL et al. was that whereas in normal knees the instantaneous centre was always placed so that the relative movement at the articular surfaces was tangential, in deranged knees there was a component of movement perpendicular to the articular surfaces), but can have only a small effect on the gross move-

ments of one limb segment relative to another. It is therefore not surprising that DENHAM and BISHOP (1978), in experiments with cadaveric knees, found that a point several centimetres along the tibial shaft described a path that was effectively circular relative to the femur within the accuracy of the observations when a pencil was attached to the tibia and a sheet of paper fixed relative to the femur.

How the Motion is Controlled

Because the articular surfaces are considerably incongruent and the menisci that reduce the incongruity are flexible and mobile, the motion of the joint cannot be controlled by these surfaces, and the ligaments must contribute. The collateral ligaments obviously serve, by elastic forces, to limit almost all the movements that can take place, but acting alone they would be inadequate to control antero-posterior gliding with any precision, and the contribution of the cruciate ligaments is therefore important.

As is well known, when viewed laterally the cruciate ligaments are crossed, and the system consisting of the femur, the tibia, and the cruciate ligaments has often been regarded in kinematic terms as a crossed four-bar chain. In such a chain the instantaneous centre is always at the intersection of the two crossed bars, and in a two-dimensional system with rigid links the positions of the instantaneous centre throughout the whole range of motion are therefore determined. Figure 5 shows the path of the instantaneous centre for a crossed four-bar chain in which the dispositions of the links are similar to those in a representative knee. The knee differs from this model in three respects: the motion is not two-dimensional, the cruciate ligaments can stretch under load, and the ligaments can be slack.

In experiments on unloaded cadaveric knees, BLACHARSKI et al. (1975) found that the instantaneous axis moved significantly both by translating and by tilting; in one knee, the instantaneous axis was inclined to the lateral horizontal axis at an angle varying from 2°–21°, and in four of the five knees tested the axis moved between 5 and 17 mm in a proximal–distal direction and between 10 and 15 mm antero-posteriorly, as measured in para-sagittal planes touching the knee medially and laterally. These observations are mentioned here partly because the authors found that cutting

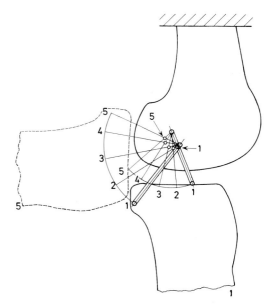

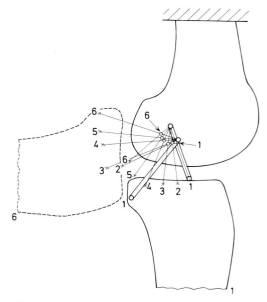

Fig. 5. The path of the instantaneous centre of the tibia relative to the fixed femur, assuming that the motion is only in the plane of the diagram and that the cruciate ligaments function as rigid links in a crossed four-bar chain, the other two members being the femur and the tibia. Five successive positions of the instantaneous centre are shown by the small circles

Fig. 6. The path of the instantaneous centre of the tibia relative to the femur, constructed on the same basis as that in Fig. 5 but with the cruciate ligaments changing in length as calculated by TRENT et al., 1976

both cruciate ligaments produced little change in the motions of the instantaneous axis. Whether this would be so with the knee under load is a different question; but the movements of the instantaneous axis with the ligaments intact are unlikely to be much larger under load than under no load, and the translations seen by BLACHARSKI et al. are likely to represent the upper limit of those that occur in normal knees under load. The translations in a plane passing through the centre of the knee could not be larger than the larger of those observed in the two planes medial and lateral to the joint, and in general they would be smaller; thus, even with the reservations arising from the use of cadaveric knees under no load, the observations of BLACHARSKI et al. suggest that the total translational movement of the instantaneous axis is a matter of about 10 mm in all in each direction. This is compatible with the observations of FRANKEL et al. (1971) in living normal knees not bearing weight (Fig. 4).

Turning to the question of ligament stretching, TRENT et al. (1976) performed tensile tests on cruciate ligaments and found extensions at rupture of about 10 mm. The same authors calculated that the cruciate ligaments increased in length by up to 5 or 6 mm in the range of knee movement from full extension to 105° of flexion (the posterior ligament being tighter in flexion and the anterior in extension). If the rigid system of Fig. 5 is modified by allowing the links representing the cruciate ligaments to stretch as calculated by TRENT et al., the effect on the path of the instantaneous centre is as shown in Fig. 6.

It appears that within the error of all such observations and the variations between individuals, the translations of the instantaneous axis can to a large extent be attributed to the action of the cruciate ligaments; but the articular surfaces and menisci must have something to do with controlling the motion.

First, the fact that the menisci are flexible and mobile means that even with the menisci in place, the tibial articular surface does not match the femoral condyles, and the motion cannot be determined by the articular surfaces alone. To take an extreme example, even if both femoral condyles were of constant curvature as seen laterally, it would not follow that the motion of the tibia relative to the femur would be one of simple rotation

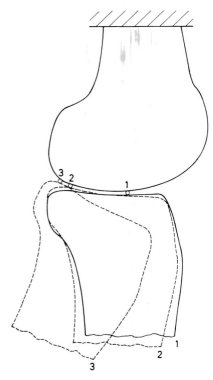

Fig. 7. If the motion of the tibia on the femur were pure rolling with no sliding, the instantaneous centre would always be at the point of contact, and would move posteriorly along the femoral and tibial condyles as the knee flexed; three positions are shown by the *small circles*

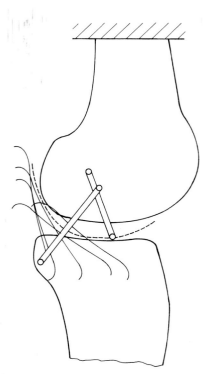

Fig. 8. If the cruciate ligaments were inextensible and always tight, and if the motion were two-dimensional, successive positions of the tibia relative to the fixed femur would be as shown, and the envelope of these successive positions (shown as a *broken line*) would be similar to a representative femoral condyle

about a fixed axis passing through the centre of curvature of the femoral condyles, because the tibia with the menisci in place is free to rock, within limits, about the point of contact. If this rocking takes place unaccompanied by sliding, the instantaneous axis passes through the contact point (Fig. 7). It is well known that the point of contact moves over a longer distance on the femoral condyles than on the tibial condyles as the knee moves from extension to flexion; this fact means that the motion of the tibia relative to the femur is not simple rotation about the point of contact and that the relative motion at the articular surfaces usually involves sliding.

Because a major function of the articular surfaces is obviously to transmit compressive force, it could be argued that their shapes are simply such as to bring a large enough area on the two bones into contact, more or less perpendicular to the direction of the resultant force, in positions dictated by the movements of the instantaneous axis

as controlled by the cruciate ligaments. KAPANDJI (1970) has shown that the shape of the femoral condyle is close to that which would be obtained by drawing the tibial articular surface in the successive positions determined by the successive positions of the instantaneous axis (supposing these to result from the operation of the cruciate ligaments). This is reproduced in Fig. 8, assuming, with KAPANDJI, that the cruciate ligaments are inextensible. If the cruciate ligaments are allowed to extend, as in Fig. 6, the corresponding condylar shape is as shown in Fig. 9. These shapes are so close to representative actual shapes as to show that the shapes of the femoral condyles are compatible with the movements imposed by the cruciate ligaments.

The question as to why cruciate ligaments are provided if the geometry of the condyles is compatible, and whether the articular surfaces cannot control the motion by themselves, may be raised. The answer is principally that incongruent articular

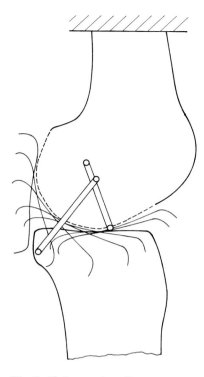

Fig. 9. If the cruciate ligaments are supposed to vary in length as calculated by TRENT et al. (1976), the envelope of Fig. 8 is modified but is still recognisably similar. (One position of the tibia must be ignored because it is incompatible with the others; the inference is that the calculations of TRENT et al. are in error at that point. Perhaps the calculated length of the posterior cruciate ligament at that point would correspond to its being slack)

surfaces with very low friction could control the motion if forces were always applied so as to be perpendicular to the surfaces at the contact point. If this condition were not met, the articular surfaces would slide and the joint would tend to be unstable. The provision of the cruciate ligaments, which can exert forces with significant components parallel to the articular surfaces, as the capsule and collateral ligaments cannot, allows the joint to remain stable even under a range of loading conditions. The tangential tibio-femoral forces calculated by DENHAM and BISHOP (1978) and the strengths of the cruciate ligaments measured by TRENT et al. (1976), referred to below, suggest that this function of these ligaments is significant in activities such as stair climbing.

The above discussion has been on the basis of the two-dimensional simplification commonly adopted. In fact, the two tibial articular surfaces

are not of exactly the same shape, and neither are the medial and lateral femoral condyles; these facts, together with the fact that the two cruciate ligaments do not lie in one plane, give rise to the three-dimensional nature of the actual motion. The macroscopic effects of this are referred to above and again below; the small-scale aspect was investigated by TRENT et al. (1976), who in their experiments on cadaveric knees found the instantaneous centre of rotation about the long axis of the tibia by a method similar to that shown in Fig. 1. At or near full extension, the instantaneous axis passed through the medial tibial condyle, usually fairly close to the centre of this condyle but sometimes medially; as flexion progressed the instantaneous axis moved laterally until in most knees it passed through the intercondylar eminence at about 100° of flexion. Antero-posteriorly, all positions of the axis were contained within a band occupying a little over the middle third of the tibial articular surface.

Movements Used in Daily Activities

The above discussion is based largely on anatomical observations and on measurements made on cadaveric knees or subjects performing special movements. It is natural, and relevant to surgery at the knee, to ask what movements are used in the activities of daily living.

In level walking, the work reported by EBERHART et al. (1947), mentioned above, was based on observations of ten subjects in the age range 19–27 years, but mostly in their early twenties. Other observations have been reported by MURRAY (1967), using interrupted-light photography, and by KETTELKAMP et al. (1970), using three-axis potentiometric goniometers. The ranges of motion reported are summarised, and quoted to the nearest degree, in Table 1. Any one of the ranges quoted can vary by several degrees between the two knees of one subject or between subjects. A vast literature has grown up around gait studies, and the influences of age, sex, and physique are being investigated; for the present purpose it is sufficient to note that three sets of observations recorded by means of essentially two noninvasive techniques have given results that for practical purposes are the same.

Activities other than level walking were included in a study by MCLEOD et al. (1975) of the knee movements of eight housewives in the age range

Table 1. Range of knee motion in level walking

Authors	Subjects			Range of motion (degrees)		
	Number	Sex	Ages	Flexion-Extension	Ad- and Abduction	Rotation
EBERHART et al. (1947)	10	M	19–27			4–19
	1	M	19	66	17	4
MURRAY (1967)	30	M	20–65	70		
KETTELKAMP et al. (1970)	16	M	21–35	68	11	13
	6	F	22	66	10	14

23–41 years. The total ranges of flexion–extension observed by means of single-axis goniometers with tape recorders were as follows:

Walking:	74°
Climbing stairs:	82°
Descending stairs:	90°
Sitting in and rising from chairs:	90°

The number of knee movements during the period of observation, including all activities, was an average of 410 movements per hour.

Rising from a chair 430 mm high was studied by SEEDHOM and TERAYAMA (1976) in two "normal athletic male students". When rising was unaided, the flexion angle varied from 8°–77°; when aided by the arms, from 6°–53°.

Forces Transmitted Through the Normal Knee

The Origin of Forces at the Knee

The knee, in common with the other joints of the lower limb, transmits force partly because of the weight which it supports, partly because of the muscles acting across it, and, sometimes, partly because at least one of the body segments connected by it is being accelerated.

If no muscles acted, in symmetrical two-legged standing each tibio-femoral joint would theoretically transmit half the weight of the part of the body above the knees, and in one-legged standing one knee would transmit the whole of the body weight less the weight of the leg segment below that knee. In fact some muscles always act, and

the effect of any muscular force, which is a tensile force between two body segments, is to increase the compressive force across the joint in question. In activities other than standing, because the moment arms of muscles about the knee (or any other joint) are smaller than the distances of the centres of gravity of the body segments, in general the muscular forces, and hence the joint forces, will be larger than the weights of the relevant body segments.

The joint forces referred to above are those applied to the system of articular surfaces, capsule, and ligaments. The forces in the last two are tensile, and tend to increase the compressive force across the articular surfaces; but because the forces in the capsule and the ligaments vary over a smaller range than muscular forces, their effect on the forces on the articular surfaces is less.

Methods of Measuring or Calculating Forces

Direct measurement of forces in a natural joint is obviously impossible within technical and ethical constraints. The closest approach to this is the measurement of forces transmitted through a joint prosthesis. This was done at the hip by RYDELL (1966), and knee prostheses incorporating force transducers and telemetry arrangements are known to be under development; but no results have so far been published. Any such results would of course relate to subjects who had needed knee replacement, and would not in general be relevant to normal subjects.

Failing direct measurement, noninvasive techniques have been used. The essential steps in any such technique are to observe the positions of all the relevant body segments, to measure the forces exerted where the body is in contact with e.g., the floor, and to discover or assume which muscle groups are acting. The calculations then made depend on whether or not there are significant accelerations. If there are, as in the swing phase of walking or in more vigorous activities, both the translational and the rotational accelerations of the relevant body segments must be found, usually by differentiating the displacements found from the record of successive positions twice with respect to time; then the corresponding inertia forces and moments can be calculated. From these, the foot–ground (or other) forces, and assumptions about the muscles acting and their lines of action, the joint forces can be calculated. If there are no significant accelerations, the inertia forces and moments are ignored but the calculation is otherwise the same.

This technique was first established by PAUL (1967) with reference to the hip, and was applied to the knee by MORRISON (1968, 1969, 1970a and b). HARRINGTON (1976) made the simplification of ignoring inertia forces, on the basis that the forces in the joints of the leg are higher during the stance phase of walking, when the accelerations are less important, than in the swing phase. For activities such as rising from a chair or stair climbing, it is customary to ignore inertia forces.

Accuracy of Calculations of Forces

The technique outlined above necessarily involves many assumptions and experimental observations, which are subject to error. Some of the major assumptions are as follows: The masses of individual body segments cannot be measured directly, and are commonly calculated by applying the coefficients of BRAUNE and FISCHER (1889), based on the dissection of the cadavers of Prussian infantrymen, to the major dimensions of the subject observed. The mass centres of body segments move as muscles change shape, but this effect is commonly ignored. If more muscle groups act than can be accommodated in the equations, those thought to be least important (often on the basis of electromyographic records) are ignored. The forces exerted by muscles are not measured directly, but are inferred by restricting their number (as just mentioned) and sometimes by assuming them to be related to the cross-sectional areas of the muscles in question. The lines of action of

the muscles are not known exactly, but are constructed from observations made on cadavers of the disposition of the areas of origin and insertion. The forces exerted by ligaments are unknown, and various assumptions are made about them.

Taking account of all these unavoidable assumptions and of the errors inherent in the experimental observations (which are chiefly the errors associated with observing the positions of targets on the skin, as mentioned under "Three-dimensional Nature of Movement", above), quoted values of joint force are likely to be in error by up to 20% in general, and sometimes perhaps by more. This is less serious than it may seem. If the information is to be applied to a large population, e.g., in the design of an implant, then the forces in the individuals in that population, if they were all calculated, would vary over a bigger range than 20% unless the population were unusually homogeneous. If the information is used in following the characteristics of one individual, e.g., a patient before and after surgery, then many of the unknown quantities about which assumptions have been made will remain reasonably constant for the one individual.

The Principal Forces at the Knee

Figure 10 shows a lateral view of the principal forces acting at a knee joint. Even this array of forces embodies some simplifications; in particular the force in each ligament or muscle is treated simply as one resultant force, although in fact the force is transmitted through a finite area of tissue and applied, not necessarily uniformly, to a finite and usually oblique area of bone, and the contact forces between cartilage surfaces are similarly treated as single resultants, although the tibio-femoral force is shared between the two compartments and the patello-femoral force is transmitted as two forces distributed over the two facets of the patellar articular surface.

There are of course many ways in which the force system could be represented. For example, some authors have referred to a tibio-femoral tangential force, and others to forces in the cruciate ligaments. The two are not completely interchangeable, since in some positions of the knee significant forces can be transmitted perpendicularly to the long axis of the tibia because the articular surfaces are significantly not flat.

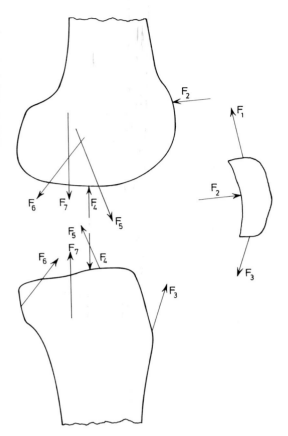

Fig. 10. Simplified array of forces acting between the femur, tibia and patella. Each force is shown as a resultant, whereas in fact each force would be distributed over a finite area of tissue

Published Values for Forces

In level walking by young adult males, BRESLER and FRANKEL (1950) found that the vertical force (not, in general, the same as the normal tibio-femoral force) rose to maxima of about 1.1 times the body weight. MORRISON (1969), observing three young adult males, found the normal tibio-femoral force to rise to between 3.05 and 3.73 times the body weight. HARRINGTON (1976), considering only the stance phase and ignoring inertial effects, found the normal tibio-femoral force to have maxima of twice to five times the body weight in four normal subjects.

JOHNSON and WAUGH (1979), using basically the techniques of HARRINGTON in a highly computerised form, found the joint force to rise to a maximum of six times the body weight in one 23-year-old normal male, and (personal communication)

to maxima of about three or four times the body weight in older subjects who walk more slowly.

MAQUET (1976) presented a calculation based on much the same kind of information as used by the other workers cited, but based less on extensive observations of particular subjects and more on detailed calculations. The compressive tibio-femoral force reached a maximum value of six times the body weight when certain assumptions were made about the position of the resultant force, or maximum values from 4.2–11.4 times body weight when different assumptions were made.

Attention has also been paid to other activities; these are important because knee forces would be expected to be higher in squatting or other activities (such as stair climbing or rising from a chair) in which body weight is supported with the knee significantly flexed than in level walking, where in the stance phase the knee is flexed by only a few degrees.

REILLY and MARTENS (1972), testing a subject with a body mass of 85 kg doing deep knee bends, found that the normal patello-femoral force rose from body weight at 60° of knee flexion to 7.6 times body weight at 130° of knee flexion. Perhaps of more general relevance are the values obtained during stair climbing by two subjects of unspecified body mass, which reached 2500–3000 N at 60° of knee flexion on a 200-mm step, and in descending stairs, 2500 N on a 200-mm step and 3500 N on a 400-mm step, both at 60° of knee flexion. If these subjects had body masses of about 70 kg (as can be inferred from the text) the maximum normal patello-femoral forces ranged up to almost five times the body weight when they were descending the 400-mm step, and 3.6–4.4 times the body weight when they were climbing the still unusually high step of 200 mm (a normal staircase having steps 150–170 mm high).

SMIDT (1973) performed experiments different from the general type described above, in that he measured the moment about the knee developed during resisted flexion and extension with no weight-bearing. With 26 subjects of body mass 57–107 kg, with an average of 82.4 kg, the average maximum normal patello-femoral force was 2160 N, or 2.7 times the average body weight; average maxima for the normal and tangential tibio-femoral forces were 2700 and 1470 N, respectively (3.3 and 1.8 times body weight). The last maximum corresponded to the tendency of the tibia to move posteriorly on the femur when the knee flexors

Table 2. Maximum forces at the knee

Activity	Authors	Maximum force as multiple of body weight		
		Tibio-femoral, normal	Tibio-femoral, tangential	Patello-femoral, normal
Knee bends	REILLY and MARTENS, 1972			7.6
	DENHAM and BISHOP, 1978	2.2	0.5	3.5
	PERRY et al., 1975 (cadaver)			2.1 [a]
Resisted extension	SMIDT, 1973	3.3	0.4	2.7
Rising from chair	SEEDHOM and TERAYAMA, 1976	2.04, 2.85	1.09, 1.04	2.36, 2.36
Climbing steps	REILLY and MARTENS, 1972			3.6–4.4
Level walking	MORRISON, 1969	3.05–3.73		
	HARRINGTON, 1976	2–5		
	JOHNSON and WAUGH, 1979	6		
	MAQUET, 1976	6	0.6	3

[a] Multiple of vertical force on femoral head, not of body weight (see text).

were acting; with the extensors acting, the corresponding value was 340 N (0.44 times body weight) in the opposite direction.

PERRY et al. (1975) used a different method again; they inserted force transducers in to the tibia, patella, and quadriceps tendon of a cadaveric leg from which soft tissues other than those about the knee had been removed, and loaded the preparation vertically through the femoral head. The normal tibio-femoral force corresponding to a load of 225 N at the femoral head was, for example, 600 N when the knee was flexed to 30°. The normal patello-femoral force, as a multiple of the vertical force applied to the femoral head, rose from 0.1 at 5° of knee flexion, through 0.6 at 30° and 1.2 at 45°, to 2.1 at 60°. In a live subject, the resultant force applied to the upper end of the femur would be the weight of that part of the body being supported, i.e., rather less than half the body weight in two-legged squatting and rather less than the body weight in one-legged squatting or climbing.

SEEDHOM and TERAYAMA (1976) studied two normal young males rising from a chair, and found the following maximum values, expressed as multiples of body weight: normal tibio-femoral force 2.04 and 2.85; normal patello-femoral force 2.36 and 2.36; tangential tibio-femoral force 1.09 and 1.04.

DENHAM and BISHOP (1978) studied three subjects doing knee bends with both legs weight-bearing. The forces calculated were presented on a basis of the angle between the thigh and the vertical,

and rose from low values to high values as this angle moved from 10°–40°. At a thigh angle of 40° the normal patello-femoral force was between 2.5 and 4 times the body weight, and it attained maxima, at thigh angles up to 80°, of 3.75–5 times body weight. In another subject, a physical training instructor, at a thigh angle of 40° the normal patello-femoral force was 3 times body weight and the normal tibio-femoral force was 1.5 times body weight, and maximum values of 3.5 and 2.2 times body weight, respectively, were reached when the thigh angle was 60°. These authors introduced some refinements and avoided the error, made by many earlier authors, of assuming the quadriceps and patellar tendon forces to be equal.

For ease of comparison, the maximum forces found by the authors quoted above are collected in Table 2.

Mode of Transmission of Force Through the Normal Knee

Tibio-femoral Joint

The basic means by which force is transmitted across the knee joint are clear: the femoral and tibial condyles are loaded in compression; the menisci are loaded in compression and, because they are wedge-shaped in cross-section, may be squeezed outwards radially and thereby stretched circumferentially; the ligaments can transmit only tensile forces, and the capsule can transmit tension and, to some extent, shear forces.

In the various investigations referred to above, the force calculated to be transmitted across the knee joint is usually that transmitted by the system including the articular surface, ligaments, and capsule but excluding any muscles. There is therefore some uncertainty about how this force is shared between the components of the joint. Because the ligaments and capsule transmit only tensile forces and the resultant force across the joint is compressive, if the ligaments transmit significant forces the articular surfaces must transmit correspondingly higher compressive forces to provide the same resultant force.

HARRINGTON (1976) considered, with various simplifying assumptions, the contributions made by the ligaments to force transmission in the stance phase of level walking. He found that in most subjects the anterior cruciate ligament transmitted force (to a maximum of about 250–400 N) during the early part of the stance phase and the posterior cruciate (to a maximum of about 300–500 N), in the later part of the stance phase. The medial collateral ligament transmitted trivial forces during the stance phase, but the lateral collateral transmitted significant force, up to about 400 N, during the second half of the stance phase. Considered against his calculated tibio-femoral forces of 2–5 times body weight (1 400–3 500 N for a typical body weight of 700 N), these values are not negligible, but they do suggest that the uncertainty surrounding any values of force calculated without knowledge of the ligamentous forces is less than the variation between individuals. The ligamentous forces that can be inferred from the observations of TRENT et al. (1976) are rather lower than HARRINGTON's. According to the results of MORRISON (1969), ignoring the forces in the cruciate ligaments leads to errors of less than 10% in the resultant joint force, which is compatible with the other findings just discussed.

MORRISON, HARRINGTON, and JOHNSON and WAUGH agree that during most of the stance phase of level walking more compressive force is transmitted through the medial than through the lateral compartment. In three of HARRINGTON's four subjects, more force was transmitted laterally than medially during about the first 10% of the stance phase, following heel strike. MAQUET (1976) states that "the load is distributed almost evenly on both plateaux".

From a knowledge of the distribution of load between the two compartments, it is natural to proceed to consideration of the contact areas in the two compartments. A few measurements have been reported. WALKER and HAJEK (1976) made methyl methacrylate castings of the joint space in cadaveric knees from which the menisci had been removed, a load of 1 500 N being applied while the cement was fluid. In three specimens, two normal and one with slight degeneration of the cartilage, the contact area on the lateral side ranged from 1–1.6 cm^2, and that on the medial side from 1.4–2.5 cm^2. The area on the medial side was fairly consistently larger, by 40%–50%, than that on the lateral side, and both areas decreased fairly consistently from full extension to 90° of flexion.

KETTELKAMP and JACOBS (1972) used a different technique, in which knee joints obtained at amputation were subjected to nominal loads of 30–80 N (up to about one-tenth of typical body weight) and were then surrounded by radiopaque liquid and radiographed along the axis of load. Thirteen specimens gave mean contact areas of 3 cm^2 laterally and 4.7 cm^2 medially at full extension, reducing to 2.4 and 3.8 cm^2, respectively, at 35° of flexion; standard deviations were about 1 cm^2. MAQUET (1976) used a similar method, but applied loads of 2 000–2 500 N after ensuring that the radiopaque liquid had penetrated to all parts of the joint. With the menisci intact, he found contact areas of 9.8 cm^2 laterally and 10.2 cm^2 medially at full extension, reducing to 4.8 and 6.7 cm^2, respectively, at 90° of flexion (most of the reduction occurred between 20° and 50° of flexion). With the menisci removed, the contact areas were reduced to about two-thirds of the above values.

Since MAQUET's contact areas at loads of 2 000–2 500 N are up to about 10 times larger than those of WALKER and HAJEK at loads of 1 500 N, there is apparently a difficulty. One would expect MAQUET's method to give a low estimate of the area, since the tendency would presumably be to expel the fluid incompletely. As MAQUET points out, when so high a load is applied the axis along which it is applied (determined by the experimenter) will influence the deformation of the cartilage in the two compartments and hence the two contact areas; but the effect on the sum of the two areas could hardly explain the difference between his results and those of WALKER and HAJEK. Those of KETTELKAMP and JACOBS pose less of a problem, because they were obtained at very low loads; they are potentially compatible with those of MAQUET.

Taking from Table 2 the highest forces estimated to act during level walking and the largest contact areas, a maximum force of about 6×700 N acts on a total area of about 20 cm^2, giving an average compressive stress of about 2.1 MN/m^2. From the information available it is not possible to say with certainty that the average stresses in the two compartments are or are not the same. Most calculations of forces agree, as reported above, that the axis of the resultant force is medial rather than lateral, and all measurements of contact area agree that the medial area is larger than the lateral; thus it is probable that the average stresses in the two compartments are roughly equal rather than considerably different. This of course refers to normal healthy subjects in level walking, and the suggested average stress under maximum load is the stress at the interface between the two cartilage surfaces, or between the meniscus and the adjacent cartilage; if one function of cartilage is to distribute stress, the stresses at the cartilage–bone junction may be more nearly uniform.

It is difficult to suppose that healthy menisci transmit no force, but how much they transmit has long been a subject of speculation or assertion. The fact that they are wedge-shaped in cross-section means that they could easily be squeezed out radially (the friction being very low) and therefore transmit very little load, but this movement is resisted by their having significant circumferential stiffness and being at least partly attached to the tibial plateau. Since they do not constitute complete rings, their circumferential stiffness would be irrelevant if their horns were not tethered, as they are. Such an arrangement, with more flexible location round the rest of the circumference, can in principle allow the menisci to change shape as required by the changing curvature of the femoral condyles, while still remaining stiff enough to carry load. Since two thicknesses of cartilage plus the thickest part of the meniscus are more compressible than two thicknesses of cartilage (unless the latter is appreciably thicker or softer than the cartilage in contact with the menisci), the menisci would transmit a share of the total load less than that commensurate with their area, unless they were preloaded. This could be achieved by arranging for the unloaded meniscus to be a little smaller than would naturally fit between the tibia and femur, so that these two bones would be held apart and under light loads the tibial plateau enclosed within the inner margin of the meniscus would not touch the femoral con-

dyle. As the load is increased, compression and outward movement of the menisci would, with this arrangement, allow load to be progressively transferred through the region of direct tibio-femoral contact. At some particular load the average stress in the region of direct contact would be the same as in the region covered by the menisci, and at higher loads the stresses in the region of direct contact would be higher than under the menisci. If the menisci do transmit significant forces, as seems inherently probable, it seems probable in turn that they do so under some such arrangement as that just outlined.

WALKER and ERKMAN (1975), using a casting technique similar to that of WALKER and HAJEK (1972) mentioned above, found that at no load virtually all contact was through the menisci; in the medial compartment some direct tibio-femoral contact was seen at loads of 500 N and upwards, but in the lateral compartment there was hardly any direct contact until the load had reached about 1000 N. SHRIVE et al. (1978) used a different method, first used by DAY et al. (1975) at the hip, in which load-bearing elements are successively removed and the proportions of the load transmitted by the several elements are calculated from load-deformation curves measured at each stage. SHRIVE et al. concluded that the menisci transmitted at least 45% of a load of 1000 N. They reported also that at loads below about half the body weight there was a gap between the tibial and the femoral condyles. BLAIMONT et al. (1975), by attaching strain gauges to the outside surface of the tibia at nine points around the circumference 5 mm below the tibial plateau, showed that at loads of up to 400 N the effect of meniscectomy was approximately to halve the strains in the cortical bone, showing that a significant fraction of the load had been transmitted to the more peripheral bone covered by the menisci.

All these observations, though incomplete and indirect, suggest strongly that at higher loads the menisci transmit a significant part, probably about half, of the total tibio-femoral compressive force, whilst at lower loads, perhaps those of below body weight or half body weight, the distribution of load is less certain but probably little or none is transmitted by direct tibio-femoral contact.

Patello-femoral Joint

The resultant patello-femoral compressive or normal force calculated by various methods is often assumed to act in a parasagittal plane but need not do so. Differences in the activity of the components of the quadriceps can impose a medial or lateral component of force on the patella, which can be transmitted in part by differing tensions in the two retinacula but is almost certain to be transmitted as unequal components of force on the two facets of the patella that contact the femur. Similarly, even small changes in alignment, which are inevitable when the knee is not a simple hinge, will result in medial or lateral components of force in some or all of the tissues attached to the patella, and it would be remarkable if in these circumstances the resultant patello-femoral force always acted precisely in the same plane, even in a normal healthy joint. The shapes of the joint surfaces (a groove instead of a surface flat from side to side on the femur, and a correspondingly two-faceted surface on the patella) allow such variations in the direction of the force to be safely accommodated, within limits.

MATTHEWS et al. (1977) measured patello-femoral contact areas by a dye-transfer method, the patella being coated with dye and pressed against the femur with a load of 893 N. The total area ranged from 170–320 mm² (average 230 mm²) at 15° of flexion and from 340–440 (average 380) mm² at 60° of flexion. At full extension the patella did not touch the femur. Combining their measurements of contact area with values for the patello-femoral force calculated from the results of MORRISON (1970a, b) and others reported by SMIDT (1973), MATTHEWS et al. calculated average contact stresses ranging up to 2.5 MN/m² in level walking, up to 7.4 MN/m² in walking down a ramp, and up to 12.6 MN/m² during resisted isometric quadriceps contracture. If the rather higher forces estimated by other workers (see Table 2) had been used, higher stresses would have resulted.

It is difficult to obtain truly comparable estimates of the contact stresses in the patello-femoral and tibio-femoral joints. Confining the discussion to level walking, if the results of MORRISON, used by MATTHEWS et al., are applied to the tibio-femoral contact area reported by MAQUET, an average stress at maximum load of about 1.1–1.3 MN/m² would result. This is appreciably lower than the 2.5 MN/m² obtained for the patello-femoral joint by MATTHEWS et al., but in view of the wide variations in tibio-femoral contact area as reported by different workers, it would be rash to conclude from these few calculations made from observations recorded by different people on different spe-

cimens and using different techniques that the patello-femoral joint is more highly stressed in level walking than is the tibio-femoral joint. Whereas in level walking the patello-femoral force is smaller than the tibio-femoral (according to MATTHEWS et al. and to MAQUET), in other activities, such as stair climbing and rising from a chair, the two forces are more nearly equal, and the patello-femoral stress is then higher than the tibio-femoral.

Average stresses in the hip under loads of 3 times body weight of about 1–2 MN/m² were reported by DAY et al. (1975), and ADAMS et al. (1978) reported local pressures of up to about 8 MN/m² with averages of 1.6–3.6 MN/m² during simulated level walking. Even with the necessary caution about comparing results from different sources, it seems clear that the average stresses in the hip, the tibio-femoral, and the patello-femoral joints are of the same order of magnitude. Presumably the local stresses in the knee vary over the contact area at least as widely as at the hip, since the hip joint surfaces are more nearly congruent than those at the knee. DAY et al. and ADAMS et al. found that at the higher loads used the maximum stress was up to about 3 times the average.

The Strength of the Normal Knee

Strength of the Intact Joint

BARGREN et al. (1978), in the course of tests on various knee prostheses, tested three natural knees by applying compressive force along the axis of the bones with the knee held in full extension. Failure was observed at 8 300, 7 600, and 7 300 N, respectively. These strengths are about 10 times a typical body weight, which suggests an adequate reserve of strength if maximum loads of about 3–4 times body weight are regularly applied, but not much reserve if the higher estimates of 6 times body weight (see Table 2) are correct. The specimens tested were from the cadavers of three persons aged 35, 36, and 36 at death.

Strength of the Bone Tissue

BARGREN et al. (1978) reported indentation tests performed on the cancellous bone of the tibia at the levels of section required by the four designs of prosthesis implanted and tested by them. A modified ROCKWELL hardness test was used, in which a conical indentor with a total angle of 120° was loaded until a force of 90 N was applied; the average stress under the indentor was calculated. The results thus represent the stresses the cancellous bone supported when indented by up to about 2.5 mm. It is not possible to obtain a knowledge of the stress that can be supported without damage when applied in the living joint directly from these results, but comparisons between different regions of one tibia and between different tibiae should be valid.

The average indentation stress for any one tibia varied from 1.1–5.2 MN/m². In general, the higher stresses were obtained at the more proximal levels of section, and the region under the intercondylar eminence was weaker than the medial and lateral regions; but at any one level of section there was wide variation between tibiae.

COLLEY et al. (1978) extended the work of BARGREN et al. to the femur. The same trends were observed (the bone was stronger with increasing proximity to the articular surface, and stronger in the condyles than in the intercondylar region), but indentation stresses measured with the same method ranged from 10–40 MN/m².

DUCHEYNE et al. (1977) tested cylindrical specimens 5 mm in diameter removed from femora. The compressive strength (taken as the stress at the point of first collapse on a stress–strain diagram) was typically 1–12 MN/m²; in five femora, the maximum values ranged from 10–17 MN/m², while in a sixth femur (65 year old female) the maximum was 35 MN/m². Specimens extracted further from the articular surface were in general weaker than those from closer to the articular surface.

Any comparison of these measurements with the estimates of the applied stresses in the tibio-femoral joint made from published estimates of the forces acting and the total contact areas should be made with great caution, because a large number of assumptions have now been accumulated. For what it is worth, the comparison suggests that even in healthy knees the margin of safety in the tibia is not very large, but that in the femur it is larger. A true comparison cannot be made until more is known of the actual stress distribution under loads, as distinct from the average stress over the whole contact area.

Table 3. Strengths of knee joint ligaments

Source	Ligament	Force (N) at rupture		
		Maximum	Mean	Minimum
TRENT et al., 1976	Lateral collateral	660	380	180
	Medial collateral	740	520	300
	Anterior cruciate	1700	620	280
	Posterior cruciate	1200	560	250

Strength of the Ligaments

TRENT et al. (1976) tested some or all of the four ligaments from each of six knees from cadavers in the age range 29–55 years. The forces at rupture were as given in Table 3. These forces are typically less than body weight (about 700 N), and the minima are about one-quarter or one-third of body weight. Since ligaments are not torn even in repeated normal activities, these results support the calculations referred to above, suggesting that the forces transmitted by the ligaments in normal walking are considerably smaller than those transmitted as compression between the articular surfaces.

Forces in Misaligned Natural Knees

Effects of Misalignment

By "misalignment" is meant an alignment, in valgus–varus or in flexion, sufficiently outside the normal range to change the distribution of forces significantly. Because the knee is a pivot roughly halfway along the leg that is loaded in compression, any misalignment is likely to produce instability and to be progressive. In a purely mechanical system, the instability could easily lead to catastrophic collapse, but in the leg any potential collapse is resisted by soft tissues whose tensile properties are time-dependent, and therefore even if muscles could not be brought into action collapse would be slow.

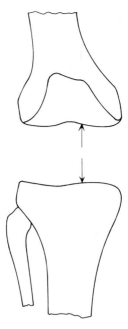

Fig. 11. Line of action of the resultant force between the femoral and the tibial condyles in a normal knee, as seen from the front. (This is not the same as the resultant force across the knee joint, which includes the forces in the ligaments, tendons and muscles)

Valgus Misalignment

In a knee whose alignment is within the normal range, the resultant force between the tibial and femoral condyles passes somewhere near the centre (in the medio-lateral sense) of the joint, as shown in Fig. 11. This is a consequence of the interactions of all the forces about the knee joint. As mentioned above, most published results agree in placing the line of action of the resultant force medially rather than strictly centrally during most of the stance phase of walking, so that more than half the total force is transmitted through the medial compartment.

If the knee is re-aligned in more than the usual valgus, the effect in an inanimate system would be to transfer force from the medial to the lateral compartment, and an alignment could be found at which all the force would be transmitted through the lateral compartment. A further increase of valgus would lead to collapse unless sufficient tensile forces could be developed in the medial tissues, principally the collateral ligament. Since the system is not inanimate, the lines of action and the magnitude of the forces can be adjusted, within limits,

and there is therefore not a determinate relationship between valgus misalignment and the medio-lateral distribution of force. JOHNSON and WAUGH (1979) have confirmed this by their finding that many patients load the medial compartment preferentially despite valgus deformity of the knee.

There must be some limit to such compensations, and if this limit is exceeded a valgus deformity or instability must be expected to increase. Whether instability or deformity results is as much a biological as a mechanical matter, but in general, if the bone is strong enough not to collapse in the lateral compartment then excessive lateral migration of the resultant force will result in stretching of the medial soft tissues and a valgus instability.

Varus Misalignment

The sequence is as for valgus misalignment, but the changes are in the opposite direction and the possibilities for compensation by changed muscular actions are different.

Flexion Misalignment

The knee can be held in flexion (or a few degrees of hyperextension) with little muscular action, but to hold it under load when flexed requires application of a significant moment by the quadriceps, with consequent forces in the patello-femoral and tibio-femoral joints. Present knowledge of the effects of sustained stress on cartilage does not permit precise statements about the effects, but it seems clear that in general they are bad. Thus a knee that had developed even a slight flexion deformity would be expected to show more degeneration of cartilage than a normal knee. Clearly, the greater the flexion, the larger the joint forces and presumably the more serious the effect on the cartilage.

Obliquity of the Joint

Obliquity is not in exactly the same category as the misalignments just considered, but can conveniently be considered here. If the joint is oblique, in the sense that the tibial plateau is significantly inclined to the long axis of the tibia as seen from the front, the effect is that the resultant force between the tibia and the femur is transmitted partly as shear instead of virtually wholly as compression. The friction between the articular surfaces is negligible, and shear forces can be transmitted only by pressure between the appropriate femoral condyle and one side of the intercondylar eminence on the tibia, since none of the soft tissues is well placed for this purpose and their stiffness is such that significant shear force would displace the femur sideways on the tibia enough to create contact of the kind described. The effect of such contact is hard to predict, but in general load-bearing contact between cartilage surfaces that have not been in contact for long periods of time is detrimental.

Biomechanics of Knee Replacement

The biomechanical considerations relevant to the design of joint replacements in general have been discussed in various publications, and have been expounded in some detail in a recent book (SWANSON and FREEMAN, 1977). The purpose of this Section is not to repeat such a detailed exposition, but merely to discuss the application of the general principles to the knee in particular.

Range of Possibilities

At the knee, there is the same choice as at any other joint, between replacing both of any two mating articular surfaces and replacing only one of them. There are additional choices, as follows: one can replace the patello-femoral joint, the tibio-femoral joint (the latter in one compartment or in both compartments), or both. Thus there is a range of possibilities, from replacing only the back of the patella or one of the tibial condylar bearing surfaces to replacing all six bearing surfaces (two femoral condyles, two tibial condyles, the patella, and the patellar groove on the femur). The choice from these possibilities and the results obtained with the different treatments are dealt with elsewhere in this book.

A closely related decision at the tibio-femoral joint is whether to replace the functions of the articular surfaces only, or those of the articular surfaces and the ligaments. This is of fundamental importance, and leads to major divergences in prosthetic design.

The selection of materials for the prosthetic components at the knee is based on the same considerations as at other joints, although the conditions

at the knee impose more stringent requirements than at, for example, the hip. Similarly, the means of fixation can be selected in much the same way as at other joints, but certain special features of the knee need to be considered.

Basic Requirements

The basic requirements are easily listed. The treatment of which the prosthesis is an essential part should:

1) Confer freedom from pain
2) Correct deformities or instabilities
3) Confer the necessary stability
4) Provide the ranges of motion needed for the activities of daily living
5) Confer the above functions for an acceptable time, preferably the remaining lifetime of the patient
6) Leave the patient in such a state that the consequences of an accident will not be unreasonably magnified
7) Allow a practicable salvage procedure if the prosthesis has to be removed
8) Cost a reasonable amount, in both money and, for example, bed occupancy.

None of the above requirements is absolutely quantifiable. Clearly, complete freedom from pain and a guaranteed working life at least equal to the remaining lifetime of the patient are desirable, but if severe pain can be reduced to mild occasional pain this is acceptable, and similarly with all the other requirements: as in most engineering design problems, the requirements are to some extent in conflict, and to satisfy one fully may be to ensure that another cannot be met fully. Perhaps the most obvious balance is that between stability and freedom from loosening (which is relevant to the working life); this is discussed in some detail below.

Taking the others briefly, in order, the following can be said.

Freedom from pain is generally assumed to require the replacement of both of two articular surfaces. Experience at the hip (HEYWOOD-WADDINGTON, 1966) and at the knee (ANDERSSON et al., 1974) with replacement of only one surface points in this direction, which is as would be expected, since in general both cartilage layers will be affected by the disease and pain may originate in either or both of the two regions of subchondral bone. An apparent exception is that many knees have been replaced with a femoral component having a continuous surface for the patella but retaining the natural patella, with satisfactory results. On the other hand, interest in replacing the back of the patella is increasing, and it seems likely that as the results of tibio-femoral replacement improve, attention will be directed to symptoms arising in the patello-femoral joint which were less important when the performance of the tibio-femoral replacement was less satisfactory.

The correction of deformities or instabilities is an obvious requirement, but complete correction is not always necessary, or even possible if there are deformities at the hip or ankle.

No range of motion can be laid down as absolutely required, because the activities that can be attempted will not be the same for different patients. A necessary part of the activities of daily living, however, is lowering oneself into a chair and rising from it, and for this the knee should be able to flex to about 90° (see "Movements Used in Daily Activities", above). If 90° of flexion is possible, this is more than is required for level walking, and will suffice for climbing and descending stairs, but this activity requires not merely flexion but the ability to transmit substantial forces from the patella to the femur in flexion. If this is not possible, climbing and descending stairs will be performed in an unnatural way. At the other end of the range, unless the knee can move into full extension and be stable there without voluntary muscular action, standing will be a tiring activity. Ad- and abduction and rotation are not necessary, but if they are prevented by the prosthesis their prevention gives rise to extra stresses, which, as discussed below, may increase the chances of loosening.

The working life may be limited by a number of factors, including loosening or breakage of the prosthetic components, wearing out, or tissue reactions to wear products.

The consequences of an accident should, if possible, be no worse for the victim with a replaced knee than for one with two natural knees. This means, in general, that soft-tissue injury is preferable to loosening or fracture of the prosthetic components or fracture of the bones. Because accidents are inherently unpredictable in nature, this consideration cannot be allowed too much importance, but it suggests prostheses that can dislocate rather than those which cannot.

Salvage may be required following failure from any cause. Formerly, infection was the commonest cause, and salvage then usually consisted of an arthrodesis, for which it is important to have available as large an area as possible of cancellous bone in the femur and the tibia, and not to have removed so much bone as to leave the leg too short. In future, it may be expected that fewer prostheses will be removed because of infection and more because of loosening, and then the implantation of another prosthesis is more likely. The requirements are still in general the same: the less tissue is removed at the first operation, the wider the range of options at any subsequent intervention.

Cost cannot be ignored, because somebody has to pay. The cost of the prosthesis is rarely more than 20% of the cost of the whole procedure, and often less, so the fact that the materials of which prostheses are made are liable to increase in cost suddenly as a consequence of war or political change (plastics are petrochemicals, and many metals, such as cobalt, are mined in some of the less stable countries in the world), though alarming in itself, is less important than it seems at first sight. It is more important that the cost of the whole procedure should be kept at a reasonable level, and this coincides with the aim of minimising the load on hospital facilities, which are becoming saturated, at least in some parts of the United Kingdom.

Tibio-femoral Joint

Replacement of Articular Surfaces and Ligaments

The most important decision is whether to replace the functions of the articular surfaces only or the functions of the articular surfaces and the ligaments. This choice has to be made at all joints (at the hip, it results in the design of either a ball-and-socket joint that is free to dislocate or one in which the ball is restrained within the socket), but at the knee it probably results in a more obvious divergence of design than at other joints.

If it is decided to replace the functions of the ligaments as well as those of the articular surfaces, then the prosthesis must restrain, to some extent, all six degrees of freedom. Flexion–extension will of course be permitted, but extension must be limited by the prosthesis; flexion may be limited by the prosthesis or by soft tissues. The other five degrees of freedom (ad- and abduction, rotation, impaction–distraction, antero-posterior gliding, and medio-lateral gliding) must be restrained by the prosthesis, and in the assumed absence of ligaments the simplest solution is to restrain all these movements completely, by using a hinge consisting essentially of a femoral and a tibial component pivoting together by means of a spindle in matching holes. All movements other than flexion–extension are then prevented absolutely (except insofar as the prosthetic components deflect elastically); flexion or extension, or both, can be limited by stops formed on the femoral and tibial components. If, as is almost inevitable for reasons of strength, the femoral and tibial components are metallic, the stiffness of all the restraints will be some orders of magnitude higher than that associated with soft-tissue constraints. This means that the joint is effectively immovable in all degrees of freedom other than flexion–extension, and that extension certainly, and flexion possibly, will be limited by impact between the prosthetic components, with high forces existing for short times. The last-mentioned effect can be significantly reduced by simply adding a buffer of soft material (e.g. silicone rubber) to one of the components so as to prevent metal-to-metal contact between the extension-limiting stops; but the former effect is less easily modified. The most notable feature of a hinged prosthesis is its simplicity, both in its construction and in the operative technique required for inserting it, and any attempt to avoid the other consequences of having a simple hinge introduces complexities. Of the five degrees of freedom that are restrained by a simple hinge, rotation of the tibia about its long axis is the one it seems to be thought most important to preserve to some extent. This can be done by modifying a hinge or by starting with a different concept. The Herbert knee, for example, uses a ball-and-socket joint, the socket being in the femoral component and the ball on the tibial component; the stem supporting the ball passes through a slot in the femoral component, and the width of this slot can be adjusted in relation to the thickness of the stem to permit or prevent ad- and abduction and rotation. In practice they are prevented near full extension and permitted in flexion; unless further complications have been introduced, to allow rotation is also to allow ad- and abduction. In the Sheehan knee, an essentially similar arrangement of a stem

passing through a shaped slot is used, although without a spherical joint.

Whatever is done to permit ad- and abduction or rotation, the three translational degrees of freedom (impaction–distraction, antero-posterior gliding, and medio-lateral gliding) remain completely restrained. This is probably not important functionally, but the fact that ad- and abduction and rotation are completely restrained at and near full extension is more likely to be important, because any such restraint means that forces must be transmitted that would not arise if the constraints were absent or less stiff. Because the system is not statically determinate, it is hardly possible to be quantitative about this, and the limited number of calculations of forces from observations made on subjects walking with replaced knees have not yet shed much light on the matter; but it can be said that every added constraint in principle introduces new forces, which must be transmitted between the prosthetic components and from them to the bones, and that the stiffer the constraint is the higher the forces will be. A separate consideration is that minor accidents that would produce soft-tissue injuries in a normal knee, or in a replaced knee in which the ligaments had been retained, may cause breakage or loosening of prosthetic components offering rigid constraints to movements other than flexion–extension. It is relevant to note that even when some rotation or ad- and abduction is allowed in flexion, this is usually limited by contact between metallic components or between one metallic and one polyethylene component, and the constraint is some orders of magnitude stiffer than would be exerted by soft tissues. Thus the components that may be termed "modified hinges" may reduce, but do not eliminate, the problems arising from stiff constraints, which are inherent in hinged prostheses.

Replacement of Articular Surfaces Only

An appreciation of the problems, mentioned above, that are inseparable from the use of hinged prostheses has led to the production of many designs in which only the articular surfaces are replaced and whose function relies to varying extents on the ligaments. The range of possibilities is still enormous, but all prostheses designed on this basis will have one feature in common distinguishing them from hinges, either simple or modified: compressive forces will be transmitted through the articular surfaces, but tensile forces will be transmit-

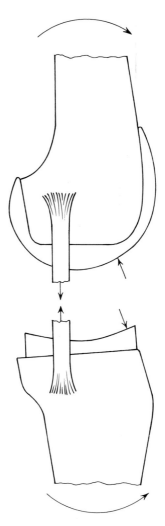

Fig. 12. In a surface-replacement knee prosthesis, a moment tending to hyperextend the knee is transmitted by a combination of tension in soft tissues posteriorly (only one collateral ligament is shown) and compression between the prosthetic surfaces anteriorly

ted through the soft tissues, principally the ligaments. This difference would be most obvious in the rare occurrence of enforced distraction, but it is important in the more frequently occurring limitation of extension, in torsion, or in any other movement. As shown in Fig. 12, in a prosthesis of the type now being considered, a moment tending to hyperextend the knee is resisted by a combination of compressive forces between the prosthetic components anteriorly and tensile forces in the collateral ligaments posteriorly (the cruciate ligaments are not shown, but if they are present

they may contribute to the tensile forces). The hyperextending moment is thus resisted in effect by two springs that act in parallel, and the stiffness of the joint in this mode (the rate of increase of applied moment with respect to the angle of hyperextension) depends on the geometry of the arrangement and on the stiffness of the two springs. In a natural knee, the anterior spring is cartilage in compression and the posterior spring is ligament in tension. The stiffnesses to be considered are those of the relevant region of cartilage (and the subchondral bone) and of the collateral ligaments; they therefore depend on the shapes and sizes of these components and not only on the Young's moduli of the materials, but in general the stiffness of the anterior and posterior springs will be of the same order of magnitude. Typical alloys used for prostheses have Young's moduli 200–300 times higher than that of ligaments. Therefore if both springs are made of metal (as in a simple hinged prosthesis) the stiffness of the joint will be 200–300 times that of the natural joint. If, however, the posterior spring is still composed of ligament, then a simple calculation shows that even if the anterior spring is made completely rigid the stiffness of the joint will be only twice that of the natural joint. Whatever the stiffness of the anterior spring, the stiffness of the joint will be between 1 and 2 times that of the natural joint, usually nearer 2 than 1 because one component is almost certainly metallic and the other, even when made of a plastic, is made of a relatively stiff plastic and is not of a shape to permit large deformations in compression. The essential point remains, though, that relying on tension in the collateral ligaments for part of the restraint keeps the stiffness of the joint in this mode at the same order of magnitude as that of the natural joint, instead of increasing it by a factor of 100 or more. The same applies in other modes; e.g. an adducting moment is resisted by compressive forces between the prosthetic components medially and tensile forces in the lateral collateral ligament.

Thus any design that depends on some ligamentous function and replaces only the articular surfaces is likely to generate lower auxiliary forces in service than a hinged prosthesis. "Auxiliary forces" is used to mean forces such as those that arise when hyperextension, torsion, etc. are resisted; all prostheses must transmit the basic forces associated with walking, rising from a chair, and other activities of daily living. Within this broad classification, particular designs may differ widely, both in shape and in the range of forces generated or transmitted. Two questions arise, the answers to which have major effects on prosthetic design. These are, first, whether the collateral ligaments only or the collateral and the cruciate ligaments are retained; and second, the amount of constraint provided by the prosthetic articular surfaces. These questions must now be considered in turn.

Retention of Cruciate Ligaments

In a severely damaged rheumatoid knee, the cruciate ligaments are often significantly attacked by the disease and of doubtful mechanical value. Therefore the design of a prosthesis intended for use in such knees should not depend on any mechanical function in these ligaments.

In osteoarthrosic knees and less severely attacked rheumatoid knees, the cruciate ligaments are usually mechanically sound, and the question as to whether or not to retain them is therefore a real one. In favour of retaining them, one can state the general view that as much healthy tissue should be retained as possible, and the particular point that since the cruciate ligaments contribute substantially to the stability of the natural knee their removal will introduce further requirements to be met by the prosthesis. Against these points, others emerge on further examination. The matter has been considered in detail by FREEMAN et al. (1977); all that need be said here from a mechanical point of view is that some mismatch between the kinematics of the prosthesis and the kinematics of the cruciate ligaments is almost inevitable and must be expected to lead, via increased forces, to increased wear or to loosening, probably in the form of posterior sinking of the tibial component.

If it is decided that better results will be obtained if the cruciate ligaments are not retained, then obviously the prosthetic components, together with the collateral ligaments, must provide the necessary constraints in all modes.

The above discussion refers to a bicompartmental replacement. Unicompartmental replacements are considered below.

Shapes of Articular Surfaces

Whether or not the cruciate ligaments are retained, the shapes of the articular surfaces must be considered in relation to the fixation of the prosthetic components and in relation to the necessary stability.

The design of joint prostheses can be regarded as deciding on the balance to be struck between instability and loosening. At one extreme, a simple hinged prosthesis is completely stable, but transmits to the bones the forces generated in resisting all the motions that it does resist. These forces raise the possibility of loosening, and all such designs have substantial intramedullary stems provided in the attempt, not always successful, to prevent loosening. At the other extreme, a prosthesis with a completely flat bearing surface on its tibial component could not transmit any forces other than compressive and the (small) shear forces due to friction, and the demands on the fixation would therefore be the least severe that are possible; but the risk of instability in some modes must be increased. Rather than invite trouble of one sort or the other (even though clinical experience with designs of the two types mentioned shows that trouble is not inevitable), it seems better to look for means of making each of the two types of trouble as unlikely as possible.

Considering first the shapes as seen from the side, the general idea of a roller in a trough is common to many designs. The roller can have a constant or a varying curvature. The trough can also have a constant or a varying curvature; if the latter, its curvature can be equal to that of the roller for part of the range of flexion–extension or it can be larger throughout (it could, in principle, be smaller throughout, but it is difficult to see any point in such an arrangement); and the trough can embrace the roller to any extent between not at all (a flat tibial plateau) to halfway up the roller. These possibilities are shown in Fig. 13. Discarding the flat tibial plateau, each of the other arrangements provides some stability in torsion and in antero-posterior gliding. The degree of stability obviously depends on the exact shapes. A constant-curvature cylindrical roller in a conforming half-cylindrical trough would be practically immovable in both these modes, and would behave similarly to a simple hinge, including the transmission of significant forces through the fixation. A roller in a less than half-cylindrical trough will react to torsion or antero-posterior gliding by climbing out of the trough, which motion will be resisted by gravity (if the knee is weight-bearing) and by tension in the soft tissues, particularly the collateral ligaments and, if present, the cruciate ligaments. This resistance, although the details differ, is the

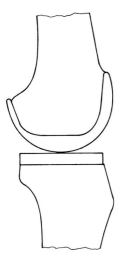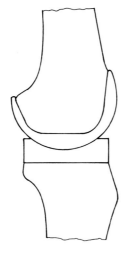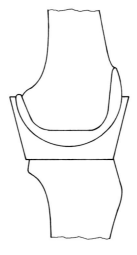

Fig. 13. Surface-replacement knee prostheses, having a cylindrical femoral component with a flat tibial component (*left*), a matching cylindrical tibial component reaching partly up the femoral articular surface (*centre*) and a matching cylindrical tibial component reaching to the diameter of the femoral articular surface (*right*)

same in principle as that of the natural knee, in which torsion or antero-posterior gliding are resisted by tension induced in soft tissues. Published measurements (WALKER and HSIEH, 1977; BARGREN et al., 1978) show that some present designs of knee prostheses have force-displacement characteristics in torsion that are quantitatively similar to those of the natural knee. The controlling factor is the way in which the roller (femur) rises in the trough (tibia) as one is made to rotate on the other, and this depends on the shapes of the two articular surfaces. Any desired torsional stiffness can be achieved by suitable arrangement of these surfaces. Whilst there is certainly nothing absolutely significant about any particular value, it seems probable that a value close to that of a natural knee will be about right; a large reduction in torsional stability might be dangerous, whilst to increase the torsional stiffness significantly would serve no useful purpose and must, in principle, increase the forces required to be transmitted through the fixation.

Any desired torsional stiffness can be achieved by using either conforming or nonconforming articular surfaces. If conforming surfaces are used, the stiffness is controlled by deciding on the angle of lap of the conforming part and then arranging nonconforming extensions of the tibial component up which the femoral component can rise. Thus when the knee is displaced in torsion (or in antero-posterior gliding) the contact is nonconforming; the difference is that in its undisplaced position a prosthesis with conforming surfaces transmits forces through a larger bearing area, which in principle should lead to a lower rate of wear.

Hyperextension is limited, as mentioned above, by a combination of compressive stresses acting anteriorly between the prosthetic components and tensile stresses posteriorly in the soft tissues. The only soft tissues that are certain to be available and effective for this purpose are the collateral ligaments, and the distance between these and the point at which compressive stresses act anteriorly between the prosthetic components is therefore significant; the longer this distance, the smaller will be the stresses required to resist any given hyperextending moment. Some designs, but not all, have included provision for increasing this distance; but since instability in hyperextension has never been reported to be a significant occurrence with any design, it must be concluded either that the precautions taken by some designers were unnecessary or that by good luck some other designs have been used only in patients with strong posterior capsules.

Considering now the shapes of the articular surfaces as seen from the front, two main possibilities emerge. Either the femoral and tibial components offer some restraint against medio-lateral gliding or they do not. In most designs they do, either by having in effect a pair of femoral condyles in a pair of concavities formed on the top of the tibial component or by having a central ridge running antero-posteriorly on a tibial component that is otherwise flat as seen from the front. The same considerations apply to the exact shape of any such constraining feature as to the shape as seen from the side; a shallower slope offers less resistance to the movement it is intended to constrain, but also induces smaller forces. At the extreme, a vertical face with a sharp transition from the horizontal would present a constraint limited only by the elastic stiffness of the system, and would transmit significant bending and shear forces to the tibial component and to its fixation. The more usual arrangement of a curved surface resists medio-lateral gliding by a combination of gravity (if weight-bearing), friction, and tension in soft tissues. The exact shapes of the surfaces are determined in part by manufacturing limitations (see below), since with the materials now used some shapes are noticeably more difficult to make than others.

Those designs in which the femoral and tibial components are free to slide medio-laterally depend for stability in this mode on tension in soft tissues. Small movements in this direction would not induce much tension in the collateral ligaments, but would induce shear in the capsule. Little restraint would be added by the quadriceps and patellar system unless the patella were located on the femur in a groove, which in at least one design it is not. It must be concluded, as about the apparently inadequate arrangements in some designs for resisting hyperextension, that something that looks not quite right in theory works in practice.

Added Constraints

It has been assumed in the preceding discussion that the prosthesis is either a hinge (simple or modified) or a replacement for the surfaces of the femoral condyles and the tibial plateau (with some attempt to replace the shapes of the menisci). Something between these two types is possible: surface replacement can be combined with some other connection between the two components, as in the spherocentric, Attenborough, Sheehan, or stabilocondylar prostheses (see other chapters of this book). Other variants are possible; the common feature is that medio-lateral gliding always, and torsion, antero-posterior gliding, and ad- and abduction to different extents, are resisted by the linkage between the two components. For the tibial component, this means that forces are applied at a finite distance above the articular surface (Fig. 14), which means in turn that extra stresses are required at the bone–prosthesis interface to transmit the bending moment constituted by such a force. This must be bad in principle; whether it is important in practice time will tell. Certainly all such designs have tibial components with longer intramedullary stems than are usual on unlinked

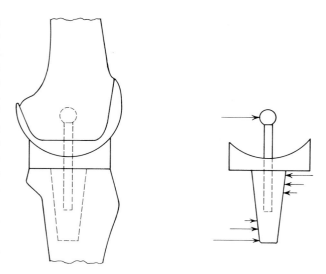

Fig. 14. Surface-replacement knee prosthesis with added constraint; if the added constraint is effective, it must transmit forces parallel to the top of the tibia and a finite distance above the articular surface, and extra stresses arise between the tibial component and the tibia to transmit the moment thus constituted

designs; again, while this may not matter much in practice it must be better in principle to invade the cancellous bone less.

The origin of linked designs lies in a belief that unlinked surface replacements are not stable enough for some knees. It must be admitted that to fit an unlinked prosthesis in a knee lacking collateral ligaments would be to invite trouble, but this is hypothetical and the question that arises in practice is whether the collateral ligaments without the cruciate ligaments confer enough stability when a suitable unlinked surface replacement is used correctly. If they do, then to add a linkage introduces more complications and, at least in theory, an increased risk of loosening, to no advantage. The rather theoretical discussion presented above suggests that there is no need for a linkage. Clinical observation will in due course provide the answer. One possible answer is that while unlinked surface replacements used correctly are adequate, when used with insufficient attention to the details of alignment they are not.

Unicompartmental Replacement

If a unicompartmental replacement is thought desirable, the general considerations discussed above apply, but with particular results.

If one compartment of the natural tibio-femoral joint is to be preserved, a hinged prosthesis with intramedullary stems is hardly possible, and even if it were possible its use would contravene the main purpose of having a unicompartmental replacement, which is to remove as little natural tissue as possible. Therefore a surface replacement has to be used. This being so, it is hardly conceivable that a unicompartmental replacement could replace the functions of the cruciate ligaments, and it follows that these ligaments must be retained (which also accords with the aim of removing as little tissue as possible), and with them the difficulties discussed above. These difficulties are if anything made worse by the presence of the other natural compartment, which reduces the options available to the designer. If a unicompartmental replacement has a geometry that is not completely consistent with the geometry of the rest of the joint, the effect may be loosening or increased wear of the prosthetic components, damage to the ligaments (cruciate or collateral), or damage to the remaining natural compartment if excessive loads are induced at certain positions. The last-mentioned effect would defeat the purpose of using a unicompartmental replacement. There is therefore little doubt that the chances of failure are higher with a unicompartmental replacement than with a total replacement.

It is clear that a primary aim must be to prevent excessive tension in the posterior cruciate ligament as the knee flexes, without inducing excessive tension in the anterior cruciate ligament in extension. This requires nonconforming bearing surfaces that will allow the instantaneous axis to move as required by the cruciate ligaments. The possibility of increased wear, not yet quantified, was mentioned above.

The fixation of unicompartmental components is not different in principle from that of bicompartmental prostheses, but it presents the same problems in a more severe form. For both the femoral and the tibial components, the area of interface with the bone is reduced in at least the same proportion as the loads, and probably by more, since the central portions of the tibia and femur cannot be used; and there is no possibility of sharing a load applied to one compartment between the interfaces behind the two compartments, as can happen in bicompartmental replacements having a single femoral component and a single tibial component. Because the tibial and femoral bearing surfaces will be nonconforming, the force transmitted between them will be more nearly a point force than that transmitted between conforming components, and the point of application of the resultant force will move over more of the bearing surfaces, in general, in a unicompartmentally replaced knee in which the motion will be controlled to a large extent by the cruciate ligaments and the remaining natural compartment. These effects are common to the tibial and femoral components, but experience with bicompartmental replacements shows that the tibial component is more likely to loosen than the femoral, partly because the cancellous bone of the tibia is weaker than that of the femur in the relevant regions (COLLEY et al., 1978), and in a unicompartmental replacement the tibial component is therefore more at risk of loosening than the femoral.

From the above, it may be concluded that a unicompartmental replacement is more likely to encounter mechanical problems than are bicompartmental replacements.

Patello-femoral Joint

Patellectomy with no measures to restore the moment arm of the patellar tendon is undesirable because it increases the quadriceps force needed for a given extending moment, and, whether or not the patient is feeble, the general aim should be to reduce rather than to increase the level of forces at the joint. With either a hinged or a surface-replacement prosthesis, a range of provision can be made for the patella. In the early years of knee replacement, the natural patella was often left to work against the patellar groove on the natural femur, or partly against this and partly against an anterior surface on the femoral component of the prosthesis. As the importance of the patello-femoral joint has become more fully appreciated, more designs have presented a smooth continuous surface over the whole of the part of the femur likely to be traversed by the patella. This is done with hinged prostheses and with surface replacement prostheses.

This having been done, the next question is whether to replace the back of the patella or to leave the natural surface, perhaps after some surgical adjustment, to work against the femoral component. Theoretically the bearing surface should be replaced, and, as mentioned above, the apparent success achieved clinically when the back of the patella has not been replaced may be less acceptable as the results of tibio-femoral replacement improve. If the natural patellar articular surface is retained, it is important that it should work against a metallic and not a plastic femoral component, because polyethylene must be expected to wear considerably faster against a degenerate cartilage surface than against metal, and the same is likely to be true of other plastics that might be used. If the articular surface of the patella is seriously degenerate but is nevertheless not to be replaced, it is obviously sensible to re-shape it to conform roughly to the shape of the relevant part of the femoral component.

If the back of the patella is to be replaced, the decision as to whether or not to make it conform to the shape of the femoral component has to be made, and this affects the shape of the bearing surfaces as seen in two views: from the side and from above.

As seen from the side, it is hardly practicable to give the femoral component a constant curvature over the whole range traversed by the patella, and the patella therefore cannot conform at all points in the range. It seems reasonable, if it is to conform anywhere, to make it do so where the forces are highest, i.e., in flexion. It is relatively easy to give the femoral component a constant curvature in this region and to increase the radius of curvature of the anterior flange as it rises up the front of the femur, so as to allow a long enough flange to lie against the front of the femur without excessive bone removal. This means that the patella will not conform when the knee is at or near full extension, but at this point the patello-femoral force is small and perhaps zero, so the bearing stress will still be low. As seen from the top, the anterior surface of the femoral component can be straight or concave. The former means that the surface is part of a cylinder (though probably not of constant curvature) and the latter is closer to the natural anatomical shape. If a part-cylindrical surface is used, it can offer no sideways restraint to the patella (except the trivial restraint due to friction). The patellar bearing surface can still be nonconforming, by being convex or concave as seen in this view, but this is pointless, and patellar components intended to work against part-cylindrical femoral components might as well have part-cylindrical concave bearing surfaces. If some sideways constraint is thought desirable, a groove can be provided on the front and bottom surfaces of the femoral component (it may run

all the way round the component, or be replaced by a gap between two condyles if the component is designed to allow the cruciate ligaments to be retained). The patellar bearing surface will then be convex as seen from the top. If the profile of the groove is constant, the bearing surfaces can conform as seen from the top; at least line contact will exist, and if the surfaces conform when seen from the side, surface contact will exist. If the groove has a varying profile, then clearly the bearing surface cannot conform at all points in the range of motion, and at some angles of flexion either single-point or two-point contact will occur. As suggested above, since the patello-femoral force is greater in flexion than at or near full extension, conformity is less important at or near full extension.

Whether or not the back of the patella is replaced, the use of a long anterior flange on the femoral component necessitates careful attention to the alignment of the extensor apparatus. If this is neglected, either the patella will be likely to sublux or, if it is restrained by formations on the surface of the femoral component, excessive wear of the patella itself or of its prosthetic surface may result.

The fixation of a patellar component is easier in some ways than that of other components, because the ways in which it can be loaded are more limited. Even if it conforms to the femoral component, the angle over which the two surfaces conform is limited by the geometry of the whole system, and the patella is effectively a shallow trough pressed against the femoral component (unless the designer goes out of his way to provide more constraint by arranging a protrusion on the patellar component to engage with a narrow groove on the femoral component); thus the twisting moment that can be applied is limited, and the fixation has effectively to transmit only compressive forces, which can of course be applied eccentrically. One potential danger in designing the fixation of this component is that if the natural patella is reduced to a shell by recessing the prosthetic component deeply into it, it may be vulnerable to accidental damage. If, to avoid this, the prosthetic component protrudes posteriorly, the effect will be to make the patella more prominent. Although this will also increase its moment arm about the axis of flexion-extension of the tibio-femoral joint, which is in general beneficial, it may also make the patella more likely to be damaged in accidents, and attention to the design of the femoral and patellar components together is needed to obtain the best balance of conflicting requirements.

Fixation

Requirements

The tibio-femoral joint must transmit compressive forces, which may be applied in a range of directions and may be eccentric to the extent of being effectively applied to the medial or the lateral condyles alone. This is the irreducible minimum. The joint must also transmit other forces and moments, whose magnitudes are determined largely or entirely by the design of the prosthesis, as has been discussed above. If a hinge is used, all possible forces and moments will arise, and the fixation must be designed to transmit them. This inevitably means long intramedullary stems, preferably of a markedly noncircular cross-section and preferably fitted, whether with or without cement, into medullary canals also prepared to a significantly noncircular cross-section. The noncircularity is needed so that twisting moments are transmitted across the interfaces mainly as compressive stresses; for a fuller discussion see SWANSON (1977). If a surface replacement prosthesis is used, the magnitudes of all the forces and moments, other than the obvious compressive force, will depend heavily on the shapes of the bearing surfaces. No general statement can be made, except that increasing freedom from subluxation is obtained at the cost of increased demands on the fixation. Since very few designs have completely flat tibial bearing surfaces, it can be said that most designs need to be able to transmit some twisting moment and some antero-posterior force.

A further general requirement is that the fixation arrangements should permit a good salvage or revision procedure if this should be necessary. In general this means removing as little tissue as possible, and in particular it means leaving continuous surfaces of cancellous bone.

Methods

Acrylic cement is now conventional, but interest in fixation by bone's being encouraged to grow into porous or roughened surfaces is increasing. These matters have been reviewed elsewhere (VERNON-ROBERTS and FREEMAN, 1977; SWAN-SON, 1977), and this is not the place to speculate on developments over the next few years. It is worth noting that one bad feature of acrylic cement (or of any other similar cement that might be introduced), namely the detachment of small particles of cement, which occurs particularly if excess cement is left at the edges of a prosthesis or if part of the cement layer is inadequately supported, is more serious in a knee prosthesis having an upwardly concave tibial component than in a hip prosthesis having a downwardly concave acetabular component; in the latter the particles of cement tend to fall away from the bearing surfaces, but in the former they tend to collect on the tibial bearing surface. With the almost universal use of a plastic for the tibial component, such particles of acrylic cement tend to abrade the surface.

Whatever interface between the prosthetic components and the bones is used, the strength of the underlying bone must not be exceeded. This means that the tibial component should engage the whole area of the sectioned tibia, including the cortices; and there is evidence (BARGREN et al., 1978) that the cancellous bone of the tibia is stronger near the subchondral bone plate than further distally. The femoral component is less critical in this respect, because in any surface replacement design it will almost inevitably be generally U-shaped when seen from the side, transmitting twisting moments as compressive stresses, and because the cancellous bone of the femoral condyles is stronger than that of the tibial condyles (COLLEY et al., 1978).

Performance

The strength of fixation can be assessed by laboratory tests, in which loads representing (so far as present knowledge permits) the loads applied in life are applied and deformations and displacements, either recoverable or permanent, are observed. Tests of this kind have been reported by NOGI et al. (1976), by BARGREN et al. (1978), and by COLLEY et al. (1978). The conclusions to be drawn from these tests are that femoral components are unlikely to loosen in the face of ordinary loads, that tibial components that engage less than the whole area of the tibia are at some risk in compression, particularly if the compressive force is applied eccentrically and the bone is weaker than average, and that in torsion and hyperextension it is perfectly practicable to design prostheses whose bearing surfaces will not transmit moments or forces sufficient to loosen the fixation. All the tests reported were performed on prostheses implanted with acrylic cement in cadaveric bones. It is certain (VERNON-ROBERTS and FREEMAN, 1977) that the strength of fixation with acrylic cement cannot increase with time in a living body, and it is as likely to decrease as to remain constant. Fixation by ingrowth of bone, if it succeeds at all, must become stronger as time goes on, but presumably it attains a steady state that, for a given shape of interface, is likely to be at least as high as that achieved with cement, since with cement failure usually occurs on the bone side of the cement–bone interface and through the soft tissue present there.

The strength of fixation can also be assessed clinically by the incidence of loosening. Systematic and strictly comparative observations are few; such published observations as have been collected by the present author (SWANSON, 1978) show loosening rates of up to about 10% with either hinged or surface-replacement prostheses. Only limited significance can be attached to such figures, because most hinged designs have been used and reported only in small numbers, and most surface-replacement designs, although used in larger numbers, have not yet been in use in large numbers for long enough for representative results to be obtained. COLLEY et al. (1978) reported a loosening rate of 5% at the tibia (with a design of tibial component that has since been improved) and of 1% at the femur; if the loosening rate for the femoral component is maintained, and if the modified tibial component loosens less frequently, as it should, then these results may show what can reasonably be expected from a carefully designed and implanted surface-replacement prosthesis.

Materials

The choice of materials for knee prostheses is basically the same as for any other joint; the requirements of sufficient strength and stiffness, compatibility with tissues, and wear performance are common. As mentioned above, the wear performance of a material combination is perhaps tested more severely in a knee prosthesis than elsewhere, because the upward-facing concave (in most designs) tibial bearing surface tends to retain both wear products and such debris as detached particles of cement. The characteristics of suitable materials, and the bases for selecting them, are discussed

fully elsewhere (WEIGHTMAN, 1977a); here it need only be stated that, of the metallic alloys that can at present be made into the required shapes at a practical cost, three groups are sufficiently compatible with the body tissues: austenitic chromium–nickel steels ("stainless steels"), cobalt-based alloys, and titanium alloys. Of these, only one cobalt–chromium alloy (65% Co, 28% Cr, 6% Mo, originally Haynes Stellite 21, now sold as "cast cobalt–chromium alloy" under various proprietory names) has been shown to be acceptable as a bearing material on itself; other cobalt-based alloys, stainless steels, and titanium alloys wear unacceptably and produce undesirably variable and high frictional forces. Some alloys from all three groups are acceptable as bearings when the other bearing surface is nonmetallic, but a limited amount of evidence suggests that titanium alloys give a higher rate of wear of a polyethylene component than either stainless steel or cobalt–chromium alloy (of the cobalt-based alloys, only the one cobalt–chromium alloy mentioned above has so far been used extensively as a bearing material; a different cobalt–chromium alloy [44% Co, 20% Cr, 15% W, 10% Ni] and a cobalt–nickel alloy [35% Co, 35% Ni, 10% Mo, 20% Cr] have been used for structural elements [e.g. stems of hip prostheses], for which their mechanical properties make them more suitable, but not as bearing surfaces, for which they are less suitable than so-called cast cobalt–chromium). Other alloys, at present regarded as exotic, may in future become practicable if a demand for their particular properties, combined with economic circumstances, makes it worth someone's while to develop means of extracting and processing them, as happened with titanium only a few decades ago.

Plastic components are made almost exclusively of high-molecular-weight polyethylene, which is compression-moulded into large blocks and then machined into the final shape from these blocks. This process is expensive, and imposes some restriction on the shapes that can be made at an acceptable cost, but direct moulding to shape in this material has not so far been practicable because of its flow characteristics. Polyesters have been used, but were withdrawn because of inadequate strength when exposed to body tissues and fluids (WEBER et al., 1974). Polyformaldehyde is currently used in at least one design of hip prosthesis (CHRISTIANSEN, 1974).

Ceramics are being used in some hip prostheses (BOUTIN, 1974), and are claimed to be less reactive than metallic alloys and to give a lower wear rate of polyethylene. This is believed to be because a ceramic surface can be polished to a more consistent finish than can a metallic surface, in which the grain boundaries are more prominent. Ceramics can be made porous, and bone will, in suitable circumstances, grow into the pores; but these attributes are not peculiar to ceramics.

The most commonly used combination is now cast cobalt–chromium alloy against high-molecular-weight polyethylene, with stainless steel against the same polyethylene also used on a large scale. With either of these combinations, fatigue fracture and wear are the limitations on working life most likely to arise from the properties of the materials.

Fatigue fracture is a danger to which all structural elements are exposed that are cyclically stressed, particularly metallic components in a corrosive environment. At the hip, fatigue fracture of intramedullary stems has been encountered at rates that are not negligible (CHARNLEY, 1971, 1973, 1975; MARTENS et al., 1974; GALANTE et al., 1975), but it is probable that metallurgical improvements, improvements to the design of stems, the use of different stem sizes matched (so far as possible) to the patient's weight and activity, and more consistent implantation techniques will reduce the incidence of fatigue fractures, even with basically the same materials. With surface-replacement designs, it should be easier to avoid such high stresses as are often encountered in intramedullary stems, and the danger of fatigue fracture should be correspondingly more remote.

With wear the problem is less simple; a full discussion is given in WEIGHTMAN (1977b). The only large-scale long-term comparative measurements of wear in service are those made by CHARNLEY and associates, using radiography and post-mortem examinations, on Charnley hips in mostly elderly patients with restricted activity. These measurements (CHARNLEY, 1974; CHARNLEY and CUPIC, 1973; CHARNLEY and HALLEY, 1975) show an average rate of wear of 0.15 mm per year, with a maximum of 0.45 mm per year, in patients operated on in 1963–65. In 547 patients operated on in 1967–68, the average rate of wear was 0.07 mm per year (GRIFFITH et al., 1978). If these wear rates remain roughly constant, a wall thickness of 5 mm would allow a wearing life of about 22 years (minimum) or about 60 years (average); many patients have of course used Charnley (and similar) hip prostheses for more than 10 years without wearing them out. Before it is concluded that

knee prostheses will wear for 20 or more years, several points must be remembered:

CHARNLEY's measurements were made on a fairly homogeneous group of elderly and handicapped patients treated by a technique that was probably more closely controlled than is usual

Knee (and hip) prostheses are now commonly implanted in younger and more active patients

Knee prostheses can be loaded in ways that are not possible with a ball-and-socket joint such as the hip, and higher local stresses are therefore almost inevitable, e.g., at opposite corners of a surface-replacement knee when torsion is applied simultaneously with compression

The dependence of wear rate on stress range in representative conditions is far from fully established

Virtually all surface-replacement knee prostheses have an upward-facing concave tibial component that is well placed to catch and retain particulate debris of cement or bone, which must tend to increase the rate of wear.

It may be concluded that a combination of favourable circumstances would be necessary for knee prostheses incorporating polyethylene to wear for as long as hip prostheses.

References

ADAMS, D., KEMPSON, G.E., SWANSON, S.A.V.: Direct measurement of local pressures in the cadaveric human hip joint. J. Physiol. (Lond.) **278**, 33 (1978)

ANDERSSON, G.B.J., JESSOP, J., FREEMAN, M.A.R., MASON, R.M.: MacIntosh arthroplasty in rheumatoid arthritis. Acta Orthop. Scand. **45**, 245 (1974)

BARGREN, J.H., DAY, W.H., FREEMAN, M.A.R., SWANSON, S.A.V.: Mechanical tests on the tibial components of non-hinged knee prostheses. J. Bone Joint Surg. (Br.) **60**, 256 (1978)

BLACHARSKI, P.A., SOMERSET, J.H., MURRAY, D.G.: A three-dimensional study of the kinematics of the human knee. J. Biomech. **8** (6), 375 (1975)

BLAIMONT, P., BURNOTTE, J., HALLEUX, P.: Rôle des ménisques du genou dans la transmission des contraintes articulaires. Acta Orthop. Belg. **41** (Suppl. 1), 143 (1975)

BOUTIN, P.: Arthroplastie totale de la hanche par prothèse en alumine. Orthop. Belg. **40**, (5–6), 744 (1974)

BRAUNE, C.W., FISCHER, O.: Über den Schwerpunkt des menschlichen Körpers mit Rücksicht auf die Ausrüstung des deutschen Infanteristen. Abhandl. Math.

Phys. Classe königl. Sächs. Gesellschaft Wissensch. **15**, 561 (1889)

BRESLER, B., FRANKEL, J.P.: The forces and moments in the leg during level walking. Trans. Am. Soc. Mech. Engrs. **72**, 27 (1950)

CHARNLEY, J.: Stainless steel for femoral hip prostheses in combination with a high density polythene socket. J. Bone Joint Surg. (Br.) **53**, 342 (1971)

CHARNLEY, J.: Biomechanical considerations in total hip prosthetic design. The hip. St. Louis: Mosby 1973

CHARNLEY, J.: Total hip replacement. JAMA **230**, 1025–1028 (1974)

CHARNLEY, J.: Fracture of femoral prostheses in total hip replacement. A clinical study. Clin. Orthop. **111**, 105 (1975)

CHARNLEY, J.: The wear of plastics materials in the hip-joint. Plastics and Rubber **1**, 59 (1976)

CHARNLEY, J., CUPIC, Z.: The nine and ten year results of the low friction arthroplasty of the hip. Clin. Orthop. **95**, 9–25 (1973)

CHARNLEY, J., HALLEY, D.K.: Rate of wear in total hip replacement. Clin. Orthop. **112**, 170–179 (1975)

CHRISTIANSEN, T.: A combined endo- and total hip prosthesis with trunnion-bearing. Acta Chir. Scand. **140** (3), 185 (1974)

COLLEY, J., CAMERON, H.U., FREEMAN, M.A.R., SWANSON, S.A.V.: Loosening of the femoral component in surface replacement of the knee. Arch. Orthop. Traumat. Surg. **92**, 31 (1978)

DAY, W.H., SWANSON, S.A.V., FREEMAN, M.A.R.: Contact pressures in the loaded human cadaver hip. J. Bone Joint Surg. (Br.) **57**, 302 (1975)

DENHAM, R.A., BISHOP, R.E.D.: Mechanics of the knee and problems in reconstructive surgery. J. Bone Joint Surg. (Br.) **60**, 345 (1978)

DUCHEYNE, P., HEYMANS, L., MARTENS, M., AERNOUDT, E., DE MEESTER, P., MULIER, J.C.: The mechanical behaviour of intracondylar cancellous bone of the femur at different loading rates. J. Biomech. **10** (11–12), 747 (1977)

EBERHART, H.D., et al.: Fundamental studies of human locomotion. Prosthetic devices research project. Berkeley, California, USA: college of engineering, University of California 1947

ELFTMAN, H.: The functional structure of the lower limb. In: Human limbs and their substitutes. KLOPSTEG, P.E., WILSON, P.D. (eds.), p. 411. New York: McGraw Hill 1954

FRANKEL, V.H., BURSTEIN, A.H., BROOKS, D.B.: Biomechanics of internal derangement of the knee. J. Bone Joint Surg. (Am.) **53**, 945 (1971)

FREEMAN, M.A.R., INSALL, J.N., BESSER, W., WALKER, P.S., HALLEL, T.: Excision of the cruciate ligaments in total knee replacement. Clin. Orthop. **126**, 209 (1977)

GALANTE, J.O., ROSTOKER, W., DOYLE, J.M: Failed femoral stems in total hip prostheses. J. Bone Joint Surg. (Am.) **57** (2), 230 (1975)

GRIFFITH, M.J., SEIDENSTEIN, M.K., WILLIAMS, D., CHARNLEY, J.: Socket wear in Charnley low friction arthroplasty of the hip. Clin. Orthop. **137**, 37 (1978)

HARRINGTON, I.J.: A bioengineering analysis of force actions at the knee in normal and pathological gait. Biomed. Eng. **11** (5), 167 (1976)

HEYWOOD-WADDINGTON, M.B.: Use of the Austin Moore prostheses for advanced osteoarthritis of the hip. J. Bone Joint Surg. (Br.) **48** (2), 236 (1966)

JOHNSON, F., WAUGH, W.: A method for routine clinical assessment of knee joint forces. Med. Biol. Eng. Comput. **17**, 145 (1979)

KAPANDJI, I.A.: The physiology of the joints, Vol. II: The lower limb. p. 120. London, Edinburgh: Churchill Livingstone 1970

KETTELKAMP, D.B., JACOBS, A.W.: Tibiofemoral contact area — determination and implications. J. Bone Joint Surg. (Am.) **54** (2), 349 (1972)

KETTELKAMP, D.B., JOHNSON, R.J., SMIDT, G.L., CHAO, E.Y.S., WALKER, M.: An electrogoniometric study of knee motion in normal gait. J. Bone Joint Surg. (Am.) **52** (4), 775 (1970)

MAQUET, P.G.J.: Biomechanics of the knee. Berlin, Heidelberg, New York: Springer 1976

MARTENS, M., AERNOUDT, E., DE MEESTER, P., DUCHEYNE, P., MULIER, J.C., DE LANGH, R., KESTELIJN, P.: Factors in the mechanical failure of the femoral component in total hip prosthesis. Acta Orthop. Scand. **45** (5), 693 (1974)

MATTHEWS, L.S., SONSTEGARD, D.A., HENKE, J.A.: Load bearing characteristics of the patello-femoral joint. Acta Orthop. Scand. **48** (5), 511 (1977)

McLEOD, P.C., KETTELKAMP, D.B., SRINIVASAN, V., HENDERSON, O.L.: Measurements of repetitive activities of the knee. J. Biomech. **8** (6), 369 (1975)

MORRISON, J.B.: Bioengineering analysis of force actions transmitted to the knee joint. Biomed. Eng. **3**, 164 (1968)

MORRISON, J.B.: Function of the knee joint in various activities. Biomed. Eng. **4** (12), 573 (1969)

MORRISON, J.B.: Biomechanics of the knee joint in relation to normal walking. J. Biomech. **3**, 51 (1970a)

MORRISON, J.B.: The mechanics of muscle function in locomotion. J. Biomech. **3**, 431 (1970b)

MURRAY, M.P.: Gait as a movement pattern. Am. J. Phys. Med. **46**, 290 (1967)

NOGI, J., CALDWELL, J.W., KAUZLARICH, J.J., THOMPSON, R.C.: Load testing of geometric and polycentric total knee replacements. Clin. Orthop. **114**, 235 (1976)

PAUL, J.P.: Forces transmitted by joints in the human body. Proc. Inst. Mech. Eng. **181** (3J), 8 (1967)

PERRY, J., ANTONELLI, D., FORD, W.: Analysis of knee-joint forces during flexed-knee stance. J. Bone Joint Surg. (Am.) **57** (7) 961 (1975)

REILLY, D.T., MARTENS, M.: Experimental analysis of the quadriceps muscle force and patello-femoral joint reaction force for various activities. Acta Orthop. Scand. **43**, 126 (1972)

RYDELL, N.W.: Forces acting on the femoral head prosthesis. Acta Orthop. Scand. **37** (Suppl. 88), 1–132 (1966)

SEEDHOM, B.B., TERAYAMA, K.: Knee forces during the activity of getting out of a chair with and without the aid of arms. Biomed. Eng. **11** (8), 278 (1976)

SHRIVE, N.G., O'CONNOR, J.J., GOODFELLOW, J.W.: Load-bearing in the knee joint. Clin. Orthop. **131**, 279 (1978)

SMIDT, G.L.: Biomechanical analysis of knee flexion and extension. J. Biomech. **6** (1), 79 (1973)

SWANSON, S.A.V.: Mechanical aspects of fixation. The scientific basis of joint replacement. SWANSON, S.A.V., FREEMAN, M.A.R. (eds.), p. 130. London: Pitman Medical 1977

SWANSON, S.A.V.: The state of the art in joint replacement. Part 3: results, problems and trends. J. Med. Eng. Technol. **2**, 16 (1978)

SWANSON, S.A.V., FREEMAN, M.A.R. (eds.): The scientific basis of joint replacement. London: Pitman Medical 1977

TRENT, P.S., WALKER, P.S., WOLF, B.: Ligament length patterns, strength and rotational axes of the knee joint. Clin. Orthop. **117**, 263 (1976)

VERNON-ROBERTS, B., FREEMAN, M.A.R.: The tissue response to total joint replacement prostheses. The scientific basis of joint replacement. SWANSON, S.A.V., FREEMAN, M.A.R. (eds.), p. 86. London: Pitman Medical 1977

WALKER, P.S., ERKMAN, M.J.: The role of the menisci in force transmission across the knee. Clin. Orthop. **109**, 184 (1975)

WALKER, P.S., HAJEK, J.V.: The load bearing area in the knee joint. J. Biomech. **5**, 581 (1972)

WALKER, P.S., HSIEH, H.H.: Conformity in condylar replacement knee prostheses. J. Bone Joint Surg. (Br.) **59** (2), 222 (1977)

WEBER, B.G., STÜHMER, G., SEMLITSCH, M.: Erfahrungen mit dem Kunststoff Polyester als Komponente der Rotationstotalprothese des Hüftgelenkes. (Experience with polyester as a component of the rotation total prosthesis for the hip-joint). Z. Orthop. **112** (5), 1106 (1974)

WEIGHTMAN, B.: Properties of materials. The scientific basis of joint replacement. SWANSON, S.A.V., FREEMAN, M.A.R. (eds.), p. 1. London: Pitman Medical 1977a

WEIGHTMAN, B.: Friction, lubrication and wear. The scientific basis of joint replacement. SWANSON, S.A.V., FREEMAN, M.A.R. (eds.), p. 46. London: Pitman Medical 1977b

Chapter 2

The Surgical Anatomy and Pathology of the Arthritic Knee

M.A.R. Freeman

The London Hospital, London E1 2AD, England

This Chapter is not concerned with the pathogenesis of rheumatoid arthritis (RA) and osteoarthritis (OA) nor with the pathology of these diseases at the cellular level, both topics that have been reviewed extensively elsewhere. The initial causes of these diseases and the associated events at the cellular level have been excluded, since at present they have little or no bearing upon the surgical treatment of these two conditions at the knee. (A partial exception to this statement is provided by the treatment of early RA by synovectomy and of early OA by osteotomy and re-alignment of the leg, topics dealt with in Chaps. 7 and 9).

This Chapter is concerned with the nature of the gross abnormalities occurring in the arthritic or arthrosic knee, since these must be understood if surgical management is to be rational. It will be argued that the fundamental element in the surgical pathology of both diseases is the destruction of the articular surfaces (i.e., of cartilage and of bone), followed usually by soft-tissue contracture and less often by soft-tissue rupture and elongation. Although the initial cause of the destruction of the articular surfaces will not be discussed (since this would be to enter into a discussion of the pathogenesis), it may be said in summary that in RA the surfaces are probably destroyed by enzymatic attack and by the mechanical action of exposed, porotic, and irregular bony surfaces moving against each other under load. In OA, in contrast, the destruction of the surfaces seems likely to be due largely if not entirely to mechanical factors. For this reason, and because the bone is not porotic, the knee is usually destroyed more slowly in OA than in RA. Although the pace of the two diseases differs, it is nevertheless the author's view that the mechanisms producing instability and fixed deformity are the same and that although in their "classic" form the diseases may be thought of as being clearly distinguishable, in reality they occupy the two ends of a spectrum,

many knees representing intermediate points in this continuum.

In this Chapter four topics will be considered: some aspects of the functional anatomy of the normal knee, the incidence of various deformities at the knee in OA and RA, some relevant observations at the hip, and the nature of the bony- and soft-tissue pathology at the knee.

Normal Alignment and Movement

A full description of the normal topographical and functional anatomy of the knee is outside the scope of this Chapter. Certain aspects of these subjects must, however, be considered if the pathology is to be understood and if modern surgical procedures for the arthritic knee, especially replacement procedures, are to be evaluated rationally. To take but one example: since one object of surgery is to correct varus and valgus deformities, it is obvious that the normal alignment of the knee must be known to the surgeon. Again: in replacement procedures some components of the knee are removed and then replaced whilst others are retained, so that it is important to establish the extent to which these components are functionally interdependent (representing elements of a single mechanism) and to what extent they are functionally separate. Thus, by analogy, the function of a motor car would be destroyed if an attempt were made to remove the crankshaft and to replace it with another of different design, because the crankshaft is functionally dependent upon other components of the engine. In contrast, it would in principle be possible to exchange the entire engine for another of different design and still have a functionally satisfactory, although different, motor car.

The description of the anatomy given in this section refers to the functionally normal Caucasian knee. It is based partly upon the author's own observations but it depends heavily upon previous descriptions, especially those of KAPANDJI (1970) and of GOODFELLOW and O'CONNOR (1978). Individual references are given only rarely since it is now difficult to determine who first made many of the relevant observations.

Alignment

In Extension

As viewed from the front with the knee in full extension, the centres of the hip, knee, and ankle lie in a straight line, the so-called mechanical axis of the limb (LANZ and WACHSMUTH, 1972). During one-leg stance, this axis is just lateral to the line of action of the body weight at the knee. Since the line of action of the body weight (which is vertical) and the mechanical axis of the limb converge at the heel, the former is inclined to the latter by about 3° in one-leg stance (Fig. 1). If the subject stands on both legs with the feet very slightly apart, the two lines obviously become parallel and perpendicular.

The transverse plane of the knee (as defined by a line drawn as a tangent to the distal extremities of the femoral condyles) is variously said to lie at right angles either to the mechanical axis or to the line of action of the body weight in one-leg stance. These planes differ from each other, the first being tilted upwards and laterally by 3° relative to the second (i.e., into valgus, as it were). It seems doubtful whether this difference is of any practical significance, especially when it is remembered that the relevant measurements are hard to make to this accuracy and that the plane of the knee relative to the horizontal will depend upon how far apart the knees are placed. For practical purposes therefore the plane of the knee can be thought of as being at right angles to the mechanical axis of the lower limb and thus at right angles to the axis of the tibia.

Because of the shape of the proximal femur and the fact that the mechanical axis is straight, the tibial shaft must lie in about 7° of valgus relative to that of the femur. This angle is remarkably constant, varying in the view of some authorities between 5° for men and 7° for women, or being 7° in both sexes in the view of others.

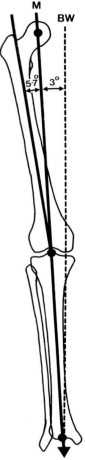

Fig. 1. A diagram to show the mechanical axis of the femur and tibia (M), the plane of the knee, and the line of action of the body weight (BW) in one-leg stance

The critical significance of these angles for the health of the knee is emphasised by the fact that if either the angle between the femoral and tibial shafts (i.e., 7°) or that between the tibial plateau and the tibial shaft (i.e., 90°) varies by as little as 4° the line of action of the body weight can be moved from its optimum position to the outer or inner thirds of the joint, whilst a variation of 10° can put the line of action of the body weight beyond the articular surface (DENHAM and BISHOP, 1978). Such malalignments will cause significant increases in the compressive stresses encountered by the bones on the concave side of the joint and in the tensile stresses encountered by the ligaments on the convex side.

The long axes of the shafts of the tibia and femur as seen in the frontal plane intersect each other in the plane of the knee. In view of this, lateral tibial shift can be said to be present if these axes intersect each other proximal to the knee.

Rotationally, the tibia is so placed that the tibial tubercle lies in the anterior midline of the tibia. This point is slightly lateral to a distal projection of the femoral shaft and hence to the presumed line of action of the quadriceps muscle. For this reason, quadriceps contraction tends to displace the patella laterally.

In Flexion

As the knee flexes with the hip in neutral rotation, the tibia deviates neither into varus nor into valgus. "Normal" tibial rotational alignment cannot be precisely defined in flexion, since active rotational movement of the tibia is possible in the flexed knee (see "Movement", below).

Patello-femoral alignment is constrained throughout the range of flexion by the bony anatomy: the patella remains in the patella groove, i.e., essentially in the anterior midline of the femur early in the range of flexion and slightly to the lateral side of the distal midline of the femur in full flexion.

A general point must be appreciated concerning the connection between tibio-femoral alignment in extension and in flexion. This is that abnormalities in the supracondylar region of the femur producing valgus or varus malalignment in extension will produce external or internal rotation, respectively, of the lower leg in 90° of flexion. It is partly because of this that the tibia lies in more external rotation in flexion than in extension: this follows from the presence of a 7° valgus angle between the femoral condyles and shaft. In contrast to this reciprocal relationship between valgus/varus and rotational alignment in extension and flexion at the femur, malalignments in the proximal tibia produce malalignments of the same kind in both extension and flexion. Thus, for example, internal rotation of the leg due to a femoral abnormality will produce lower leg valgus in flexion, whilst internal rotation of the leg due to a tibial abnormality will produce internal rotation in flexion also.

Movements (see also Chap. 1)

Arcs of Movement Permitted

Extension is limited by the ligaments of the knee (see below) at a position about 5° "over-straight"

as judged by the axes of the distal femur and proximal tibia. When the knee is fully extended, its axis of rotation lies behind the line of action of the body weight in the erect posture. The body weight then tends to hyperextend the knee, a movement that can be resisted by ligament tension without the support (over short periods) of extensor muscle action. Thus the erect posture can be maintained at the knee without the expenditure of energy. Although this position can be maintained without muscle action, the quadriceps muscle can actively extend the knee up to the limit of extension.

It should be noted that although the knee hyperextends, the posterior aspect of the lower limb (i.e., the buttock, thigh, knee, calf, and heel) is approximately straight. Thus a normal subject lying on his back with the knee braced into full extension can raise his heel little if at all from a flat examination couch.

In full extension the ligaments and bones of the knee permit a negligible arc of tibial rotation and ab- and adduction, such of these movements as occur being due to tissue elasticity. As flexion proceeds the tibia rotates externally (see elsewhere in this Chapter), and because the attachments of the ligaments approach each other as the knee flexes (i.e., because these attachments lie for the most part behind the axis of rotation) the tibia becomes increasingly free to rotate and to abduct or adduct. The former movement is under active muscular control but the latter is not. At 90° of flexion the range of rotation is about 30° (MARKOLF et al., 1976), and that of abduction and adduction about 20°. The latter arc is difficult to measure, since rotation of the hip gives the appearance of tibial abduction and adduction in the flexed knee.

Flexion is limited at about 130° by contact between the soft tissues of the calf and thigh. In this position the posterior overhang of the femoral and tibial condyles provide an arch within which the neurovascular bundle can lie without risk of compression. In contrast to extension, the last few degrees of flexion are not under active muscular control.

Nature of Tibio-femoral Movement During Flexion and Extension

The extent to which rolling and/or gliding occur at the tibio-femoral joint during flexion has been a subject of discussion for nearly a century. The matter is fully considered by KAPANDJI (1970). In

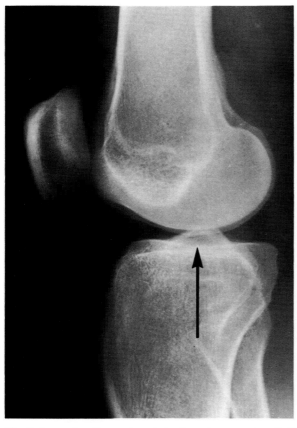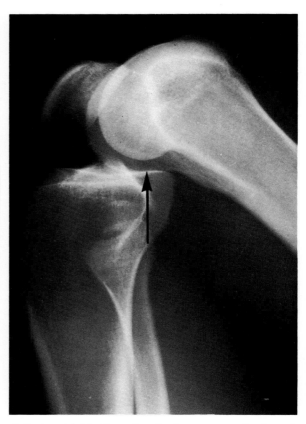

Fig. 2. Lateral radiographs of the knee in extension (*left*) and flexion (*right*). Note that the femur moves backwards across the tibial condyles as the knee flexes

the present author's view the movements and the relevant anatomy can be described with reasonable accuracy as follows.

The profiles of the femoral condyles are almost circular throughout the part of their articular surfaces that contacts the tibia between about 10° and 120° of flexion. From 0° to 10° the femoral facet have a greater radius of curvature (i.e., they are flattened), whilst at the extreme of flexion the radius diminishes.

In full extension the relatively flattened distal aspects of the femoral condyles make area contact with the anterior halves of the tibial facets, thus tending to extrude the anterior horns of the menisci from between the bone ends. As flexion progresses, contact between the femur and the tibia moves posteriorly (Fig. 2). As a consequence, by about 10° of flexion anterior contact has been lost and the femur and tibia now contact each other over a much smaller area, located roughly at the midpoint of the tibial facets. Thus the anterior halves

of the tibio-femoral joint hinge open like a book as flexion commences. Conversely, they close like a book — to prevent further movement — near full extension. This behaviour suggests that the femur might act as a cam to limit extension (see Section: "The Limitation of Extension", below).

From 10° to 120° of flexion the circular portions of the femoral facets roll backwards (and thus, because of the slope on the tibial facets, downwards: Fig. 3; MOORE and HARVEY, 1974) across the posterior halves of the tibial facets.

During the final degrees of flexion the posterior edges of the tibial facets contact, and slide round, the sharply curved posterior extremes of the femoral condyles.

Axis of Flexion and Extension

For some years it has been accepted that the position of the axis about which the tibia rotates as the knee flexes varies throughout the range of

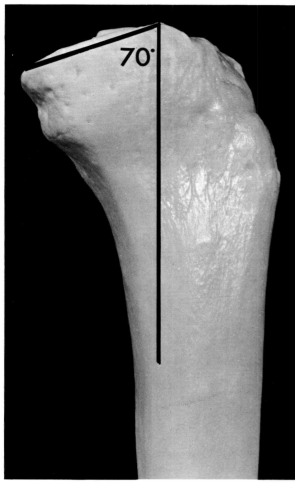

Fig. 3. A lateral view of the tibia to show the backward and downward slope of the tibial articular facets

of the cadaver knee has now been reported, which suggests that the tibia in fact rotates around a single unmoving axis, rather than about a migrating one (DENHAM and BISHOP, 1978). In this experiment a cadaver knee was fixed by the femur to a sheet of paper. The knee was placed on its side so that during flexion the tibia moved in the plane of the paper. A pencil was now passed through a hole drilled in the tibia perpendicular to the paper so that the tibia and the pencil acted as a protractor. As the knee was flexed from full extension, the pencil was found to draw a circle on the paper, thus demonstrating (directly and apparently without the possibility of misinterpretation) that the tibia rotates around a single, unmoving axis at the knee. This apparent conflict may be resolved when it is realized that the total movement of the instant centre is only a matter of a few millimetres, so that the area within which it moves can be viewed as a point in the context of the experiment described by DENHAM and BISHOP (see Chap. 2, Section on "Two-dimensional Simplifications").

Antero-posterior Tibio-femoral Movement

As described above, antero-posterior movement of the tibia on the femur always occurs during flexion and extension. Since in everyday clinical practice antero-posterior tibial movement in the flexed knee is thought to reflect the integrity of the cruciate ligaments, the obvious possibility arises that these structures play an essential role in governing this normal movement at the knee.

The relevant mechanism appears to have been described first by KAPANDJI (1970) and will be summarised here. The posterior cruciate ligament is attached to the femur, *distal* to the centre of rotation of the knee (be that a line connecting instant centres or a point). If the femur is thought of as flexing across the top of a fixed tibia without antero-posterior movement, the point on the femur to which the posterior cruciate ligament is attached would therefore tend to move first forwards and then upwards. Such movement cannot of course occur because the posterior cruciate ligament is inelastic for practical purposes: instead the femur must move bodily first backwards and then downwards relative to the tibia, the latter movement being permitted by (and presumably accounting for) the backward and downward slope of the tibial articular surfaces (Fig. 3).

movement. The method used by FRANKEL et al. (1971) to determine the path of the centre of rotation from instant to instant (i.e., the "instant centres") consisted of observing (from radiographs) the relative movement of two points upon the tibial shaft as the tibia moved on the femur through a series of arcs subdividing the full range of flexion. Perpendiculars were drawn to lines connecting each pair of points at either end of these arcs. The intercept between each pair of perpendiculars (now viewed as radii of the arc under study) was regarded as being the centre of rotation for that part of the range of movement, i.e., as being the instant centre. A line connecting the intercepts for each of the arcs taken in turn was drawn to show the path of the instant centre.

Although there appears to be no obvious flaw in FRANKEL's methodology, an experimental study

The anterior cruciate ligament contributes to the reverse movement during extension (and helps to limit hyperextension; see below).

Although forward and backward translation of the femur across the tibia is due largely to the action of the cruciate ligaments, these movements occur in the absence of the ligaments, partly because the femoral condyles roll backwards and forwards like wheels across the top of the tibia as the knee flexes and extends, and partly because the collateral ligaments act in the same way as do the cruciate ligaments (because, like the cruciate ligaments, their long axes are also crossed: KAPANDJI, 1970).

The force with which the knee can be extended, i.e., the extensor turning moment, is given by the product of the force generated by the quadriceps muscle and the length of the lever arm through which this force acts. The lever arm may be represented by the distance between the attachment of the patellar tendon to the tibia anteriorly and the point of contact between the tibia and the femur posteriorly. Because this point of contact moves backwards as the knee flexes, the length of the lever arm, and hence (for a quadriceps contraction of given force) the magnitude of the extensor moment, both increase as the knee flexes, reaching a maximum at about 90° of flexion when the femur contacts the posterior extremity of the tibial articular facet.

In view of this phenomenon and the fact that backward migration of the femur across the tibia depends on the posterior cruciate ligament, it follows that to achieve a given extensor movement at 90° of flexion, a more powerful quadriceps contraction would be required in the absence of the posterior cruciate ligament than in its presence. Since the patello-femoral compressive force is proportional to the force generated by quadriceps contraction, it follows in turn that for a given extensor moment the patella will be driven less forcibly against the femur in the presence of the posterior cruciate ligament than in its absence. In view of this it would not be surprising if the loss of the posterior cruciate ligament resulted in patellar pain.

When they are thought of as levers, there is an interesting similarity between the proximal tibia and the proximal femur: the distance from the centre of the femoral head to the greater trochanter (i.e., the length of the abductor lever arm) is approximately the same as the distance from the back of the tibial articular facets to the tibial tubercle

(i.e., the length of the extensor lever arm when the knee is extended from 90° of flexion).

Limitation of Extension

The elliptical shape of the femoral condyles is of some significance in the limitation of extension: the femur represents a section of a cam having a circular profile virtually throughout the range of movement, but with a nearly flat area meeting a corresponding flat surface on the front of the tibial facets at full extension. When these "flats" meet, further extension can only occur if the bones hinge apart around the anterior edge of their area of contact. Such separation (and hence hyperextension) is prevented by tension in all the ligaments lying behind the axis of rotation of the knee (a group that includes the collateral ligaments), by muscle actions, and by the body weight. It is for this reason that a cadaver knee with the collateral ligaments intact, but with the posterior capsule divided, will not hyperextend, provided that forward subluxation of the tibia is prevented by the anterior cruciate ligament (and the menisci; see below). It is primarily, if not entirely, by this mechanism that the anterior cruciate ligament acts to limit extension, since in the cadaver knee hyperextension will occur in the presence of an intact anterior cruciate ligament if the structures lying posterior to the axis of rotation are divided.

Extension is also limited by contact between the femoral intercondylar notch and the tibial intercondylar eminence, a subject discussed below.

Rotation of the Tibia About a Vertical Axis ("Tibial Rotation")

The femoral intercondylar notch is wider posteriorly than anteriorly. As a consequence, the sides of the tibial intercondylar eminence articulate with the walls of the notch in the fully extended knee but they do not do so beyond about 10° of flexion. As flexion increases the eminence becomes an increasingly loose fit in the notch.

In view of the loose fit between the tibial intercondylar eminence and the femoral intercondylar notch, tibial rotation on the femur cannot be, and is not, limited by bony contact, save possibly in full extension. Rotation is in fact limited by the tension in all the tibio-femoral ligaments, which develops as they are "wrung out" by the movement. In full extension all the major ligamentous structures are already tight, and thus they are immediately wrung out by any attempt at tibio-femoral rotation. No such movement can therefore occur in the fully extended knee (both for this reason and because the movement is limited by bony contact in the midline).

At full extension the eminence is driven into the narrowing anterior end of the notch. As a consequence, firstly further extension is prevented; and secondly, the femur is prevented from sliding forwards across the medial tibial facet, because the anterior margin of this facet runs upwards onto the intercondylar eminence to constitute a "wall" across the front of the facet. In contrast, the lateral femoral condyle is free to continue to slide forwards across the top of the tibia, because the anterior edge of the lateral tibial facet is flat. This continuing forward movement of only the lateral femoral condyle on the tibia manifests itself as tibial external rotation during the last few degrees of extension. As flexion is initiated the tibio-femoral joint is "unlocked", perhaps by tibial internal rotation produced by contraction of the popliteus muscle.

Beyond 10° of flexion the increasingly loose fit between the tibial intercondylar eminence and the femoral intercondylar notch allows more and more tibial rotation to occur. This motion occurs around an axis passing through the lateral side of the medial tibial condyle (i.e., nearly through the centre of the tibia) and thus involves backward translation of one femoral condyle across the tibia and equal and opposite forward translation of the other condyle. If, for any reason, the translational movement permitted in one compartment were to increase (or diminish) relative to that permitted in the other compartment, the permitted range of rotation would increase (or decrease) and the axis about which the movement was occurring would shift towards the less mobile compartment. This fact may have some bearing upon so-called "pivot shift" and tibial rotational instability.

As the femur moves backwards across the tibia during flexion, the anterior halves of the menisci must be placed under tension and hence must to some extent regulate backward movement of the femur relative to the tibia. The posterior halves of the menisci will act in a similar way during extension to limit forward movement. Thus in general, each meniscus restricts antero-posterior movement of one femoral condyle on the tibia. The loss of this mechanism in one compartment only would tend to increase the range of tibial rotation and displace its axis (i.e., it would tend

to produce tibial rotational instability and "pivot shift").

At full extension the femur meets the tibia, leaving no gap for the anterior horn of the meniscus to occupy. The anterior horns of the menisci must therefore be sufficiently mobile to move forwards completely out of the articular area at the end of extension. Similarly the posterior horns are "extruded" from the knee in full flexion.

Side-to-Side Translational Movements

In theory, side-to-side translational movement could occur between the femur and tibia and between the femur and patella. The former is prevented by the tibio-femoral ligaments and by the presence of the tibial intercondylar eminence between the femoral condyles. Similarly, the latter is prevented by the patellar ligaments and the presence of the wedge-shaped posterior surface of the patella between the femoral condyles. Since the patella must move with the tibia during flexion and extension, these two bones can be thought of as one unit having a central keel located in a central femoral groove.

Incidence of Deformity

Before considering the morbid anatomy underlying the various deformities seen clinically in the arthritic knee, it is appropriate to consider their incidence and nature. Although clinical impressions abound as to the incidence of these deformities in the two sexes, there do not appear to have been any studies specifically devoted to this subject. Therefore, for the purpose of this Chapter, CAMERON and FREEMAN (unpublished) studied a population of patients with disorders of the knee seen in several centres throughout the United Kingdom and in Sweden. The population was a selected one, since all the patients were thought to have knees sufficiently damaged to merit total replacement. Thus the various incidence figures presented below for particular deformities should be understood to be incidences in severely damaged knees, not in all knees affected by these diseases.

Deformity, or malalignment, at the knee can affect both the tibio-femoral and the patello-femoral joints. Unfortunately, we have precise data only for the former.

The overall incidence of involvement of the knee in OA and RA has been reported on by a number of workers. Thus the knee has been said to be the commonest site for OA (HEINE, 1926; COLLINS, 1949; ALLANDER, 1977) and for RA (KUHNS and POTTER, 1963; GSCHWEND, 1977). In a recent survey GSCHWEND (1977) reported that the knee joint was involved in 74% of 300 patients with RA, whilst in a study of patients with RA attending a rheumatological clinic at The London Hospital, KING et al. (1978) found that of patients whose arthritis interferred with their ability to walk the knee was the principal cause of this disability in 53%. Thus deformities at this joint represent a numerically and functionally important problem.

Material

Prior to ICLH total knee replacement at The London Hospital and in certain other hospitals in Britain and Sweden, all patients had, for some years, a standard preoperative assessment performed, the records of which were kept at The London Hospital. As part of this assessment, fixed flexion deformity and the tibio-femoral angle in varus and valgus were recorded. Regrettably, the position of the patella was not recorded until 1977. An analysis of these records has been carried out.

The records were considered adequate in 338 cases of RA and 137 cases of OA. Clearly prior operative intervention might alter the pattern of deformity in the knee and therefore knees in which previous surgery had been performed were excluded. There remained 256 cases of RA and 102 cases of OA without previous surgical intervention for analysis.

Definitions

The terms used in this study have been defined as follows.

Valgus/Varus Alignment

Neutral
5°–10° valgus when the tibia is stressed first medially and then laterally

Varus
0°, or more than 0°, varus when the tibia is stressed medially

Valgus
More than 10° valgus when the tibia is stressed laterally

"Loose"
More than 10° valgus when the tibia is stressed laterally and 0°, or more than 0° varus when it is stressed medially

Fixed deformity
Fixed deformity was said to be present if the knee could not be passively stressed into the neutral range, i.e., if the malalignment was fixed, at least in part

External rotation
No precise definition by measurement. The tibia was classified as being in external rotation, neutral (i.e., normal alignment), or internal rotation as judged by eye in the flexed knee

Fixed flexion deformity
A knee which could not be placed in full extension passively. (Any additional extensor lag, i.e., an inability to maintain extension actively, was ignored for the purposes of this study)

Examples

Tibio-femoral angle with tibia stressed laterally	Tibio-femoral angle with tibia stressed medially	Description
20° valgus	20° valgus	Valgus. Fixed deformity present
25° valgus	15° valgus	Valgus. Fixed deformity present, combined with instability
25° valgus	5° valgus	Valgus. No fixed deformity, i.e., an unstable valgus knee
5° valgus	15° varus	Varus. No fixed deformity, i.e., an unstable varus knee
10° varus	25° varus	Varus. Fixed deformity present, combined with instability
5° valgus	5° valgus	Neutral. Stable
15° valgus	15° varus	Loose, i.e., an unstable knee in valgus and in varus

Results

The incidence of valgus and varus malalignment, the presence or absence of fixed valgus and varus deformity, of fixed flexion deformity, and of external rotation deformity are set out in Tables 1–5 in relation to the sex of the patient and the diagnosis.

We have no precise data relating to the incidence of patello-femoral malalignment. It is our impression, however, that medial subluxation is rare or nonexistent but that lateral subluxation is common, especially in the valgus, externally rotated knee.

Table 1. Sex vs diagnosis

	Male[a]	Female[a]	Total
OA	47 (46)	55 (54)	102
RA	56 (22)	200 (78)	256

[a] Absolute numbers (% of total in total column)

Table 2. Valgus or varus malalignment vs sex and diagnosis

Sex	Vg[a]	N[a]	Vr[a]	Loose[a]	Total
OA					
Male	15 (32)	17 (36)	13 (28)	{2 (4)}	47
Female	18 (33)	15 (27)	19 (55)	{3 (5)}	55
RA					
Male	19 (34)	23 (41)	13 (23)	{1 (2)}	56
Female	128 (64)	59 (30)	{5 (2)}	{4 (4)}	200

[a] Absolute numbers (% of figure in total column)

Table 3. Valgus and varus contractures

			Total	Present
OA	Male	Valgus	15	12 (80%)
		Varus	13	11 (84%)
	Female	Valgus	18	13 (72%)
		Varus	19	14 (74%)
RA	Male	Valgus	19	12 (63%)
		Varus	13	9 (69%)
	Female	Valgus	128	89 (69%)
		Varus	5	{0 (0%)}

Table 4. External rotation deformity

	Vg[a]	N[a]	Vr[a]	Loose[a]
OA				
Male	1/15 (7)	0/17 (0)	3/13 (23)	{0/2 (−)}
Female	5/18 (28)	1/15 (7)	5/19 (26)	{0/3 (−)}
RA				
Male	4/19 (21)	5/25 (20)	2/13 (15)	{0/1 (−)}
Female	54/128 (42)	7/59 (13)	{1/5 (−)}	{4/8 (−)}

[a] $\dfrac{\text{Number with ER}}{\text{Total in that category}}$ (%)

Table 5. Valgus, varus, and flexion contractures

			% with Vg or Vr contracture	% with flexion contracture
OA	Male	Vg	80	15
		Vr	84	46
	Female	Vg	72	67
		Vr	74	74
RA	Male	Vg	63	74
		Vr	69	69
	Female	Vg	69	60
		Vr	(0)	(20)

Discussion

Two preliminary points must be stressed. First, the figures in this study are based upon a population of patients thought suitable by a number of surgeons for replacement of the knee. The precise indication for this operation may vary a little from surgeon to surgeon, but in general it is reserved for severely damaged knees. Broadly speaking, therefore, these results can be thought of as depicting the end result of the osteoarthrosic and rheumatoid processes. Having said this, we believe that the progress of the disease (and hence case selection of the kind we have employed) will affect the magnitude of the various deformities we have seen but not their nature. Once a knee has developed valgus or varus malalignment it is unknown in the author's experience for the deformity to diminish to neutral and then to increase, but in the opposite direction. In contrast, it is commonplace for a deformity to remain in the same direction but to increase in magnitude. (Loose knees are a partial exception to this general rule and are mentioned below.) For these reasons we have not recorded the magnitudes of the valgus and varus malalignments seen in this series, since it seems likely that these would only reflect the intervals of time that had elapsed between the onset of the disease and referral for surgery, rather than any more fundamental variable. For what the information is worth, the greatest valgus angle encountered in the knees we studied was 70°, and the greatest varus 30°. In the case of flexion contractures we have included an intermediate group of 5°, between "absent" and "present", since "contractures" of this magnitude are hard to measure, are occasionally seen in normal, symptomless knees, and even in arthritic knees cause little disability (PERRY et al., 1975). The greatest flexion deformity encountered was 70°. External rotation, in contrast to the other deformities, has not been measured in degrees and has simply been recorded as present or absent, as judged by eye.

Secondly, it seems likely that the pattern of deformity and the incidence of contractures would be different if a different genetic stock were to be studied. Thus for example INSALL (personal communication, 1977), studying a population containing a larger number of people of Southern European origin, who initially had a more stocky build with a tendency to a more varus knee, has encountered 20 varus female RA knees in 64 female RA knees treated: an incidence of 31%, as against our incidence of 2%. INSALL's corresponding figure for RA female valgus knees was 45% (as against ours of 64%), and that for neutral knees, 23% (as against ours of 30%). Thus it appears that the initial tibio-femoral alignment has an important effect upon the nature of the deformity a knee may develop in RA.

Having made these preliminary points, the essential findings in this study may be summarised as follows.

1) *Severely damaged knees* usually occur in women with RA (Table 1). Amongst the remainder, women with OA, men with OA, and men with RA appear with equal frequency. Thus for every seven severely damaged knees included in this study, four were in women with RA, and one each in women with OA, men with OA, and men with RA. To some extent this distribution may reflect case selection rather than differences in the effect of the disease. Nevertheless, it is probably true that RA causes severe damage more commonly than does OA (perhaps especially in women).

2) *The three smaller groups (women with OA, men with OA, and men with RA)* are similar to one another with respect to the incidence within any one group of valgus, neutral, and varus knees: about one-third are in each category (Table 2). In contrast, in women with RA in this population, varus knees virtually did not occur: two-thirds of these patients had knees in valgus and one-third, knees in neutral.

3) *Some degree of fixed valgus or varus deformity* was present in about 75% of knees (Table 3). Fixed deformity was most frequent in men with OA, less frequent in women with OA, and least frequent in both sexes in RA. The differences between these groups were not great, however.

4) *External rotation* had a scattered incidence of around 10%–20%, save in valgus rheumatoid female knees, where the incidence was 42% (Table 4). Only in this last group were our numbers in fact large enough to give a meaningful figure for the incidence.

5) *The presence or absence of valgus and varus malalignment*, whether in the form of instability or of fixed deformity, did not have any clear-cut relationship to the presence of fixed flexion. In all male OA knees and in female RA valgus knees, fixed flexion was less common than fixed valgus or varus (Table 5). In other knees, however, the frequency with which valgus or varus malalignment became fixed was about equal to the frequency with which flexion became fixed, and the incidence of the latter was unchanged even if there was neither valgus nor varus malalignment present.

6) *Loose knees*, i.e., knees displaying both valgus and varus instability were rare (Table 2). Their apparent incidence in this study was 4%, but of the fourteen knees concerned, five had fixed flexion deformities in excess of 20° and in such knees rotation at the hip during stressing of the tibia might have been mistaken for medio-lateral instability.

7) We have no precise data regarding *patello-femoral alignment*, but it is our impression that medial subluxation occurs rarely if at all. In contrast, lateral subluxation is common, especially in knees that are in valgus with an externally rotated tibia. It does, however, occur in neutral and varus knees.

These findings suggest the following generalisations. In a North European population, severe damage to the knee is equally likely to affect men with OA, men with RA, and women with OA. These groups are equally likely to develop a valgus, varus, or neutral knee with or without external rotation and fixed flexion (a possible exception to this last point being men with OA, who are unlikely to develop fixed flexion). In contrast, women with RA represent a special group: they are numerous (because RA is common in women and probably because severe damage is more common in RA), and the pattern of deformity differs in that (1) varus is rare, (2) valgus (specifically valgus associated with external rotation and lateral patellar subluxation) is twice as common as in other groups, and (3) if the knee does not develop valgus malalignment it almost always develops a flexion contracture instead.

The question as to what anatomical abnormalities cause these deformities remains.

Relevant Observations at the Hip

Arthritis of the hip has been treated surgically for many years, and there is now little controversy as to the nature of the gross changes taking place. Since it seems reasonable to think that the essential pathological processes in both OA and RA at the hip and at the knee are broadly similar, it is worth recapitulating the well-known changes at the hip before considering the knee. They consist of bone and cartilage loss and soft-tissue contracture.

Bone and Cartilage Loss

Bone and cartilage are lost from the zenith of the femoral head and acetabulum. This accounts for the "wandering acetabulum", for a break in Shenton's line, and for true shortening of the leg. As measured by the latter, a loss of 2 cm of bone, especially in RA, is not rare: Figure 4 shows an example of OA in a post-mortem specimen from which 10 cm³ of bone and cartilage had been lost from the hip.

Soft-Tissue Contracture

It is particularly the structures on the anterior and medial aspects of the hip (accounting for fixed flexion and fixed adduction) and the short external rotators and posterior capsule (accounting for fixed external rotation) that are affected by soft-tissue contracture. The most dramatic, well-known

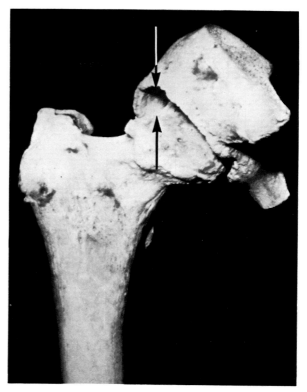

Fig. 4. The bones in OA of the hip. Note that destruction of the zenith of the femoral head and of the acetabulum has created a space between the bones superiorly. The measured volume of this space was 10 cm³

example of this is a contracture of the adductor muscles (especially of adductor longus), accounting for the persistence of an adduction deformity after hip replacement unless corrected by adductor tenotomy.

Osteophyte Formation

Osteophytes are formed particularly in OA where peripheral cartilage persists, since only in such circumstances can osteophytes grow by endochondral ossification (FREEMAN, 1972). Osteophytes grow only into soft-tissue spaces (the best example being the space created in the cavity of the hip inferomedial to the femoral head by bone loss at the zenith), and although they may limit movement mechanically (and thus help to maintain deformity) it is difficult to conceive that their growth could actually produce deformity by "pushing" the bones into an abnormal position.

Ligamentous Elongation

Ligamentous elongation appears never to occur to any significant extent in the arthritic hip, even in RA: hypermobility and dislocation, which would be expected if gross elongation did occur, are never seen.

Ligamentous Rupture

The only intra-capsular ligament in the hip (the ligamentum teres) is subject to ligamentous rupture. Whether the ligament is destroyed by enzymatic digestion or mechanical attrition is unclear: in RA both seem possible, whilst in OA the latter is more likely.

Summary

At the hip, the processes responsible for the development and maintainance of deformity appear to be tissue loss (affecting first cartilage and then bone) and soft-tissue adhesions and contracture (affecting ligaments and muscles, respectively). Ligamentous elongation either does not occur or is only slight. Ligamentous rupture affects the ligamentum teres: probably it is usually due to mechanical attrition. Although this view is not well documented, it is the present authors' impression that it is generally accepted amongst orthopaedic surgeons.

If bone loss and soft-tissue contracture are the cause of deformity at the hip, and if significant ligamentous elongation does not occur at this joint, it would not be unreasonable to expect that the same would be true of the knee. This view is controversial, however: valgus and varus instability in the arthritic knee are frequently attributed (presumably by analogy with similar instability after ligamentous injury) to "elongated" or "defective" medial and lateral collateral ligaments, respectively. However, although instability in the arthritic knee might in theory be due to elongation, it is equally possible (in theory) that it might be caused by bone loss on the concave side of the joint, a view that would be consistent with the morbid anatomy of the arthritic hip. According to this view, valgus or varus instability at the arthritic knee could be accounted for by postulating the presence of bone loss, and fixed valgus and varus deformity by postulating a combination of bone loss and soft-tissue contracture.

This controversy is not simply of academic, pathological interest, since the object of surgical procedures in the arthritic knee is to reverse the gross anatomical abnormalities. For this to be done, the nature of these abnormalities must be understood.

The Nature of the Morbid Anatomical Changes Responsible for Deformity of the Knee in OA and RA

The nature of the changes responsible for knee deformity in OA and RA will be dealt with by considering first instability in a varus and valgus direction, and then the same two malalignments but with the addition of fixed deformity. The other abnormalities of alignment to be seen in the arthritic knee will then be considered.

Varus Instability

Theoretically, varus instability might be due to: (1) rupture and/or elongation of the lateral soft tissues (as after soft-tissue trauma), and/or (2) a loss of cartilage and bone medially. Both these pathological processes would produce the same physical sign on the examination couch, i.e., it would be possible to displace the tibia from neutral to varus alignment and back again. In contrast, if the knee were to be compressed axially (as on bearing weight or during muscular contraction), a knee with normal bones would tend to be stabilised in normal alignment, whereas a knee with bone loss would tend to be driven into the position of deformity (Fig. 5). It is a commonplace radiological observation in the arthritic knee (1) that bone loss is present (Fig. 6) and (2) that the affected knee falls into a position of deformity on bearing weight (Fig. 7). (Hence the near-irrelevance of non-weight-bearing X-rays in the arthritic knee.) It may be concluded — even without visual inspection of the articular surfaces of the knee — that bony defects are responsible, at least in part if not wholly, for varus instability.

The possibility remains that lateral collateral ligament elongation or rupture may also play a part in the genesis of varus instability. However,

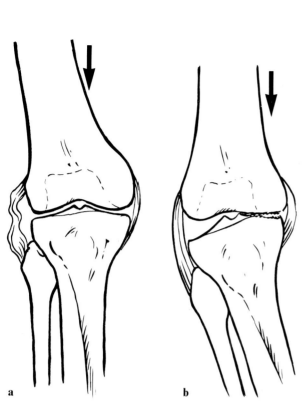

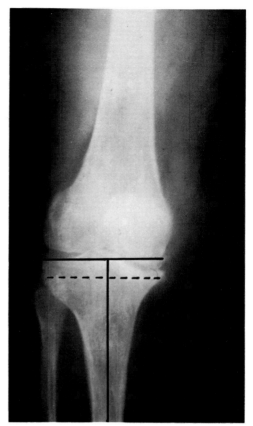

Fig. 5. **a** A diagram to show a knee without bony defects but with laxity of the lateral collateral ligament loaded in compression, as during one-leg stance. Because the line of action of the load on the knee passes through the area of contact between the femoral and tibial condyles, there is no tendency for the joint to open laterally and normal alignment is maintained. **b** A diagram to show a knee with a medial bony defect during one-leg stance. The load now acts to close the defect, causing the knee to buckle into varus malalignment

Fig. 6. An antero-posterior radiograph of the knee, taken with the patient supine. The *vertical line* over the tibia represents the tibial axis, i.e., this line passes from the centre of the knee to the centre of the ankle (the latter is not seen). The *horizontal solid line* has been drawn perpendicular to this axis. Laterally this line passes through the upper surface of the undeformed lateral tibial condyle. Medially it passes approximately 1 cm above the medial tibial condyle. The *horizontal dotted line* passes through the articular surface of the medial tibial condyle. The distance between these two horizontal lines represents the size of the medial tibial defect

the present author has never observed a frank rupture of the lateral collateral ligament and lateral capsule at operation in uninjured knees. This finding does not exclude the possibility that this lesion occurs, but it must mean that if it does, it is rare.

Elongation of a collateral ligament (as against rupture) seems to be a likely possibility: indeed its existence is strongly suggested by X-ray appearances such as those shown in Fig. 8. It is necessary to ask, however, what mechanism might be responsible for elongation, especially in OA, where damage to the ligament by distension secondary to a prolonged synovitis or by collagenase — both

conceivable in RA — seens very unlikely. A probable answer is that as the deformity on bearing weight increases, a point is reached (at about 10° of malalignment; see above) at which the line of action of the resultant of the forces acting on the knee passes medial to the most medial point of bony contact in the joint. At, or a little before, this stage the knee will tend to hinge open, thus subjecting the lateral soft tissues to persistent tension (Chap. 2). Since it seems most unlikely that the collateral ligaments are persistently subjected to tensile forces in the normal knee, the result may well be that the ligament is overstressed and

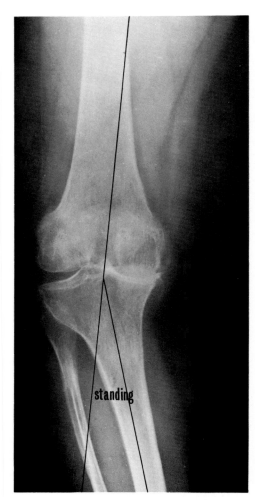

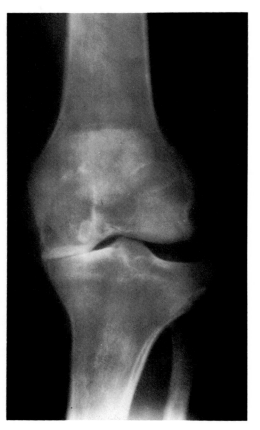

Fig. 7. A radiograph of the same knee as that shown in Fig. 6, now taken with the patient standing. Note that the medial tibial and femoral condyles approach each other so that the knee falls into varus malalignment. Compare this X-ray with the diagram shown in Fig. 5b

Fig. 8. An antero-posterior radiograph of a weight-bearing varus knee, to show the appearance of opening of the lateral compartment of the joint. This appearance suggests that the lateral collateral ligament has been elongated, perhaps as a consequence of tensile stresses developing in it secondary to the varus malalignment. Although the lateral compartment appears to have opened, the radiological space between the lateral femoral and tibial condyles is in fact partly occupied by articular cartilage and the meniscus. The actual elongation of the lateral collateral ligament is therefore much less than it appears on this X-ray

Fig. 10a. The Tenser in place, with its blades opened, in a knee having no bony defect, but an elongated lateral collateral ligament (such as that shown in Fig. 5a). The blades of the Tenser could be opened more widely in the lateral compartment than in the medial compartment of the knee, turing the joint into varus

Fig. 10b. The Tenser in place, with its blades opened, in a joint having pre-operatively a medial tibial and femoral defect such as that shown in Fig. 5b. The blades can now

be opened more widely on the medial than on the lateral ▶ side of the joint. When the medial and lateral soft tissues are equally tense, this knee will lie in normal alignment

Fig. 10c. A Tenser in place, with its blades opened, in a knee having pre-operatively a ruptured lateral collateral ligament. In such a knee the lateral blade could theoretically be opened indefinitely, turing the knee into progressively increasing varus

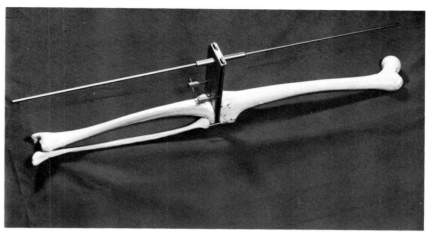

Fig. 9. The Tenser, an instrument used in ICLH arthroplasty of the knee, with which the presence or absence of soft-tissue contractures can be demonstrated at operation. Before insertion of this instrument, the cruciate ligaments are divided and the tibial plateau is sectioned at right angles to the anatomical axis of the bone. The Tenser is then inserted into the extended knee with the solid plate on the transected surface of the tibia. Two blades can be screwed away from this solid plate to separate first one and then the other femoral condyle from the tibia and thus tense the medial and lateral soft tissues in turn. A bar passes through the tibial plate at right angles to the latter. The distal end of this bar must lie over the centre of the ankle. The proximal end of the bar will lie over the hip when the soft tissues are tensed only when there is neither contracture nor elongation of these tissues on either side of the joint. Thus by tensing the tissues, and then noting the relationship of the proximal end of the bar to the hip, the surgeon can judge the presence or absence and magnitude of soft-tissue contracture or elongation

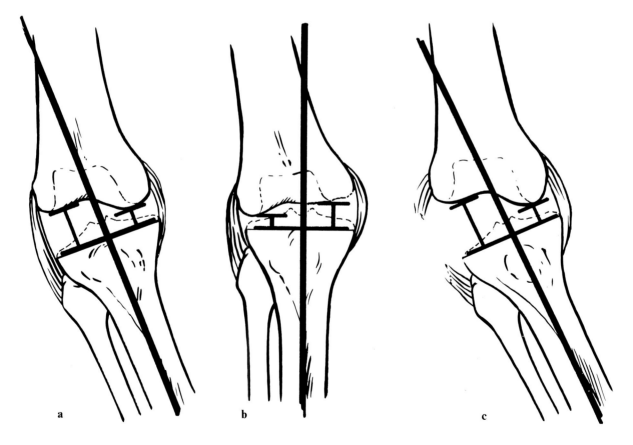

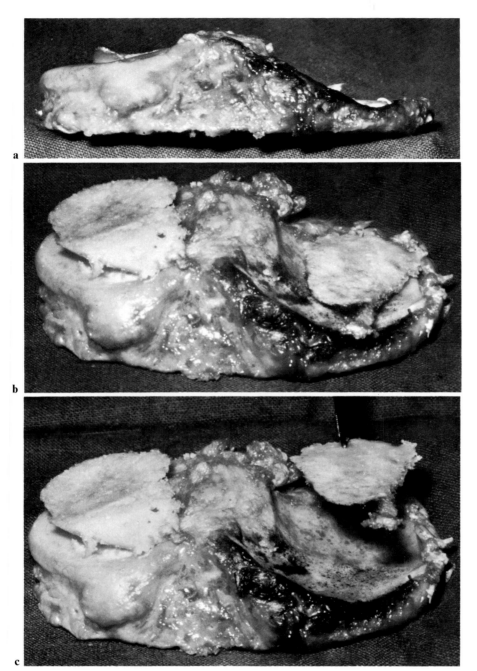

Fig. 11 a–c. The operative specimen taken from the knee shown in Figs. 6 and 7 **a** The appearance of the anterior aspect of the bone removed from the tibia. This bone was sectioned just distal to the *dotted horizontal line* in Fig. 6. Note that more bone has been removed laterally than medially, because of the pathological loss of bone from the medial tibial condyle. The anterior edge of this defect has been stained with methylene blue. **b** The fragments of bone resected from the distal aspects of the femoral condyles have now been added to the tibial specimen shown in Fig. 11 a. The distal femoral condyles have been sectioned at right angles to the anatomical axis of the femur, i.e., in 7° of valgus relative to the axis of the femoral shaft. In this photograph the medial femoral and tibial condyles are in contact, i.e., the pathological specimen represents the situation shown in the weight-bearing knee seen in Fig. 7. **c** The same specimen as shown in Fig. 11 b. The medial femoral bone fragment has now been lifted to place it on the same horizontal level as the lateral femoral fragment. This has created a gap of rather over 1 cm on the medial side of the joint. This gap represents the defect in the medial side of the knee produced by cartilage and bony loss. The joint in this position is approximately the same as that seen in Fig. 5. Closure of this defect creates the varus malalignment shown in Fig. 7

that it therefore stretches. On this analysis, ligamentous elongation might be expected to increase the malalignment in a knee that is already significantly malaligned as a consequence of bone loss, but not to initiate the malalignment.

That this is indeed the case may be demonstrated at operation by using a special surgical instrument known as a Tenser (an instrument used routinely in ICLH arthroplasty). This instrument and its mode of action are illustrated in Figs. 9 and 10. It will be seen that if a Tenser were used to tighten the two collateral ligaments in a knee that before operation had been unstable (i.e., fully correctable to neutral alignment passively), three possibilities would theoretically arise. First, if the lateral collateral ligament had elongated but not ruptured, the collateral ligaments would tighten, leaving the knee in persistent varus (Fig. 10a). Second, if only a medial bone defect were present, the medial blade of the Tenser would need to be opened more than the lateral one, but the two collateral ligaments would then tighten with the knee in anatomical alignment (Fig. 10a). Finally, if the lateral collateral ligament had ruptured, it would not be possible to tense it, so that the lateral compartment of the knee could be opened indefinitely, turning the knee into ever-increasing varus (Fig. 10c). The author has never observed the last of these possibilities. The first possible outcome has occurred but has been unusual and the degree of residual deformity has been slight, suggesting only slight elongation of the ligament on the convex side of the deformity. The usual outcome is the second.

It may be concluded that material elongation of the lateral collateral ligament is an uncommon, late event and that rupture occurs rarely or never. Thus varus instability in OA (and, when it occurs, in RA) is mainly, if not entirely, due to medial bone loss. Simple trigonometry shows that, roughly speaking, 1 cm of medial bone and cartilage loss will result in 10° of varus malalignment. Since 2 cm of tissue loss is commonplace at the hip, 13° of varus (i.e., 20° of deformity relative to an initial 7° valgus) might be commonplace at the knee.

The appearances produced by such bone loss in the tibial and femoral condyles of an OA varus knee are shown in Fig. 11. As usual in a varus knee, the defect is mainly tibial. In contrast to the usual femoral defect in a valgus knee, the femoral defect in the varus knee is, typically, small. This may perhaps be attributed to the fact that the bone of the distal femur is stronger than that

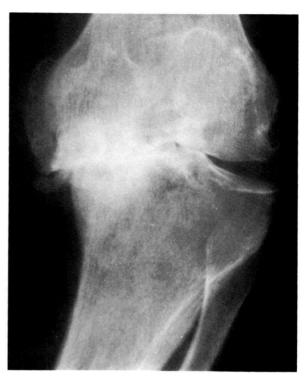

Fig. 12. An antero-posterior radiograph of a weight-bearing knee in varus, to show contact between the intercondylar eminence of the tibia and the midline of the femur, resulting in load-carriage through the medial and central bone but not the lateral bone in the knee. Note that the areas of bone carrying load are relatively sclerotic and that the tibial intercondylar eminence has tilted laterally (see also Fig. 8).

This knee and that shown in Fig. 8 appear to display lateral tibial subluxation. However, in Fig. 8 the medial side of the medial femoral and tibial condyles are in line, whilst in this figure the apparent overlap of the medial femoral condyle is largely due to the presence of an osteophyte. On the lateral side of the joint, the lateral tibial condyle is normally more prominent than the lateral femoral condyle. To what extent is the appearance of lateral tibial subluxation in these knees a radiological illusion?

of the tibia (and hence less likely to be crushed), whilst medial patellar subluxation (leading to damage to the medial femoral condyle by the patella in a way analogous to that which occurs laterally in a valgus knee; see below) is rare, if it occurs at all.

As bone is lost from the medial side of the joint, the intercondylar eminence of the tibia (1) moves upwards relative to the femur and (2) tilts (as the tibia as a whole tilts) so that its apex moves laterally (Fig. 12). The combined effect of these two

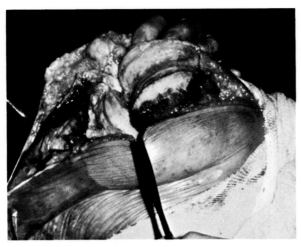

Fig. 13. An operative photograph of an osteoarthrosic knee in which osteophytes growing on the edges of the intercondylar eminence have fused to convert the knee into a "switch-back". The whole of the proximal surface of the tibia was ebernated and articular

to the formation of a false midline joint in the knee. The latter does indeed occur, so that the knee comes to transmit load medially and centrally, but not laterally (Fig. 12).

The formation of a false midline joint in OA is encouraged by the formation of osteophytes at the margins of the femoral intercondylar notch. Such osteophytes are possibly formed by "crushing over" of the articular margins of the notch rather than by endochondral ossification, the process by which osteophytes normally grow (FREEMAN, 1972). Whatever their origin, the osteophytes on the medial and lateral edges of the notch eventually fuse to bury the cruciate ligaments and to produce a continuous, false, central articular surface. Progressive destruction of the weight-bearing medial and central areas of the knee may eventually re-establish weight-bearing contact between the lateral condyles, so that finally the lateral surfaces also become eburnated to produce the "switch-back" knee (Fig. 13).

displacements is to produce impingement within the knee between the normally nonarticular central parts of the femur and tibia. By analogy with such abnormal bony contact elsewhere (e.g., between the fibula and the os calcis), this process might be expected to be painful, and to lead gradually

Valgus Instability

All the arguments and observations applied above to varus instability apply to valgus instability, save that the bony defects are now lateral and the soft-

Fig. 14. a–e The knee in RA displaying fixed valgus deformity. **a** An antero-posterior radiograph of the knee in the supine patient. The valgus deformity persists because it is held, whether the knee is weight-bearing or not, by the presence of a lateral soft-tissue contracture. Note the obvious tibial defect. The femoral defect is less obvious but is nevertheless present: (see Fig. 14b). **b** The same radiograph as in Fig. 14a, with the mechanical axis of the femur added. This line passes from the middle of the femoral condyles to the middle of the femoral head (not seen on this radiograph). A *perpendicular* has been drawn to this axis, passing through the most distal point on the medial femoral condyle. The distance between the lateral half of this line and the lateral femoral condyle represents the femoral defect in this knee. Note that the defect extends on to the distal–lateral as well as the distal aspects of the lateral femoral condyle. This is because the defect is produced partly by the tibia (destroying the distal end of the femur) and partly by the laterally subluxated patella (destroying the distal and lateral aspects of the femur: see Fig. 18). **c** An operative photograph of the knee shown in Fig. 14a. The hip and the proximal end of the incision are beyond the top of this photograph. An instrument with a plate attached to it at right angles has been passed into the medullary canal of the femur.

This plate can be seen in the lower part of the photograph. The medial side of the plate touches the medial femoral condyle. The approximate extent of the lateral defect (seen in Fig. 14b) can be judged by noting the distance between the lateral femoral condyle and the lateral side of the plate. In fact, the true defect is not quite as great as that shown here, since the lateral femoral condyle normally lies on a line perpendicular to the mechanical axis of the femur (drawn in Fig. 14b) which, unlike the plate on this instrument, is not perpendicular to the medullary canal and hence to the shaft of the femur. **d** The operative specimen removed from the distal femur shown in Fig. 14c by resection of the bone at 83° to the long axis of the shaft (i.e., at 90° to the mechanical axis). A significant amount of bone has been removed from the medial condyle (*left*). On the lateral side, little or no bone has been removed because of the pre-existing defect. **e** The specimen removed from the tibia (seen in Fig. 14a) by transecting it at right angles to the axis of the shaft. Note that here again a significant amount of bone has been removed from the medial side but little or none from the lateral side. Indeed, posteriorly no bone whatsoever has been removed, because the defect was distal to the line of section. Note that the tibial and the femoral defects are particularly evident posteriorly

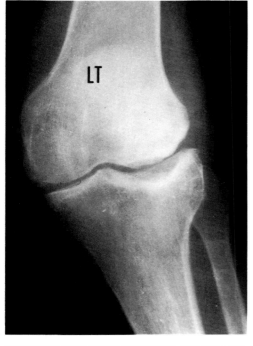

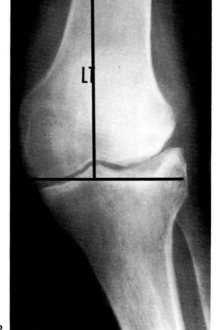

a

b

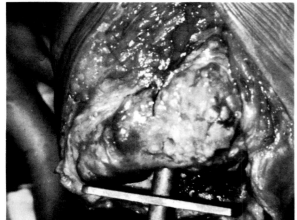

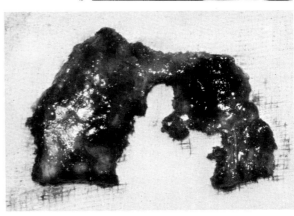

c

d

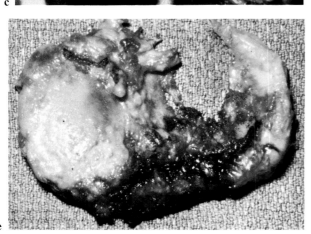

e

tissue defects (if they occurred) would be medial. Such bony defects are illustrated in an RA knee in Fig. 14. It should be noted that the tibial defect involves particularly the posterior three-quarters of the condyle, the anterior margin being relatively spared (Fig. 14e). This may be attributed to the fact that the femur does not articulate with, and thus will not mechanically damage, the anterior part of the tibial condyle. The lateral femoral condyle is often more grossly destroyed than the lateral tibial condyle (Fig. 14), which may be attributed to the fact that it is exposed to damage not only from the tibia but also from the laterally subluxed patella. (Lateral patellar subluxation is often present in such knees: its cause and its consequences are discussed under "Lateral Patellar Subluxation", below).

As with varus instability, it may be concluded that valgus instability is mainly (if not entirely) due to bone loss laterally, and that this loss is explicable mainly on simple mechanical grounds. With the Tenser, the author's experience in knees displaying valgus instability has been the same as that in knees displaying varus instability. This suggests that elongation of the medial collateral ligament is a relatively rare, late, secondary event.

Fixed Varus Deformity

Theoretically, a fixed varus deformity could be due only to one of two possible events: (1) ligamentous elongation laterally combined with "growth" of the lateral condyles, or (2) collapse of the bone medially combined with contracture of the medial soft tissues (Fig. 15). The former seems inconceivable: growth (as distinct from marginal and intracartilaginous surface osteophytosis) of the condyles is never seen in RA nor in OA. Contractures (e.g., at the hip, causing fixed adduction, and at the knee, causing fixed flexion), in contrast, are commonplace. It may be concluded that contracture formation, not growth, is at work, a conclusion that reinforces the view put forward above that instability is due to bone loss rather than to soft-tissue elongation.

The nature of the contractures that may be responsible must now be considered. Surgeons will be familiar with the concept of a contracture at the hip, as already discussed in this Chapter. Although such lesions are clinically commonplace, the precise nature of the pathological events responsible for them is unclear: presumably they are due to a mixture of shortening and fibrosis in muscles and adhesion formation around muscles and ligaments. Whatever their exact pathological nature, it is now suggested that similar contractures occur in the arthritic knee (and indeed in all arthritic joints) and that they are responsible for the maintenance of fixed tibio-femoral deformities in varus, valgus, flexion, external rotation and lateral subluxation, for fixed patellar subluxation, and in part for an inability to flex the knee fully.

In fixed varus deformity the presence of such contractures can easily be demonstrated at operation. With the Tenser in place and the condyles

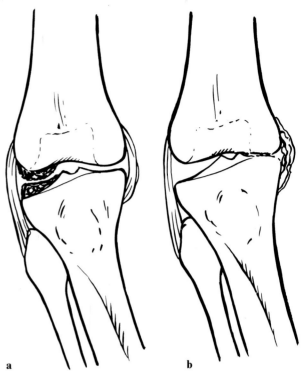

Fig. 15 a and b. Diagrams to show two mechanisms that might theoretically produce a fixed varus deformity. **a** The varus deformity has been produced by growth of the lateral femoral and tibial condyles combined with elongation of the lateral collateral ligament. This seems impossible. **b** The fixed deformity has been produced by a medial tibial defect similar to that shown in Figs. 5, 6, 7, and 11, combined with a medial soft-tissue contracture. This seems likely in reality

fully separated in such a knee, a varus deformity persists and the contracted tissues can be felt and seen to be tight. These tissues include the medial collateral ligament, the medial half of the posterior capsule, the cruciate ligaments, and the muscles crossing the medial side of the knee. In addition, medial osteophytes may "tent" the medial collateral ligament and hence contribute to the maintenance of the deformity by effectively shortening this ligament. (The contracted structures are more easily displayed on the lateral side and they are illustrated therefore under "Fixed Valgus Deformity", below.)

Fixed Valgus Deformity

Lateral contractures affecting most obviously the ilio-tibial tract and the tendonous part of the biceps

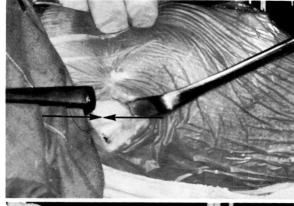

a

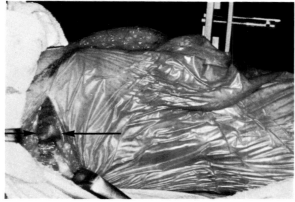

b

Fig. 16. a A lateral view of a knee with fixed valgus deformity during operation. A second incision has been made over the ilio-tibial tract (*arrow*). At this stage of the operation, the leg lay in valgus even though the medial and lateral soft tissues had been tensed. This implies the presence of a lateral soft-tissue contracture. **b** The ilio-tibial tract has now been incised and the lateral blades of the Tenser (seen *top right*) have been opened further, to correct the valgus deformity. This has caused the cut edges of the ilio-tibial tract to separate and to be out of sight in this photograph. A contracture of the ilio-tibial tract (perhaps involving particularly the Tensor fascia lata muscle) was mainly responsible for the fixation of valgus malalignment in this knee

maintain fixed valgus deformity. If these structures are divided, their cut ends spring apart (Fig. 16) to allow separation of the lateral femoral and tibial condyles with consequent correction of the valgus deformity. In addition to the contractures mentioned above, a fixed valgus deformity may be maintained by adhesions between the lateral femoral condyle on the one hand and the posterior capsule and lateral ligament on the other. Contracture of, or adhesions around, the cruciate ligaments may also prevent full correction of the defor-

mity. It should be appreciated that both in valgus and in varus, the extent of the contracture may be less than that of the bone loss: such a knee will display some degree of instability super-imposed upon an element of fixed deformity. Only the latter is due to contracture, whilst the bone defect underlies both the instability and the fixed deformity.

Fixed Flexion

The position of comfort in the knee (i.e., the position of maximum intrasynovial volume) is one of about 15° of flexion. If, because of pain, the knee is never voluntarily extended beyond this point, contractures (in this case probably due particularly to adhesion formation) involving the posterior capsule (becoming adherent both to itself and to the posterior femoral condyles), the hamstring muscles, and, to a lesser extent, the cruciate ligaments may develop and physically prevent full extension. Weight-bearing on the flexed knee then loads the distal and posterior femoral condyles where they articulate with the posterior half of the tibial condyles, and it does so at loads significantly greater than those borne by the weight-bearing extended knee (PERRY et al., 1975). If, as commonly happens in RA, the loaded bone collapses, the femur in effect "sinks" downwards into the posterior part of the tibial condyles until the tibial intercondylar eminence comes to abut against the roof of the femoral intercondylar notch (Figs. 12 and 13). Eventually a groove is formed, running across the antero-distal aspect of the femoral condyles into which the anterior margin of the tibia locks as the knee is extended (Fig. 17). Both these bony impingements prevent extension. Midline impingement may cause an attrition rupture of the anterior cruciate ligament — especially in RA, when the ligament may be weakened enzymatically and is rarely protected by osteophytes. Such ruptures might be considered as being analogous to ruptures of the ligamentum teres at the hip.

Loss of Flexion

Loss of flexion is simply the reverse of a flexion deformity, but it is not usually thought of as such. Viewed in this light, however, it may be regarded as being due to (1) a contracture of the quadriceps muscle and cruciate ligaments, (2) adhesions be-

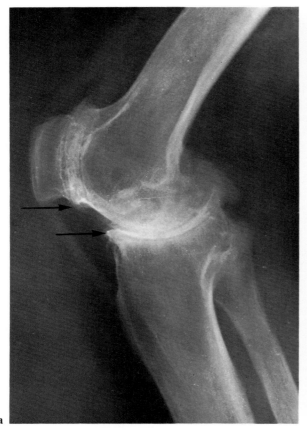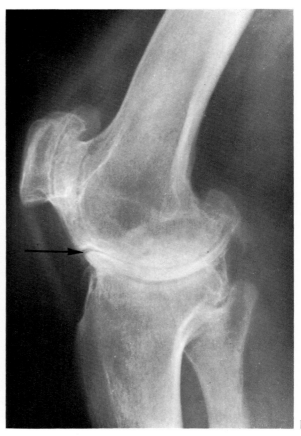

a

b

Fig. 17a and b. Lateral radiographs of an osteoarthrosic knee having a fixed flexion deformity. **a** Note the anterior osteophyte on the tibia (*arrow*) and the groove on the distal end of the femur (*arrow*) in the slightly flexed knee. **b** Note that the tibial osteophyte and the femoral groove contact each other (*arrow*) to limit extension

tween the collateral ligaments and the sides of the femoral condyles, and, perhaps (3) to posterior osteophytosis.

Lateral Subluxation of the Patella

Lateral subluxation of the patella is seen particularly in valgus, externally rotated RA knees, and is presumably caused by the action of the quadriceps muscle, which must tend to pull the patella laterally if the knee is in valgus with external rotation of the tibia (Fig. 18). It is permitted by bone loss (as are valgus and varus tibio-femoral deformities), bone being lost in this case from the antero-lateral femoral condyle and from the patella (Fig. 19). In the author's experience the deformity is usually fixed, because the lateral patellar retinaculum becomes contracted.

External Rotation of the Tibia

Usually seen in RA female valgus knees (Table 4), external rotation of the tibia is most obvious in the flexed, rather than in the extended, joint. There appear to be two possible sources for a deforming external rotation force: the laterally subluxed extensor mechanism and the biceps muscle. It seems possible that this external rotation thrust is exacerbated by a loss of the internal rotation power of the popliteus muscle since (in the author's experience) the intra-articular tendon of this muscle is usually absent from the rheumatoid (but not from the osteoarthrosic knee). The tendon is presumably ruptured by being ground between the collapsing lateral femoral and tibial condyles. (So-called posterior ruptures of the knee are probably in fact due to the discharge of synovial contents through the hole left in the posterior capsule by the retrac-

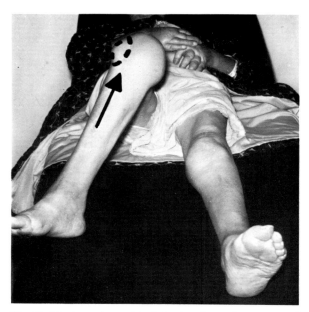

Fig. 18. The knee (*arrow*) in RA, showing valgus, external rotation, and lateral subluxation of the patella (*dotted*) in the flexed knee

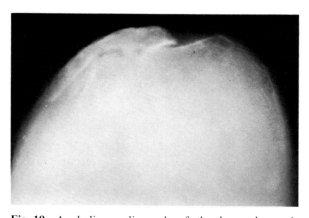

Fig. 19. A skyline radiograph of the knee shown in Fig. 18. Note the lateral subluxation of the patella permitted by destruction of the patella itself and of the lateral femoral condyle. It will be recalled that the anterior prominence of the lateral femoral condyle is normally greater than that of the medial femoral condyle, the reverse of the situation seen in this knee

tion of this tendon from the joint rather than to a rupture of the capsule: the capsule itself is very strong and is never found to be ruptured at operation, and arthographically the synovial leak in posterior ruptures is lateral, i.e., it corresponds

in position to the point of exit of the popliteus tendon.)

Such unbalanced external rotation forces would themselves be capable of rotating the tibia only to its normal extreme and not beyond. In the author's view, the hyperexternal rotation that occurs in these knees is permitted by the lateral tibial and femoral bone loss in the valgus knee, since this will effectively relax posterior cruciate control over the lateral but not over the medial compartment of the knee. As a consequence, the equivalent of a posterior drawer sign can occur laterally but not medially; i.e., the lateral but not the medial tibial condyle is free to sublux posteriorly. Thus the tibia rotates externally. Once rotated, the same contractures that maintain fixed valgus in the extended knee (i.e., contractures of the ilio-tibial tract and of the biceps) will maintain fixed external rotation in the flexed knee. Finally, the whole circumference of the tibia may become adherent to the capsule in its new position of external rotation.

Hyperextension

Hyperextension is uncommon but when it occurs it usually accompanies a fixed valgus deformity, i.e., it occurs in knees with contractures of the ilio-tibial tract (Fig. 20). For the first 5°–10° of flexion, the ilio-tibial tract passes in front of the axis of rotation of the knee and therefore acts as an extensor. Its contracture in the absence of a fixed deformity may therefore lead to hyperextension. The tendency for this deformity to develop should theoretically be exacerbated by bone loss from both sides of the knee, since this would loosen all those ligaments that lie behind the axis of tibiofemoral rotation and thus normally prevent hyperextension. If, as is frequently the case in the rheumatoid knee, the anterior cruciate ligament has been ruptured, its contribution to the limitation of extension will also be lost.

The Stable Neutral Knee

From what has been said above, it can be seen that a stable arthritic knee in neutral alignment might be due either to the absence of both significant cartilage and bone loss and soft-tissue abnormality, or paradoxically to the presence of both bone loss (medially and laterally) and soft-tissue contracture (medially and laterally).

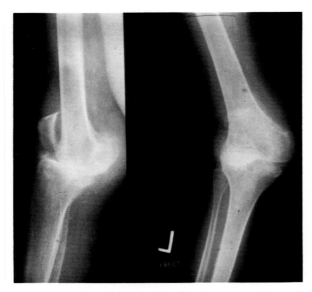

Fig. 20. The knee in RA, showing hyperextension and valgus malalignment, the latter being fixed. It has been suggested elsewhere in this Chapter that hyperextension is permitted by a rupture of the anterior cruciate ligament, which in turn allows the tibia to sublux forwards. Note that such subluxation is present in this knee, and at operation a rupture of the anterior cruciate ligament was found. It is also suggested that hyperextension is contributed to by a contracture of the ilio-tibial tract in the absence of fixed flexion. Such a contracture must have been present in this knee, as evidenced by the fixed valgus deformity: at operation the use of the Tenser demonstrated that such a contracture was present (see also Figs. 10 and 16)

The Loose Knee

In loose knees, which are rare (Table 2), there is both medial and lateral bone loss without soft-tissue contracture. Theoretically, in such a knee both collateral ligaments might elongate. They are, however, never absent; all the knees of this kind that the author has treated could be stabilised in neutral alignment with the Tenser.

Lateral Subluxation of the Tibia

Although lateral subluxation of the tibia, usually combined with varus, is a well-recognised clinical entity, possibly illustrated in Figs. 8 and 12, it is not clear why in some (but not in all) knees the tibia tends to shift laterally on the femur as the loss of medial cartilage and bone turns the knee into varus. (Indeed to some extent the appearance of lateral subluxation may be illusory, Fig. 12.) Perhaps in such knees, prior to the onset of degenerative changes, the long axis of the tibia intersects that of the femur not in the plane of the knee but further proximally, i.e. perhaps the tibia is congenitally somewhat laterally placed in these knees. Whatever the initial cause of lateral tibial subluxation, it is permitted (as are all other abnormalities of alignment) by bone and cartilage loss — in this case from the tibial intercondylar eminence and/or the medial side of the lateral femoral condyle. Precisely what contracture then holds the tibia laterally is unclear but theoretically the popliteus muscle might be responsible, since it runs from the tibia medially to the femur laterally. In support of the view that a popliteus contracture is responsible, division of the popliteus tendon in knees displaying lateral tibial subluxation eliminates the tendency otherwise seen after replacement of the surface with an unconstrained prosthesis for the tibia to move laterally relative to the femur as the knee nears full extension.

A connection exists between subluxation of the patella and of the tibia. Both occur in a lateral direction and they might be causally connected since the extensor mechanism must be carried laterally with the tibia. Thus, at least in theory, a vicious regress may be initiated as follows. The tibia subluxes laterally carrying the patella with it. The resulting increased lateral thrust in the patello-femoral joint promotes the destruction of the anterior aspect of the lateral femoral condyle and of the patella, thus allowing the patella to sublux even further laterally. Once the patella has moved laterally, quadriceps activity must tend to pull the tibia laterally. If such a knee already has a medial tibio-femoral defect (as a consequence of which it is in varus), this lateral patellar pull would displace the proximal tibia bodily laterally, rather than turning the bone into valgus, i.e. there would be increasing lateral subluxation of the tibia in a varus knee.

Alternatively, it seems conceivable that the lateral shift of the tibia is not due, as suggested above, to some congenital variation in the tibial and femoral axes but rather to prior lateral patellar subluxation (i.e. on this view varus malalignment and lateral patellar subluxation precede a lateral shift of the tibia, rather than that the initial tibial shift precedes the patellar subluxation). In this connection, it is the author's impression that such knees are more common in women, a finding which would fit with this view since clinical experience suggests that the patella is more likely to lie laterally in the female than in the male knee. Hypothetically, varus might cause lateral patellar subluxation if it became sufficiently severe to generate tension in the lateral soft tissues acting not just in the long axis of the limb but also transversely to it. If this were to happen, the lateral patellar retinaculum would draw the patella laterally until the patello-femoral joint subluxed. The pathology would now be self-perpetuating and the deformity progressive.

Finally, it is perhaps significant in this context that for practical purposes the tibia always subluxes laterally, not medially, and that both the commonly occurring bone defects (a medial defect in the tibia and a lateral defect in the femur) produce a joint line that slopes upwards and laterally, an abnormality that might well lead to lateral tibial subluxation (J.R. LOUDON, personal communication, 1978).

Conclusions

The fundamental pathological event, on the gross scale, in the knee in OA and RA is the destruction first of cartilage and then of bone. If, as is usual, this happens asymmetrically, it manifests itself as malalignment: lateral tibio-femoral defects causing valgus, medial tibio-femoral defects causing varus, and lateral patello-femoral defects causing lateral patellar subluxation.

When the tibio-femoral or patello-femoral joints become malaligned, the lines of action of the forces acting on both joints are altered — unfortunately in such a way as to increase the forces acting on the destroyed area of the knee. As a consequence, bone destruction tends to be progressive.

The most important pathological processes affecting muscle–tendon units and ligaments are contracture and adhesion formation. Such contractures hold the bones in a position of deformity — converting, for example, varus instability into fixed varus deformity. They also limit movement.

The ligaments of the knee are rarely, if ever, destroyed in arthritis: the only exception to this is the anterior cruciate ligament, which is sometimes destroyed by attrition between the tibia and

femur in RA. The collateral ligament on the convex side of a valgus or varus deformity may stretch if the deformity is sufficient to generate tensile forces on its convex side. Such elongation is, however, secondary to the bone defect, and, in the author's experience, relatively slight in extent.

It can be argued that the objective of surgery in the treatment of significantly damaged knees should be to restore alignment, either by releasing contractures and the reconstituting the destroyed bone or by introducing a compensating deformity in either the tibia or the femur, adjacent to the knee. Such procedures can only be carried out appropriately if the details of the morbid anatomy are understood. For this reason, the present author believes that consideration of, and hopefully agreement upon, the views set out in this Chapter must precede a discussion of the merits and demerits of any surgical procedure at the knee.

References

ALLANDER, E.: Nordiskt Rundabordssamtal om Reumatikervarden. Nord. Med. **92**, 111 (1977)

COLLINS, D.H.: The pathology of articular and spinal diseases. London: Arnold 1949

DENHAM, R.A., BISHOP, R.E.D.: Mechanics of the knee and problems in reconstructive surgery. J. Bone Joint Surg. (Br.) **60**, 345 (1978)

FRANKEL, V.H., BURSTEIN, A.H., BROOKS, D.B.: Biomechanics of internal derangement of the knee. Pathomechanics as determined by analysis of the instant centres of motion. J. Bone Joint Surg. (Am.) **53**, 945 (1971)

FREEMAN, M.A.R.: The pathogenesis of primary osteoarthrosis: An hypothesis. In: Modern trends in orthopaedics. APLEY, A.G. (ed.), p. 40. London: Butterworths 1972

GOODFELLOW, J., O'CONNOR, J.: The mechanics of the knee and prosthesis design. J. Bone Joint Surg. (Br.) **60**, 358 (1978)

GSCHWEND, N.: Die operative Behandlung der kronischen Polyarthritis. Stuttgart: Thieme 1977

HEINE, J.: Arthritis deformans. Archives of pathological anatomy. **260**, 521 (1926)

KAPANDJI, I.A.: The physiology of the joints. Lower limb, Vol. II. London, Edinburgh: Churchill Livingstone 1970

KING, T., BURKE, D., FREEMAN, M.A.R.: The incidence of in the rheumatoid hindfoot and the significance of calcaneo-fibular impingement. International Orthopaedics **2**, 255 (1978)

KUHNS, J.G., POTTER, E.A.: Problems of the knee joint in rheumatoid arthritis of the knee. Current practice in orthopaedic surgery. ADAMS, J.P. (ed.), p. 65. St. Louise: Moseby 1963

LANZ, T., WACHSMUTH, W.: Praktische Anatomie, Bol. I/4: 2nd ed. Berlin, Heidelberg, New York: Springer 1972

MARKOLF, K.L., MENSCH, J.S., AMSTUTZ, H.C.: Stiffness and laxity of the knee — the contributions of the sup-porting structure. A quantitative in vitro study. J. Bone Joint Surg. (Am.) 58, 583 (1976)

MOORE, T.M., HARVEY, J.P.: Roentgenographic measurement of tibial-plateau depression due to fracture. J. Bone Joint Surg. (Am.) 56, 155 (1974)

PERRY, J., ANTONELLI, D., FORD, W.: Analysis of knee-joint-forces during flexed-knee stance. J. Bone Joint Surg. (Am.) 57, 961 (1975)

Chapter 3

Clinical Assessment

R.C. Todd
Essex County Hospital, Colchester, Essex, England

M.A.R. Freeman
London Hospital, London E1 2AD, England

N. Gschwend
Schulthess Stiftung, Neumünsterallee 3, CH-8008 Zürich, Switzerland

The assessment of joint function is, as yet, essentially a clinical rather than a laboratory procedure. Unfortunately there are no universally accepted methods for the collection, recording, analysis, and presentation of the required clinical information. Indeed, almost every centre working in the field has its own methods. As a consequence, results from different centres are not always easily compared, so that the relative merits of the different surgical procedures used in the treatment of the arthritic knee are almost impossible to assess.

In attempts to overcome this difficulty, two groups have recently met to seek agreement, at least on the nature of the data that should be recorded. One of these groups, chaired by Professor GSCHWEND, is the Sub-committee on the Surgical Treatment of Rheumatoid Arthritis of the European League Against Rheumatism (EULAR).

When this Chapter was written (June 1978) this group was still at work. Its Chairman, however, read the text of this Chapter, and finding himself in personal agreement with its contents, agreed to allow his name to appear as a co-author, thus emphasising the extent of the agreement that now exists.

One of us (MARF) was a member of the second group, set up by the British Orthopaedic Association in 1977. This group, chaired by AICHROTH, sought agreement as to the categories of information that should be recorded and presented by surgeons working in this field. This Committee has now completed its work, and its conclusions have been published in the *Journal of Bone and Joint Surgery* (AICHROTH et al., 1978).

Since the information required by the British Orthopaedic Association is covered by the forms used at The London Hospital, since the Chairman of the EULAR group is in personal agreement with the London Hospital procedures, and since the form used at the London Hospital is derived from that devised in the Mayo Clinic, there seem

to be grounds for hoping that international agreement on this subject may not be far away.

Thus in this Chapter we present the results and conclusions reached at The London Hospital after 8 years of practical experience in the management of computer-aided prospective studies of knee surgery. We venture to suggest that these conclusions might form a possible starting point for general agreement on this topic.

Collection of Data

General Considerations

For an operation to be reliably assessed the review of patients must be prospective and complete. Accurate and comprehensive information is more likely to be obtained if the patients are seen in a special clinic, staffed by experienced surgeons; but the methods of collecting and recording clinical data should be applicable (if necessary in a simplified form) to routine practice. In either situation it is an advantage if at least some of the surgeons involved in the review are independent of the knee replacement service, so as to minimise problems of observer error and patient's loyalty to one particular surgeon. The work load should be such that thorough assessment is possible, though this need not, indeed should not, be time-consuming. A simple index of patients, or rather knees, is necessary, filed preferably by trial number, i.e., a number specially allocated to each knee under review. The index records the date of operation and of subsequent follow-up examinations, so that missed appointments can be easily detected and rearranged (Fig. 1). It may be an advantage to record additional information on the index, such as the diagnosis, type of operation

Trial number and name	Hospital number	Clinic Reg. number	Side	Date of operation	Follow up					
					6/12	1 year	2 years	3 years	4 years	5 years
0258 Mary JONES	21	568723	R	6.12.73	4.6.74	10.12.74	9.12.75	—	10.12.77	—
0259 John SMITH	19	047326	L	14.12.73	—	20.1.75	10.12.75	Died 3.3.76	—	—

Fig. 1. A suggested lay-out for an index of operated knees

performed, etc., depending on the other facilities that may be available for the recording and retrieval of this information (see "Storage, Retrieval, and Analysis of Data").

Specific Considerations

The information required about a particular knee can be considered under two headings, Function and Structure. Under Function may be included pain, the subjective stability of the knee, the range of movement, and the patient's ability to carry out various activities. Structure covers tibio-femoral deformity (fixed flexion, valgus/varus, lateral subluxation, and rotational deformity), tibio-femoral instability (extensor lag, valgus/varus, and antero-posterior), and the alignment and stability of the extensor mechanism.

Pain is notoriously difficult to quantify. Most authors use a simple classification of Mild, Moderate, and Severe but many do not define these categories, or if they do, do so in an overelaborate way that can cause confusion. We have tried to minimise this difficulty by using the following definitions. A mild pain is one that does not require analgesics, over and above those that the patient may be taking for other joints. A moderate pain is one that does require simple analgesics but does not then significantly limit activity. Any other pain is severe. Because of the importance of the patello-femoral joint in relation to knee replacement, and in particular to post-operative pain, it is desirable to distinguish pain arising from the tibio-femoral and patello-femoral joints. Pain from the patella is likely to be particularly bad on stairs, and we therefore enquire specifically about this.

For research purposes we believe it is important to enquire about the subjective stability of the knee, since this is not necessarily the same as the instability demonstrated on examination. It is possible for a knee to be unstable on examination but for the patient to feel secure when he walks. Conversely, a knee may feel grossly insecure to the patient without there being any demonstrable instability. However, as symptomatic insecurity will probably manifest itself as an interference with walking there is little need to record subjective instability for routine purposes.

It is possible to compile a long list of activities that may be restricted by an unsatisfactory knee; for example, the ability to walk, climb and descend stairs, reach the foot, bathe, use public transport, drive, and pursue one's normal occupation, and this can be further qualified by defining the aids required to carry out those activities, the method used (for climbing stairs, for example), and the degree of limp on walking. However, all these things may be affected by factors other than the knee in question, and even if the knee is the sole cause of disability it is difficult to assign relative importance to each feature and to condense the various features into one concise overall assessment of function. It therefore becomes impossible to compare different knees on this basis. Many patients undergoing knee replacement are severely handicapped by multiple joint problems, and the ability to walk, with or without aids, is of paramount importance. We therefore limit our enquiries to the patient's ability to walk and to climb and descend stairs. In respect of walking ability we believe it is sufficient to distinguish among four levels of function, and we record whether the patient is able to walk at all, and if he is, whether he can walk outdoors or is confined to the house. For patients who walk outdoors we record the time for which they are able to walk. We find that patients are better at assessing time rather than distance. Most authors record distance, and many North American surgeons use a block as their unit of distance, which may not have much meaning for surgeons in other parts of the world. We record the walking aids used and the degree of limp, but we find the latter very difficult to assess and we have not taken either factor into account in assessing function.

An inability to climb or descend stairs is frequently due to complex circumstances and may be compounded of weakness, instability, pain, stiffness, habit, and fear at the prospect of falling. A number of patients deliberately avoid stairs, living in one-level accommodation. It is thus very difficult to design a questionnaire that will fully reflect not only the fact that a patient has difficulty on stairs but also the reason for his difficulty.

The remaining parameter of function, range of movement, and most of the parameters relating to structure are fortunately more or less capable of objective measurement. To ensure maximum accuracy, range of movement and valgus and varus deformity and instability should always be measured with a long-limbed goniometer and with the patient sufficiently undressed. Errors are particularly likely in patients with short, fat legs. We measure both the passive and the active range of movement. The presence of an extensor lag gives a crude indication of quadriceps function. Attempts to grade quadriceps function more precisely, as is done by some workers (WILSON, 1972; INSALL et al., 1976), seem to us to be prone to error, and they do not contribute much to the overall assessment of the knee. Valgus and varus deformity and instability are measured as deviation from straight alignment, in degrees.

Terms such as "gross valgus instability" and "minor varus deformity" are not sufficiently precise for accurate evaluation and comparison of results.

Lateral subluxation, rotational deformity, and antero-posterior instability are more difficult to quantify, and we simply note their presence or absence. We also note the alignment of the extensor mechanism with the knee flexed, as either anterior, antero-lateral, lateral etc.

Radiological and Ancillary Methods of Examination

Examination by radiological and ancillary methods is considered in Chap. 4.

Recording of Data

Special forms are valuable in ensuring that full and accurate information is recorded at each examination. For research purposes these forms may be extremely detailed, but if they are too complicated they are likely to be inadequately completed and for routine clinical use such a form should be as simple as possible. In either situation attention should be given to the overall design and lay-out of the form so that it is easy to complete accurately and quickly. Where necessary it should be made to conform to hospital note size. Forms for use in connection with knee arthroplasty have been published by COVENTRY et al. (1973), by AMSTUTZ and FINERMAN (1973), by INSALL et al. (1976), and by FREEMAN et al. (1977a). At The London Hospital a form has been devised upon which the relevant data can be recorded numerically (Figs. 2–5) and hence transferred via punch cards to a computer. However, the form is equally suitable for use without a computer. It is divided into three parts, each corresponding to one punch card. For reasons of space these parts are spread over eight pages in the form. Each page is laid out in the same way. A list of questions, each identified by a number, is arranged on the left. A number of possible answers, also identified by number, are provided for each question. The form is completed by ringing the appropriate item or by placing the number corresponding to the appropriate answer in a box or a series of boxes, on the right of the form, opposite the question. For the sake of the computer the boxes (or "columns") are also numbered. So far as possible the answers have been designed to be mutually exclusive and collectively exhaustive. Where this has not been possible an opportunity has been provided to write in a specific answer.

Each of the three parts of the form is headed by information essential to the identification of the knee concerned (i.e., trial number and patient's name and registration number).

Part 1 (entitled General Information, p. 1.1 of the form, Fig. 2) records the patient's age, sex, diagnosis, duration of disease, and previous operations. This information is obviously recorded only once, pre-operatively.

Part 2 (entitled Pre-operative/Post-operative Function, pp. 2/4.1, 2/4.2, 2/4.3, and 2/4.4, Fig. 3a, b, c, d) is used both pre-operatively and post-operatively, and records the patient's symptoms

Item		Columns	Code
1	Card number	1–2	
2	Trial number	3–6	
3	Hospital record number	7–16	
4	Surgeon under whom the patient is admitted	17–18	
5	Date	19–24	
6	Hospital (enter code number)	25–26	
7	Patient's name (Surname first, initials only second)	27–41	
8	Age	42–43	
9	Sex 1=male 2=female	44	
10	Side 1=right 2=left 3=right; left already replaced 4=left; right already replaced	45	
11	Diagnosis 1=OA 2=RA 3=post-traumatic 4=other, specify	46	
12	Duration of disease in the patient (in years) specify		
13	Duration of disease in the knee (in years) specify		
14	Previous operation on the knee		

If YES specify interval in years between a previous operation and the present time in second and third columns (e.g. MacIntosh 4 years previously to be coded as 204)

		Columns
MacIntosh or similar	100=no 2––=yes	51–53
Osteotomy (any kind)	100=no 2––=tibia 3––=femur 4–=Benjamin	54–56
Patellectomy	100=no 2––=yes	57–59
Synovectomy+/–spring clean	100=no 2––=yes	60–62
Meniscectomy	100=no 2––=yes	63–65
Arthrodesis	100=no 2––=yes	66–68
Total replacement	100=no 2––=yes, specify type..........	69–71
Other	100=no 2––=yes, specify..........	72–74

Fig. 2. The first page of the form completed before operation at The London Hospital
The word "SKIP" is an instruction to the punch card operator

LEFT KNEE
RIGHT KNEE
(circle side form refers to)

Item		Columns	Code
1	Card number 03=Pre-Operative 04=6 months Post-Operative 05=1 year Post-Operative 06=2 year Post-Op 07=3 year Post-Op 08=4 year Post-Op 09=5 year Post-Op 10=6 year Post-Op 11=7 year Post-Op 12=8 year Post-Op 13=9 year Post-Op 14=10 year Post-Op 15=11 year Post-Op 16=12 year Post-Op 17=13 year Post-Op	1-2	☐☐
2	Trial number	3-6	☐☐☐☐
3	Night pain 1=none 2=mild 3=moderate (awakens) 4=severe	8	SKIP ☐
4	Day pain sitting in a chair 1=none 2=mild 3=moderate 4=severe	9	☐
5	Pain walking 1=none 2=mild 3=moderate 4=severe 5=severe immediately on standing 6=cannot stand	10	☐
6	Location of most severe pain 1=pain-free 2=medial 3=lateral 4=anterior 5=posterior 6=general		
7	Other important pain features (e.g. pain rising from a chair, 'stiffening up', etc.) 1=absent 2=present, specify..........................		SKIP
8	Use of aids 1=none 2=stick, out of doors, long walks 3=stick, full-time 4=crutch 5=two sticks 6=two crutches 7=walking frame 8=furniture 9=unable to walk		
9	Distance walked without stopping (1, 3 & 4: enter 000 in columns 15-17) 1=unlimited 2=outdoor but limited (specify time in mins. in cols.15-17) 3=indoors only 4=unable to walk	14-17	☐☐☐☐
10	Ability to get out of a dining chair or its equivalent 1=able with ease 2=able with difficulty but without push-off 3=able but only by push-off 4=unable		

Fig. 3a. The subsequent pages of the form completed before, and after, operation. Information is recorded by ringing the appropriate answer and writing where necessary. For transfer to the computer the numbers signifying the answers to certain questions are entered in the boxes on the right. This information is essential to the review and represents the information acquired on the abbreviated form suggested for routine use, set out in Fig. 7

Item

11   Climbing stairs
   1 = leads with affected leg, no pain, no hands
   2 = leads with affected leg, no pain, uses hands
   3 = any other method/or question inapplicable, specify ....

12   Descending stairs
   1 = leads with unaffected leg, no pain, no hands
   2 = leads with unaffected leg, no pain, uses hands
   3 = any other method/or question inapplicable, specify ....

13   Does the knee feel stable? ('instability' = 'insecurity', 'unsteadiness' or equivalent complaint)
   1 = yes   2 = no   specify complaint ....

14   Bath
   1 = normal   2 = with difficulty +/− aids   3 = unable

15   Stockings/toenails
   1 = normal   2 = with difficulty +/− aids   3 = unable

16   Work
   1 = heavy manual   2 = light manual   3 = sedentary/or semi-sedentary
   4 = retired   5 = unable   6 = Q.17 applies

17   Housework, gardening, etc.
   1 = full   2 = partial   3 = not attempted (i.e. has full domestic support)
   4 = Q.16 applies

18   Is the above disability due to the affected knee?
   1 = entirely   2 = mainly   3 = partially
   4 = scarcely at all
   If 2, 3 or 4, specify cause of disability ....

SKIP

Fig. 3b

Item		Columns	Code

EXAMINATION

19   Gait without aids   **SKIP**

       1 = normal   2 = slight limp   3 = grossly abnormal,
       specify nature of abnormality ....

20   Range of passive movement; extension in columns 23–25 (full extension = 000°)   **23–28**   ☐☐☐☐☐☐
       flexion in columns 26–28

21   Extensor lag   100 = absent   2–– = present (specify degrees in cols. 30 & 31)   **29–31**   ☐☐☐
       If fixed flexion is present in addition to an extensor lag, specify only the lag here

22   Hyperextension   **SKIP**

       100 = absent   2–– = present, specify degrees ....

23   Crepitus   1 = absent   2 = present

24   Alignment of tibial and femoral shafts as patient stands (normal, i.e. 7° of valgus = 207)   **36–38**   ☐☐☐
       100 = 0°
       2–– = valgus (specify degrees in cols. 37 & 38) (normal = 207)
       3–– = varus (specify degrees in cols. 37 & 38)

25   Alignment of tibial and femoral shafts when the tibia is stressed laterally (i.e. valgus-producing stress)   **39–41**   ☐☐☐
       100 = 0°
       2–– = valgus (specify degrees in cols. 40 & 41) (normal = 207)
       3–– = varus (specify degrees in cols. 40 & 41)

26   Alignment of tibial and femoral shafts when the tibia is stressed medially   **42–44**   ☐☐☐
       (i.e. varus-producing stress)
       100 = 0°
       2–– = valgus (specify degrees in cols. 43 & 44) (normal = 207)
       3–– = varus (specify degrees in cols. 43 & 44)

27   Position of patella at 90° flexion   **SKIP**

       1 = anterior and midline (i.e. normal)   2 = antero-medial   3 = antero-lateral
       4 = medial   5 = lateral
       6 = other, specify (e.g. patellectomy, stiff knee, patella subluxed even in extension) ....   **80**   **G**

Fig. 3c

Item

28 Antero-Posterior instability at 90° flexion
    1 = absent (i.e. 0–0.5 cm.)   2 = present, specify direction and magnitude of
                                    tibial movement ....

29 Antero-Posterior instability in full extension
    1 = absent   2 = present, specify direction and magnitude of
                                    tibial movement ....

30 Tibial subluxation
    1 = absent   2 = lateral   3 = medial   Specify (a) if in flexed knee, extended knee or both and
    (b) extent of subluxation ....

31 Rotational position of the tibia at 90° (as judged by tibial tubercle)
    1 = midline or very slight external rotation (i.e. normal)
    2 = abnormal external rotation, specify degrees if possible ....
    3 = internal rotation, specify degrees if possible ....

32 Synovial thickening
    1 = none   2 = slight   3 = moderate   4 = severe

33 Synovial fluid
    1 = none   2 = slight   3 = moderate   4 = severe

34 State of opposite knee, specify...

35 State of left hip, specify...

36 State of right hip, specify..

37 State of left foot & ankle, specify...

38 State of right foot & ankle, specify..

39 State of spine, specify..

40 State of left upper limb, specify...

41 State of right upper limb, specify..

42 Weight of patient in Kilograms, specify...

43 Any other important feature(s) in the history or examination, specify...........................

SKIP

Fig. 3d

and the findings on clinical examination. We record the severity of pain in different circumstances, at night, by day at rest, and on walking. Regarding walking ability, the group into which the patient falls is recorded as a number (e.g. '2' for outdoors, '3' for indoors, '5' for unable) and for those able to walk outdoors the time they can walk is recorded in minutes. Range of movement is recorded as two three-figure numbers denoting maximum extension and maximum flexion. Separate categories are provided for hyperextension and extensor lag. If one of these is present it is recorded by placing a '2' in the appropriate box, followed by the magnitude of the instability in degrees in the two following boxes. Tibio-femoral alignment and instability are recorded as a series of three three-figure numbers, denoting the alignment of the knee at rest, with the tibia stressed laterally and with the tibia stressed medially. Straight alignment is recorded as '100', valgus alignment as '2' followed by the deviation from straight alignment in degrees, and varus alignment as '3' followed by the number of degrees. A final page records in summary the state of the lumbar spine and other lower-limb joints.

Part 3 (entitled Operative Details and Post-operative Course, pp. 3.1 and 3.2, Figs. 4 and 5) is used to record the details of the operation and post-operative course, including any complications occurring before the patient's discharge from hospital. A separate form (Fig. 6) is completed for any major complication that requires special management after the patient's discharge from hospital. Such complications are divided into the following categories:

— Those requiring conservative treatment or operative treatment not involving permanent removal of the prostehesis
— Those requiring permanent removal of the prosthesis
— Those leading to amputation of the limb
— Those causing death of the patient or withdrawal of the knee from further follow-up for any other reason.

This form is also used following hip and ankle replacements and a code letter has to be written on the form to enable the computer to identify the joint concerned.

We claim no particular originality for this form. It is derived from that used at the Mayo Clinic (and for this we are indebted to Dr. Mark Coventry). Once the surgeon is familiar with the layout of the form it takes only a few moments to complete, and since in general the number '1' has been used to indicate normality the general state of the knee can be determined from the form at a glance.

We have deliberately included information that can be used retrospectively for investigations that may not have been precisely defined at the outset of any particular study, and in its present state the form is unnecessarily long for routine (as distinct from research) purposes. Indeed, in the 7 years that it has been in use we have used only some of the recorded information to evaluate our results, and this information is contained in the boxes on the forms. Since the value of the review of an operative procedure depends on the percentage of patients for whom the relevant data are recorded, and since this percentage depends in turn on the ease of making the record, we believe that for everyday purposes it would be desirable to shorten the form, even if this meant omitting some information of value in a research context. For this purpose the first and last parts of the form recording the general features of the patient's condition and past operations and the operative procedure and post-operative management could be omitted entirely. The first half of the second part, which records the symptomatology, could be abbreviated to two questions, one concerning pain and the other the ability to walk. Although in the research form we have separated pain at night, pain on walking, and pain when not weight-bearing, and have set questions concerning pain on stairs and the location of pain, we have evaluated our results by reference to only the most severe pain, regardless of its location or the activity that provokes it. Thus the information with respect to pain could be reduced to the answer to one question: "What is the severity of the worst pain felt by the patient?" This could be answered as "none", "mild", "moderate", or "severe".

In the second half of the second part of the form dealing with the findings on examination of the knee and, in outline, of the lumbar spine and the other lower limb joints, four questions cover the most important features. These features are the only ones that we have used in evaluating our results to date, and are range of movement and flexion deformity (both given by recording the arc of passive movement), extensor lag combined with flexion deformity (given by recording the angle of the knee during "straight leg raising"), and the valgus and varus alignment of the knee when

Item		Columns	Code
1	Card number	1–2	0 2
2	Trial number	3–6	☐
	OPERATIVE DETAILS		
3	Date of operation	7–12	☐
4	Prophylactic antibiotics		SKIP
	1 = no 2 = yes, specify..........		
5	Type of femoral prosthesis. Use numerical code and specify size & type in writing	14–15	☐
6	Method of femoral fixation	16	☐
	1 = fully cemented 2 = partially cemented		
	3 = no cement		
	Specify where cement used		
7	Type of tibial prosthesis. Use numerical code and specify size & type in writing	17–18	☐
8	Method of tibial fixation	19	☐
	1 = fully cemented 2 = partially cemented		
	3 = no cement		
	Specify where cement used		
9	Patella	20	☐
	1 = untouched		
	2 = patellectomy at time of arthroplasty		
	3 = previous patellectomy		
	4 = posterior surface and/or osteophytes trimmed		
	5 = posterior surface replaced – specify type of prosthesis		
10	Method of patellar fixation	21	☐
	1 = fully cemented 2 = no cement 3 = no prosthesis		

the knee is stressed first towards and then away from the midline. From a knowledge of these alignments it is possible to calculate the extent of any fixed deformity and/or instability that may be present. Thus we believe that this section of the form could be reduced to these four questions.

In summary, we now think that a satisfactory form for routine purposes might consist of only seven questions, namely those relating to pain, walking ability, range of movement (including fixed flexion deformity), extensor lag, valgus or varus deformity, valgus or varus instability, and the alignment of the extensor mechanism. These questions, two relating to history and five to examination, could easily be contained on one sheet of the record paper used in most hospitals (Fig. 7).

Storage, Retrieval, and Analysis of Data

The form described above has been designed to allow the transfer of information, via punch cards,

Item		Columns	Code
11	Medial tibio-femoral release 1 = not required 2 = required, specify procedure		
12	Lateral tibio-femoral release 1 = not required 2 = required, specify procedure		
13	Lateral patellar retinacular release 1 = not required 2 = required, specify procedure		
14	Other release procedures 1 = not required 2 = required, specify		SKIP
15	Operative difficulties (e.g. residual instability, deformity etc.) 1 = none 2 = present, specify		
16	Skin incision and method of skin closure, specify		
17	Other comments 1 = no 2 = yes, specify		
18	Operating surgeon (complete cols. 27–28 as 00 if surgeon has no code number). Specify name in writing	27–28	☐☐ SKIP Ⓖ

Fig. 4. The pages of the form used to record details of the operation

to a computer, but it is equally suitable for use in a department that does not have access to a computer or where the volume of work does not justify the use of one. The forms are in any case kept and filed, preferably in order of trial number.

The computer program at The London Hospital includes built-in checks so that forms that have been improperly or inadequately completed are rejected. They are brought to the attention of the surgeon in charge of the knee follow-up program, who is then able to correct and resubmit them. Periodically the computer prints out a list of data on file, including a list of errors and a table showing the completeness of the follow-up. Missing records can be detected at a glance and enquiries made to complete the necessary form or to identify the reason for failure of follow-up. Obviously this checking of the forms and of the completeness of follow-up can be done manually.

The analysis program will extract from the file those records satisfying certain constraints such as date of operation, hospital, surgeon, diagnosis, and type of prosthesis, though any or all of these constraints can be set to neutral, in which case

Item

POST-OPERATIVE COURSE

19 Splintage
     1 = plaster of paris, specify duration..
     2 = other, specify...

20 Day on which flexion started ....

21 Day on which weight bearing started..

22 Infection
     1 = no   2 = superficial   3 = deep. 2 & 3 specify basis for diagnosis, bacteriology and
                                    treatment ....

23 Venous thrombosis
     1 = no   2 = yes, specify basis for diagnosis and treatment..

24 Pulmonary embolism
     1 = no   2 = yes, specify basis for diagnosis and treatment ....

25 Haematoma
     1 = no   2 = yes, describe state of knee and treatment required ....

26 Failure of primary wound healing
     1 = no   2 = yes, describe state of knee and treatment required ....

27 Other complications
     1 = no   2 = yes, specify...

28 Manipulation under anaesthesia
     1 = no   2 = yes, specify number of days post-operative and range of movement obtained
     ....

29 Range of movement on discharge from hospital, extension to flexion, full extension = 000......

30 Days in hospital ....

31 Other comments
     1 = no   2 = yes, specify..

SKIP

Fig. 5. The page of the form used to record details of the post-operative course

Item		Columns	Code	
1	Card Number	1–2	**0** **0**	This form applies to: (Circle as appropriate)
2	Trial Number	3–6		Right

Left

3 Complications and technical failures requiring special management or a revision operation but not requiring permanent removal of the prosthesis

Columns 7–8

This form applies to:
Knee
Hip
Ankle
Elbow
Shoulder
Other (specify)

10 = complications and technical failures absent
2– = complications or technical failures present:
    21 = treatment not involving the prosthesis itself.
        Specify date of onset, nature of complication, treatment:
        ....
    22 = treatment involving removal of the prosthesis and replacement by another ICLH prosthesis. Specify date of onset, nature of complication, treatment: ....

4 Complications and technical failures requiring permanent removal of the prosthesis

Columns 9–10

10 = complications and technical failures absent.
2– = complications or technical failures present:
    21 = joint converted to fibrous ankylosis. Specify reason and date of operation ....
    22 = joint successfully converted to arthrodesis. Specify reason, date, method of arthrodesis, final shortening:
        ....
    23 = joint unsuccessfully converted to arthrodesis. Specify reason for operation, date, method of arthrodesis, reason for failure, final state:
        ....
    24 = joint converted to an arthroplasty other than ICLH. Specify reason, date, nature of prosthesis:
        ....
    When the patient has fully recovered from the conversion procedure, complete Part 2/4 on one final occasion to describe the state of the joint and withdraw from the trial.

5 Amputation

Column 11

1 = no   2 = yes. Specify level, reason and date of operation:
    ....

6 Lost to follow-up

Columns 12–13

10 = no   21 = death, specify cause and date..............................
22 = lost for reasons other than death. Specify reason
    ....

7 Patient withdrawn from the trial for any reason other than those listed above

Column 14

1 = no   2 = yes. Specify reason and date of withdrawal..............
    ....

8 Code the joint to which this form applies:

Column 80

D = Knee; E = Hip; F = Ankle
K = Other joints in the foot, specify ....
L = Shoulder   M = Elbow
N = Joint in the hand, specify ....

Fig. 6. The form used to record post-operative complications

1   What is the severity of the worst pain felt by the patient?
    1 = None   2 = Mild   3 = Moderate   4 = Severe

2   Distance walked without stopping
        1––– = Outdoors (specify time in minutes in the last 3 boxes)
        2000 = Indoors only   3000 = Unable

3   Range of passive movement, extension to flexion. Full extension = 000

4   Extensor lag, plus flexion deformity
        100 = absent
        2–– = present (specify degrees in last 2 boxes)

5   Valgus/varus deformity with tibia stressed medially
        100 = 0°
        2––– = valgus ⎫
        3––– = varus ⎭ (specify degrees in last 2 boxes)

6   Valgus/varus deformity with tibia stressed laterally
        100 = 0°
        2––– = valgus ⎫
        3––– = varus ⎭ (specify degrees in last 2 boxes)

7   Position of patella in the flexed knee
        1 = anterior and midline (i.e. normal)
        2 = antero-medial   3 = antero-lateral
        4 = medial   5 = lateral
        6 = other, specify (e.g. patellectomy, stiff knee,
        patella subluxed even in extension)

Fig. 7. A suggested knee assessment form abbreviated for routine use. This form contains the data set out in the boxes of the research form and the item describing the position of the patella

operations of any date, at any hospital, by any surgeon etc., will be accepted. It then produces standard tables regarding age, sex, previous operations, etc. extracted from these records. It also extracts and graphs certain other data, comparing the pre-operative value of the parameter in question (pain, range of movement, etc.) with the post-operative value for each knee in the series. The post-operative value used may be the latest available or that relating to a particular examination, e.g., that at 2 years after operation. Finally the program computes a pre-operative score and a post-operative score for each knee and graphs these along with a mean score for all the knees on the graph (see "Presentation of Results"). Without a computer this analysis must be done by hand, and it is then a great help if the master index carries information relating to operation date, diagnosis, prosthesis inserted, etc.

Presentation of Data

Tables

The age, sex, diagnosis, details of previous operations, and complications are most conveniently presented as printed by the computer, in the form of conventional tables. Another table shows the completeness of follow-up (Fig. 8). In this the knees, identified by trial number, are listed on the left and opposite each number a line is formed of numbers, each of which corresponds to a completed follow-up examination. A gap in the line or a line that contains too few entries for the date of operation indicates an incomplete follow-up. The numbers in the line represent the overall score for the knee at that particular examination, and the progress of the knee can be seen from any change in the overall score with time.

Trial Number	Year of operation	Overall functional score						
		Pre-op	6 mths.	1 year	2 year	3 year	4 year	5 year
262	1971	30	80	85	75	85	85	85
264	1971	40	85	90	95	90	90	95
266	1972	30	95		100		100	
273	1972	30		90	95	90	100	
274	1973	40	100			100		
275	1974	45	100	95	60			
278	1975	25	85	90				

Fig. 8. A follow-up for seven knees. From a lay-out of this kind, it can be seen that: 1) Knees 262 and 264 attended regularly for 5 years, were improved by surgery by about 50 points and remained functionally unchanged over the period of follow-up. 2) Knees 266, 273 and 274 were operated on 4, 4 and 3 years ago and have attended irregularly. 3) Knee 278 was operated on a year ago and has attended regularly. 4) Knee 275 had a satisfactory result for the first post-operative year but then deteriorated. Creation date: 31st December, 1976

Graphs

The parameters that we have elected to graph are pain, walking ability, range of movement, deformity (both in flexion and in valgus/varus), and instability (as extensor lag and in valgus/varus), but in principle any variable could be treated in this way. In each graph (Fig. 9) pre-operative values are plotted on the vertical axis and post-operative values on the horizontal axis to the same scale. The values ascend in magnitude on the pre-operative axis and increase in magnitude from left to right on the post-operative axis. Entries on the graphs take the form of a number representing the number of knees falling on that point. Thus the results for any number of knees can be shown on one graph.

On such a graph, points falling on a 45° diagonal represent knees that have not changed as a result of surgery. Points to one side of the diagonal correspond to knees that have been improved by operation and points on the other side of the line correspond to knees that have deteriorated. In some

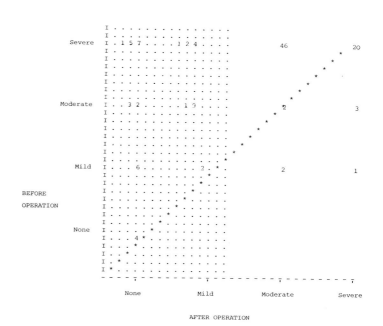

Fig. 9. A representative graph (in this case for pain) as printed by the computer. The pre-operative values are on the vertical axis, the post-operative on the horizontal. The figures on the graph show the number of knees. Thus for example 157 knees had severe pain pre-operatively and no pain post-operatively

graphs the improved knees will be above the line while in others they will be below. If desired the improved knees could be made to lie above the diagonal on every graph, by reversing the scale of the axes of certain graphs. The extent of an individual joint's improvement or deterioration can be read precisely from the graph. A quick visual impression of the extent of any change in a knee can be gained by noting the distance between the point in question and the diagonal (the greater the distance, the greater the change), while the general quality of the results in a group of knees can be seen by their distribution about the "no change" line.

Subdivision of Results in Any One Graph

To simplify the presentation of results, knees are divided post-operatively into two broad categories, the unsatisfactory and those that are acceptable. The term "acceptable" is used to indicate a level of function, perhaps less than perfection, that has been chosen for each parameter, bearing in mind that the majority of patients requiring knee replacement are either handicapped by polyarthritis or are elderly, so that surgery cannot be expected to restore them or their knees to complete normality. It seems reasonable to seek instead to improve the function of the knee so that this joint does not itself constitute a disability. Thus by this definition an acceptable result is not necessarily perfection, but implies a knee that is funtioning acceptably within the context of the life-style imposed by the patient's general condition.

By drawing a vertical line on each graph corresponding to the threshold of Acceptable Function for the parameter in question (e.g., between mild and moderate pain, see Fig. 9) it is possible to separate at a glance those knees that are acceptable post-operatively from those that are not.

Although it is possible to see from each graph whether or not a knee with acceptable function has been improved or worsened by surgery, we believe that it is an allowable simplification to ignore such changes when presenting the results. (If, for example, a patient preoperatively has 130° of movement but such severe pain that he cannot walk, it is of little consequence to him that he loses 20° of movement if his pain is abolished by surgery.) On the other hand, for joints that are not functionally acceptable after operation, it is important to distinguish those that are finally unsatisfactory because they have been made worse

Absent or Mild		82%	—93% Worthwhile
Moderate or Severe	but improved	11%	
	and unchanged		—7% Not Worthwhile
	and deteriorated		

Fig. 10. A table setting out the results for pain shown in Fig. 9. Note that the percentages are calculated and printed by the computer

POINTS SCORING SYSTEM

Pain	None —	50
	Mild —	40
	Moderate —	15
	Severe —	0
Ability to Walk	Outdoors, 30+ minutes	20
	Outdoors, 0–30 minutes	15
	Indoors —	5
	Unable —	0
Range of movement	90°+ —	30
	60–89° —	20
	30–59° —	5
	0–29° —	0
Acceptable function	Pain —	40–50
	Function —	15–20
	Movement —	30
	If "acceptable" in all the above categories	10
	Overall Assessment	95–110

EXAMPLE

	Pre-operative State		Post-operative State	
Pain	Severe	= 0	Mild	= 40
Ability to walk	Indoors	= 5	Outdoors 30+	= 20
Range of movement	90°	= 30	90°	= 30
Overall Assessment	+0	= 35	+10	= 100

Fig. 11. The points scoring system used to form an overall assessment of the function (not the structure) of the knee at The London Hospital

by surgery from those that, although improved, are still unsatisfactory because they were severely abnormal in the first place.

Four kinds of result can therefore be distinguished post-operatively, and these are displayed in separate areas of each graph:

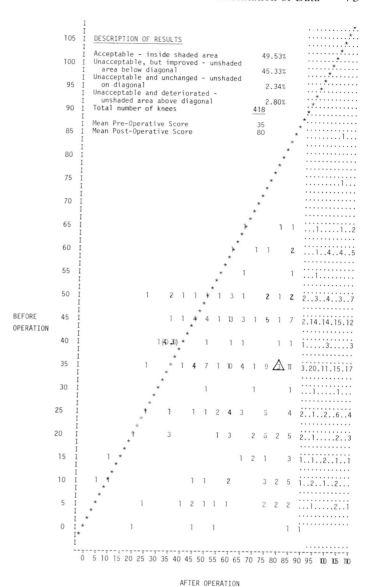

Fig. 12. A graph as printed by the computer for overall scores (calculated as shown in Fig. 11) for a group of 418 knees. The categories used are the same as those in Fig. 9. Knees in the shaded area are regarded as having had an acceptable postoperative result. The remainder are unacceptable but may be improved (i.e., below the diagonal), unchanged (i.e., on the diagonal), or deteriorated (i.e., above the diagonal). The computer calculates and prints the percentage of knees falling into each of these four categories and in addition shows the mean pre-operative and post-operative score (identified by a triangle on the graph)

1) Function is acceptable after operation (in these cases it is immaterial whether the knees have improved, undergone no change, or deteriorated)

2) The knee is not acceptable but has improved following operation

3) The knee is not acceptable and has remained unchanged, and

4) The knee is not acceptable and has deteriorated.

The computer prints out the number and percentage of knees falling into each of these categories below each graph.

Exactly the same classification as that applied to factors describing the functions of the knee (such as pain) has been applied to those describing structure (such as valgus deformity).

To simplify the presentation of the results even further, the result of surgery in the first two groups (acceptable and improved) can be grouped as "worthwhile" and the remainder as "not worthwhile". A table showing the results in Fig. 9 presented in this way is shown in Fig. 10.

Identification of Individual Results in a Graph

In association with each graph, the computer prints a list showing the trial number of each knee in the graph and its position on the graph, as given by its values on the two axes. Thus it is possible to identify the position of any particular knee on each graph, or alternatively to identify the knee (or knees) represented by any particular entry on a graph.

Overall Functional Assessment

In a further attempt to summarise the effect of surgery upon the function (not the structure) of the knee, we have used a points scoring system, the basis for which is set out in Fig. 11. The score has been based on as small a number of parameters as possible for two reasons: first to minimise the difficulty of deciding — on essentially arbitrary grounds — how to weigh one variable against another, and second because as the number of variables used as a basis for a score increases, so too does the number of possible combinations that can result in the same score. Thus, the more complex the scoring system, the more easily it can produce the same score for widely different knees. We have chosen as the basis for the score the three variables that are of most interest to the patient, namely pain, the ability to walk, and the range of movement, giving pain the highest weighting. In practice most other variables are subsumed under these three: for example material instability or deformity will result in a limited ability to walk and will hence be reflected in the score.

To accentuate the difference between knees that are excellent on two counts but poor on the third (such as an arthrodesis might be) and the knees that are good on all three counts, a further ten points are awarded to knees in the latter category. Thus, as reference to Fig. 11 shows, a score between 95 and 110 represents a knee that has acceptable function on all three counts and thus has acceptable function on overall assessment.

The scores for each knee pre- and post-operatively are plotted on a final graph. The mean pre- and post-operative scores and the numbers and percentages in the four categories of result mentioned above are printed at the head of this graph (Fig. 12).

Other scoring systems have been devised by KETTELKAMP and THOMPSON (1975), CONVERY and BEBER (1973), WILSON (1973), POTTER et al., 1972; EVANSKI et al. (1976), MARMOR (1976) and INSALL et al. (1976). We claim no special advantages for ours and describe it merely for the sake of illustration.

Discussion

It is our impression that much of the controversy surrounding this subject stems from a failure to distinguish its separate component parts clearly. In our view these are:
1) A decision as to what items of clinical information need to be recorded
2) The necessity for, and the lay-out of, any special forms that might be needed to ensure that this information is accurately recorded
3) The storage of this information
4) Its presentation in a standardised manner.

In connection with this last matter a particular topic arises, which tends (perhaps because of its essentially arbitrary nature) to generate endless, inconclusive debate: namely, the attempt to characterise a given knee numerically by giving it a "score".

A decision as to what information needs to be recorded cannot be made until it is known for what purpose the information is required. For the purpose of prospective research there is something to be said for recording everything that is known about the joint. The disadvantage of doing this is that in the real world time is limited and the more information that has to be recorded, the greater is the likelihood that errors and omissions will occur. It has been our experience at The London Hospital that an enormous amount of time and effort is required to check and correct forms: had we not been able to do this the length of our form would have rendered it much less useful than it has been in practice. As it is, experience over nearly 10 years, leading to publications based on observations recorded in the forms, has suggested to us that for the great majority of research purposes, and certainly for day-to-day quality control, a nucleus of information will suffice. A form setting out this nucleus can be surprisingly short: one such is shown in this Chapter. (It will be noticed that the questions in the research forms that provide this information are picked out from the rest by recording the data in boxes.)

Once it is known what information is required, an appropriate method of recording it can be devised. This must take the form of a sheet of paper containing the relevant questions, since otherwise the examining surgeon will usually forget to elicit or to record some of the data. The phrasing of the questions is a matter requiring the utmost care if they are to be brief and unambiguous. This matter is of course bound up with the storage and retrieval of the data, since if this is to be done by computer the data has to be coded numerically, a fact which greatly influences the way in which the questions and answers are presented.

In some cases, e.g., the range of movement, a numerical answer is relatively simple to obtain, but in other cases it necessitates the provision of alternative answers from which the patient and surgeon must choose. The difficulty here is to design a reasonably short list of alternatives that are mutually exclusive and exhaustive. In the case of the use of stairs, for example, this is almost impossible, and the opportunity must then be provided for specifying the patient's particular circumstances in writing.

In designing the answer and consigning a numerical value to them we have found it helpful to use '1' for normality and to signify increasing abnormality by ascending numbers. A surgeon can then get an impression of the severity of a patient's disability from the form at a glance.

We have not recorded radiological data on our form, and this Chapter is not concerned with this subject. Obviously it can be done, but not until the essential features of the pre- and post-operative radiographs have been agreed upon — by no means an easy matter.

If any significant number of knees are to be handled, some form of mechanical aid is required to analyse the data. A computer can be used to do this but appropriate programs must then be devised, the data must be transferred to punch cards, and the questions and answers on the form must be designed in an appropriate, and often apparently cumbersome way. All this creates difficulties as well as solving them: devising programs is a costly, professional matter; once devised they cannot readily be modified for special circumstances; computer time may be hard to obtain; and transferring the data to punch cards introduces scope for error. Nevertheless we have found the programs devised at The London Hospital (by Mr. A. CUNDY, to whom the authors (RCT and MARF) are greatly indebted) to have stood the practical test of time. They have proved easy to extend to the hip, foot, and elbow, and we would not now consider evaluating a group of say 50 joints without their aid. Nevertheless, they are only an aid, and the data presented by the computer needs to be constantly scrutinised for error.

As an alternative to a computer, cards in which holes are punched can be used to record the data, and these may then be analysed by passing rods or light through the cards. Our research form is too long to be analysed by this method, but it could easily be used for the short form. Because of the limit on the number of possible answers, a range of movement, for example, could not be recorded as a precise number of degrees, but instead as falling within one of a limited number of categories: 10° for example could be recorded as falling in the category '0°–30°', not precisely as '10°'. The British Orthopaedic Association's form is in fact set out in this way, and for the day-to-day purposes of most hospitals a short form, answered by punching holes in a card, might well be ideal.

With regard to the presentation of results, we feel that two innovations at The London Hospital have been of special value. These are firstly the presentation of results with respect to certain variables such as pain, movement, etc. as graphs of the pre-operative versus the post-operative state, and secondly the construction of a follow-up table based on overall scores.

The advantages of a graphical presentation of certain data have already been mentioned: in summary we would only say that no other method we have tried has proved to be capable of compressing so much information into a limited space whilst at the same time enabling individual knees to be identified in the overall data. (Histograms, for instance, do not make this possible.) Graphs can of course be constructed by hand, but their real convenience is only felt when a computer has been programmed to produce them automatically.

The urge to devise a method of designating an individual knee by a numerical score arises from the need to characterise a population of knees and then to compare one population with another. Once a knee has been given a score, the scores can be handled statistically to characterise a population. The difficulty is deciding what variables shall be included in the score and how they shall be weighted. Our own feeling has been that a score based on both function and structure is probably meaningless, since it covers two dissimilar aspects of the knee. We therefore treat these two separately and score only function. The reasoning behind our particular system has already been discussed: here all that need be said is that our system, like any other, is essentially arbitrary, so that extended argument over its merit is not likely to be fruitful (any more than would be a debate as to the "right" colour for a motor car). If, by a miracle or by executive fiat, the world of orthopaedic surgery were to agree on a particular scoring system, encapsulated comparisons between groups of knees would become possible, although they would necessarily be approximate only. In the meantime, and in our view probably more usefully, valuable and direct comparison can be made of individual features of different groups of knees, such as pain, valgus or varus malalignment, etc. without the need to devise a score at all.

Where a score — however arbitrary — is certainly useful, however, is in the monitoring of changes in a given knee or in a particular group of knees with the passage of time. Provided the scoring system is reasonably sensitive, a gradual post-operative deterioration in a given knee or an improvement in the results to be obtained by surgery as the years go by (to give but two examples) can then be detected. A computer programmed to produce a score for a given knee and then to print out both a graph of pre- versus post-operative scores and a follow-up table of the kind shown in Fig. 12 is an invaluable aid in this connection.

References and Bibliography

AICHROTH, P., FREEMAN, M.A.R., SMILLIE, I.S., SOOTER, W.A.: A Knee Function Assessment Chart. J. Bone Joint Surg. (Br) **60**, 308 (1978)

AMSTUTZ, H.C., FINERMAN, G.A.M.: Knee joint replacement — Development and evaluation. Clin. Orthop. **94**, 24 (1973)

BARGREN, J.H., FREEMAN, M.A.R., SWANSON, S.A.V., TODD, R.C.: I.C.L.H. (Freeman-Swanson) arthroplasty in the treatment of arthritic knee. Clin. Orthop. **120**, 65 (1976)

BRADY, T.A., GARBER, J.N.: Knee joint replacement using Shiers knee hinge. J. Bone Joint Surg. (Am.) **56**, 1610 (1974)

British Orthopaedic Association Research Sub-Committee: Knee function assessment chart. J. Bone Joint Surg. (Br.) **60**, 308 (1978)

CHAO, E.Y., STAUFFER, R.N.: Biomechanical evaluation of geometric and polycentric knee arthroplasty. Conference on total knee replacement, Institution of mechanical Engineers, London 1974

CONVERY, F.R., BEBER, C.A.: Total knee arthroplasty. Clin. Orthop. **94**, 42 (1973)

COVENTRY, M.B., UPSHAW, J.E., RILEY, L.H., FINERMAN, G.A.M., TURNER, R.H.: Geometric total knee arthroplasty. Clin. Orthop. **94**, 177 (1973)

EVANSKI, P.M., WAUGH, T.R., OROFINO, C.F., ANZEL, S.H.: UCI knee replacement. Clin. Orthop. **120**, 33 (1976)

FREEMAN, M.A.R., SWANSON, S.A.V., TODD, R.C.: Total replacement of the knee using the Freeman-Swanson knee prosthesis. Clin. Orthop. **94**, 153 (1973)

FREEMAN, M.A.R., CUNDY, A., TODD, R.C.: The presentation of the results of knee surgery. Clin. Orthop. **128**, 222 (1977b)

FREEMAN, M.A.R., CUNDY, A., TODD, R.C.: A technique for recording the results of knee surgery. Clin. Orthop. **128**, 216 (1977a)

FREEMAN, M.A.R., SCULCO, T., TODD, R.C.: Replacement of the severely damaged arthritic knee by the I.C.L.H. (Freeman-Swanson) arthroplasty. J. Bone Joint Surg. (Br.) **59**, 64 (1977c)

HASTINGS, D.E., HEWITSON, W.A.: Double hemiarthroplasty of the knee in rheumatoid arthritis. J. Bone Joint Surg. (Br.) **55**, 112 (1973)

ILSTRUP, D.M., COMBS, J.J., BRYAN, R.S., PETERSON, L.F.A., SKOLNICK, M.D.: A statistical evaluation of polycentric total knee arthroplasties. Clin. Orthop. **120**, 18 (1976a)

ILSTRUP, D.M., COVENTRY, M.B., SKOLNICK, M.D.: A statistical evaluation of geometric total knee arthroplasties. Clin. Orthop. **120**, 27 (1976b)

INSALL, J.N., RANAWAT, C.S., AGLIETTI, P., SHINE, J.: A comparison of four models of total knee replacement prostheses. J. Bone Joint Surg. (Am.) **58**, 754 (1976)

KETTLEKAMP, D.B., THOMPSON, C.: Development of a knee scoring scale. Clin. Orthop. **107**, 93 (1975)

KETTLEKAMP, D.B., JOHNSON, R.J., SMIDT, G.L., CHAO, E.Y.S., WALKER, M.: An electrogoniometric study of knee motion in normal gait. J. Bone Joint Surg. (Am.) **52**, 775 (1970)

MACINTOSH, D.L., HUNTER, G.A.: The use of the hemiarthroplasty prosthesis for advanced osteoarthritis and rheumatoid arthritis of the knee. J. Bone Joint Surg. (Br.) **54**, 244 (1972)

MARMOR, V.: The modular (Marmor) knee. Clin. Orthop. **120**, 86 (1976)

POTTER, T.A., WEINFELD, M.S., THOMAS, W.H.: Arthroplasty of the knee in rheumatoid arthritis and osteoarthritis. J. Bone Joint Surg. (Am.) **54**, 1 (1972)

SKOLNICK, M.B., BRYAN, R.S., PETERSON, L.F.A., COMBS, J.J., ILSTRUP, D.M.: Polycentric total knee arthroplasty. J. Bone Joint Surg. (Am.) **58**, 743 (1976)

SKOLNICK, M.D., COVENTRY, M.B., ILSTRUP, D.M.: Geometric total knee arthroplasty. J. Bone Joint Surg. (Am.) **58**, 749 (1976)

WATSON, J.R., HILL, R.C.J.: The Shiers arthroplasty of the knee. J. Bone Joint Surg. (Br.) **58**, 300 (1976)

WILSON, F.C.: Total replacement of the knee in rheumatoid arthritis. J. Bone Joint Surg. (Am.) **54**, 1429 (1972)

WILSON, F.C.: Total replacement of the knee in rheumatoid arthritis. Clin. Orthop. **94**, 58 (1973)

WILSON, F.C., VENTERS, G.C.: Results of knee replacement with the Walldius prosthesis. Clin. Orthop. **120**, 39 (1976)

Chapter 4

Radiological Examination of the Knee Joint and Other Special Investigations

R.A. DENHAM

Queen Alexandra's Hospital, Cosham, Hampshire, England

In the past the orthopaedic surgeon has often relied upon small antero-posterior and lateral radiographs for the planning and control of treatment in rheumatoid and in degenerative arthritis of the knee (Fig. 1). These are not adequate. A full range of pictures showing the three parts of the joint is required for proper diagnosis and assessment.

Antero-posterior (AP), lateral, intercondylar, and patello-femoral radiographs should be taken. Lateral views in full extension and in 90° of flexion are necessary. Patello-femoral skyline pictures are needed at 30°, 60°, and 90° of flexion (Fig. 2). As will be emphasised later, the angle the tibia makes with the femur while the patient is standing is of the greatest importance to the long-term function of the knee. Therefore, the large cassette normally reserved for chest films is used to take the AP radiographs while the patient is standing trying to take equal weight through each hip. In this way, sufficient femoral and tibial shaft is seen to enable axial lines to be drawn and to compare with reasonable accuracy the existing angle with the normal 7° of valgus. Only weight-bearing AP radiographs are of value in the planning and control of treatment. Pictures taken while the subject is supine are misleading, for the cooperative radiographer often corrects some of the deformity by positioning the limb on the table before the film is exposed (Fig. 3).

Pictures in full extension with valgus or varus strains upon the knee are often required. The leg is stressed by the surgeon while the patient lies on the X-ray table.

Special Radiographs

Leg Alignment

Although the simple pictures described above are needed for diagnosis, they may not be sufficient for the planning and control of surgery in degenerative arthritis in the knee. MAQUET (1972) has stressed the importance of a normal straight leg in the AP plane, for only with normal anatomy are normal force transmission and normal function possible. If a severe varus or valgus deformity exists it is impossible for the patient to reposition the centre of gravity of the body above the middle third of the knee joint by simple changes in posture (DENHAM and BISHOP, 1978) (Fig. 4). This abnormality leads to a great increase in force transmission in the knee.

A most important guide to normal anatomy is the "leg alignment" radiograph. In this long AP picture, which shows the whole lower limb on one film, the centres of the femoral head, knee, and ankle should be in a straight line (Fig. 5). This does not mean that the shafts of the femur and the tibia are themselves in line. The femoral neck makes an angle with the femoral shaft, so that the gluteal muscles can abduct the hip. This offset means that the femoral shaft joins the tibia at the knee at an average angle of 7°. Against all expectations, I have not been able to show that there is a significant difference between adult male and female patients in this measurement, nor does the patient's height make any difference. The line has been called the "mechanical axis", for it runs its course within the tibia and alongside the femur, but the danger in this name lies in the false assumption that it can be used as a reference for calculations of force transmission in the knee during function in a living subject. Normal anatomical alignment of the leg simply means that

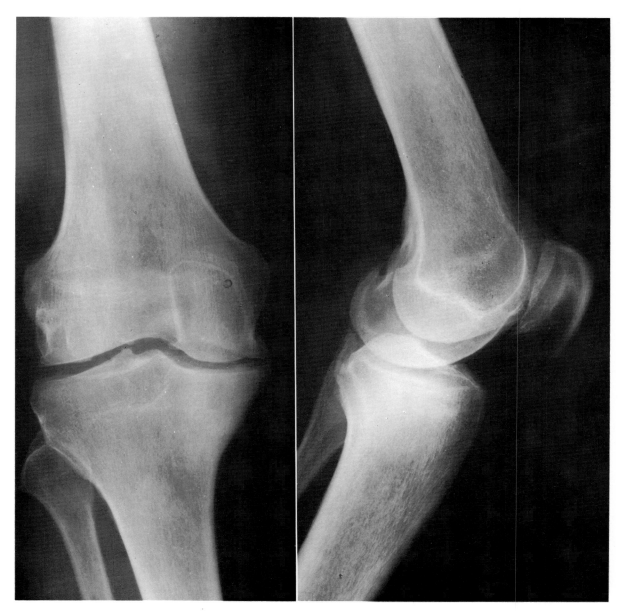

Fig. 1. An antero-posterior and lateral radiograph of an osteoarthritic knee. These pictures are not extensive enough for the planning of operative treatment

normal physiological function can be expected. When the centres of the three joints are not in line in this AP plane, function will be abnormal (Fig. 6).

Technique

The patient stands upon a strong, stable platform, trying to put equal weight through each leg. The knee, and the ankle if possible, should present a true AP view, and the X-ray tube should be centred at the level of the knee and about 9 ft (3 m) in front of it. For old and disabled patients it is useful to have a handrail at chest height to give them some stability. A cassette holding a 112×30 cm film is put behind the leg to be examined so that the hip, knee, and ankle can be seen on this one long picture taken with one exposure. To do this

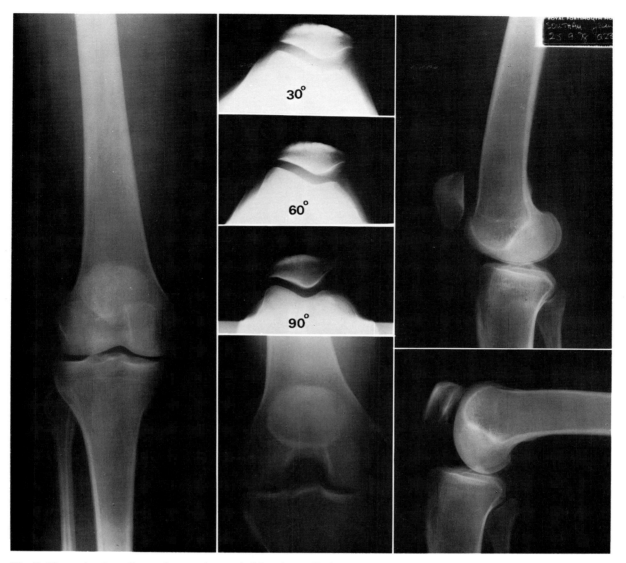

Fig. 2. These simple radiographs may be needed for the preliminary assessment in disorders of the knee joint

it is necessary to have a cassette with screens of graded intensity. For the hip and thigh a 30 × 40 cm Dupont Lighting Plus screen is needed, for the knee a 30 × 40 cm Ilford standard, and for the tibia and ankle a 30 × 24 cm Ilford High Definition screen. A standard Ilford 112 × 30 cm film is used, but if this is not available it is very important that the three single films should be loaded exactly into the long cassette with their edges touching so that after processing they can be taped into a complete picture of the leg. Single 112-cm films are easy for the radiographer but they present a storage problem. They should be cut into three, fixed with transparent sticky tape, and stored in the normal envelopes after the leg alignment line has been drawn upon them. This straight line passes from the centre of the femoral head to the centre of the body of the talus. In the normal adult it passes between the tibial spines of the knee (Figs. 7–18).

While the radiograph is being taken it is important that the knees are not pressing together, for if this is allowed to occur a true picture will not be obtained (Fig. 19).

Fixed flexion at the knee only complicates the leg alignment radiograph if the picture is taken

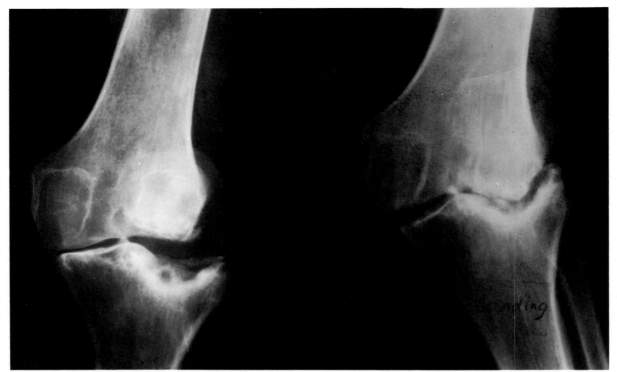

Fig. 3. These two radiographs were obtained within a few minutes of each other. The picture on the right was taken while the patient was weight-bearing. On the left the radiographer has tried to obtain the anatomical position with the patient supine on the X-ray table

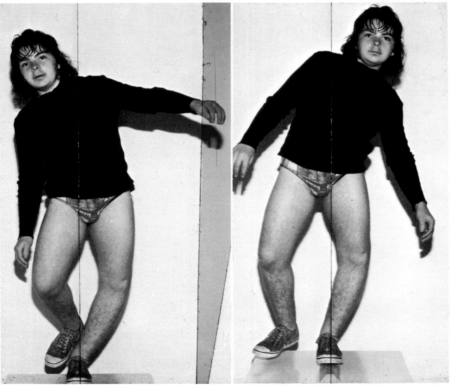

Fig. 4. This patient has bow legs. When he stands on one leg, in spite of leaning as far as he can to one side or the other, he is unable to bring the line of body weight up to the knee joint

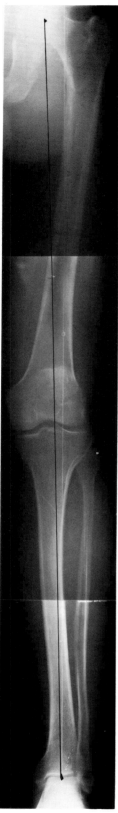

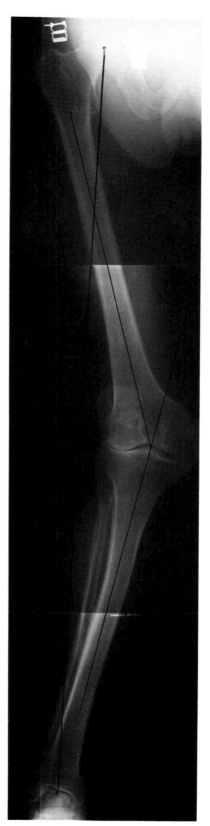

Fig. 5. In the normal subject, the straight line that passes from the centre of the femoral head to the centre of the talus should pass between the tibial spines

Fig. 6. This leg alignment radiograph shows the extent of a severe valgus deformity

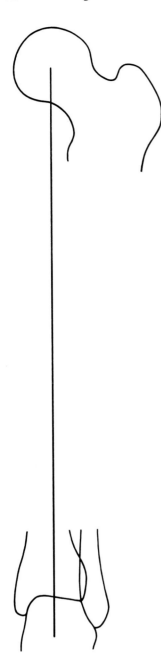

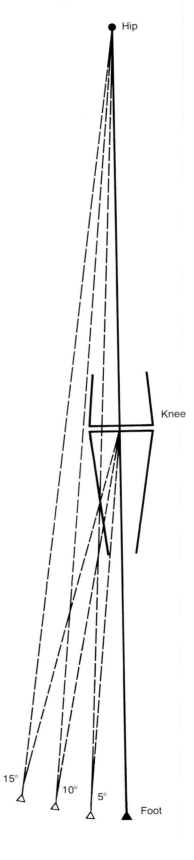

Fig. 7. This format will be used to save space in subsequent illustrations. The relevant part of the radiograph, which includes the knee and the leg alignment line, will be mounted in the appropriate position

Fig. 8. This graph shows how small variations in the tibiofemoral angle produce substantial changes in the position ▶ of the line of leg alignment

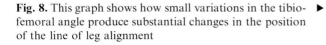

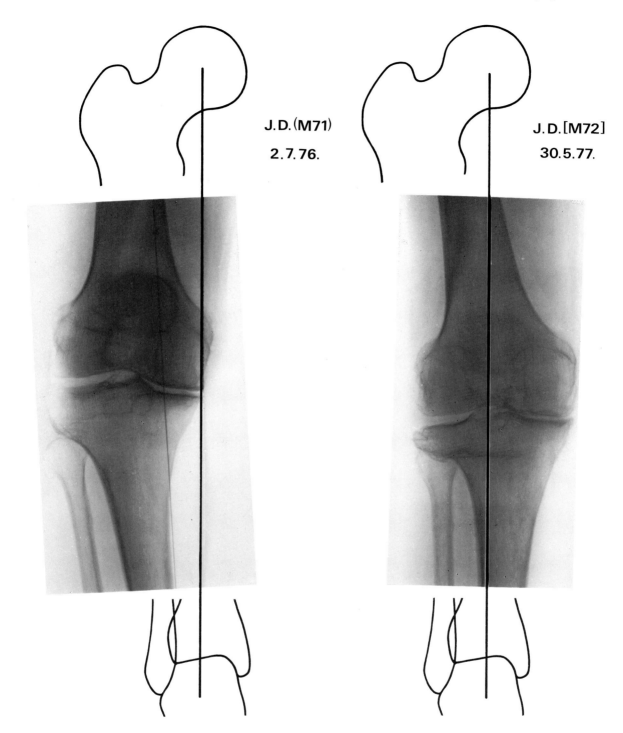

J.D.(M71)
2.7.76.

J.D.[M72]
30.5.77.

Fig. 9. The pre-operative radiograph shows a varus deformity. Tibial osteotomy has corrected this exactly

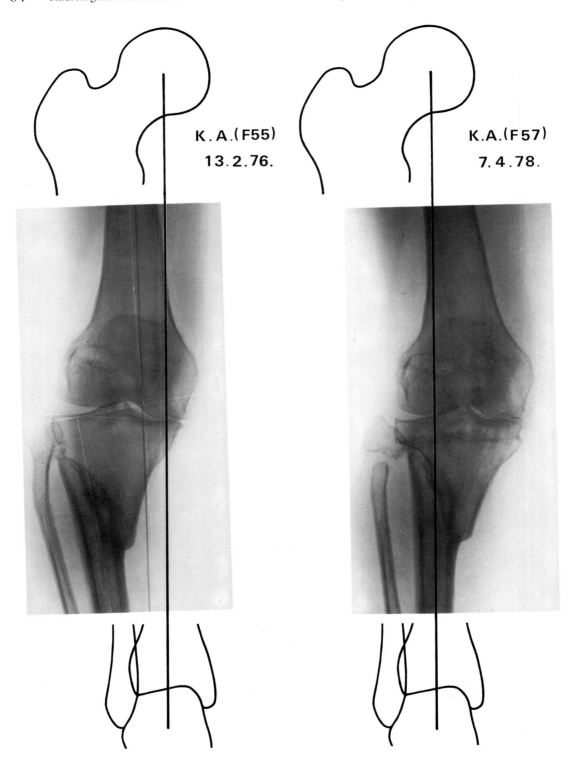

Fig. 10. The fracture in the upper tibia has resulted in a varus deformity. This has produced degeneration in the medial compartment of the knee. Slight overcorrection has been obtained by a tibial osteotomy

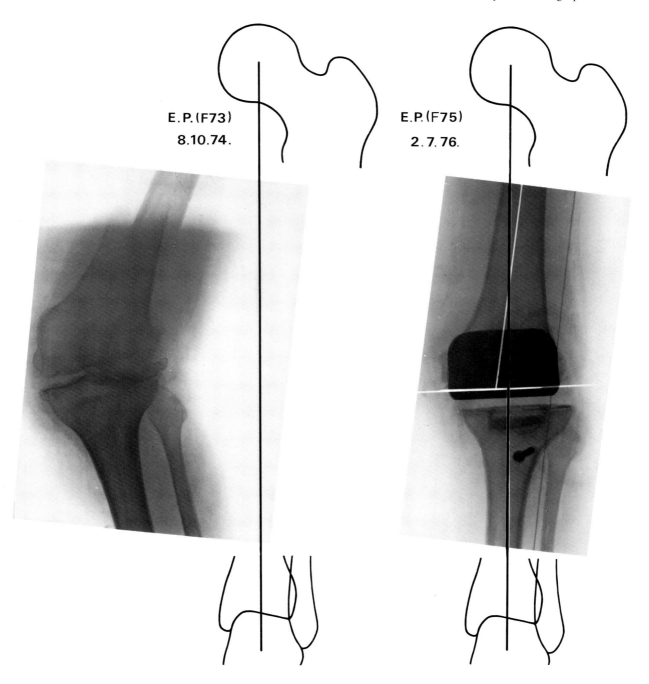

E.P. (F73)
8.10.74.

E.P. (F75)
2.7.76.

Fig. 11. The radiograph of 8.10.74 shows a severe deformity. Knee replacement has corrected the leg alignment but both surfaces of the new joint have been placed obliquely

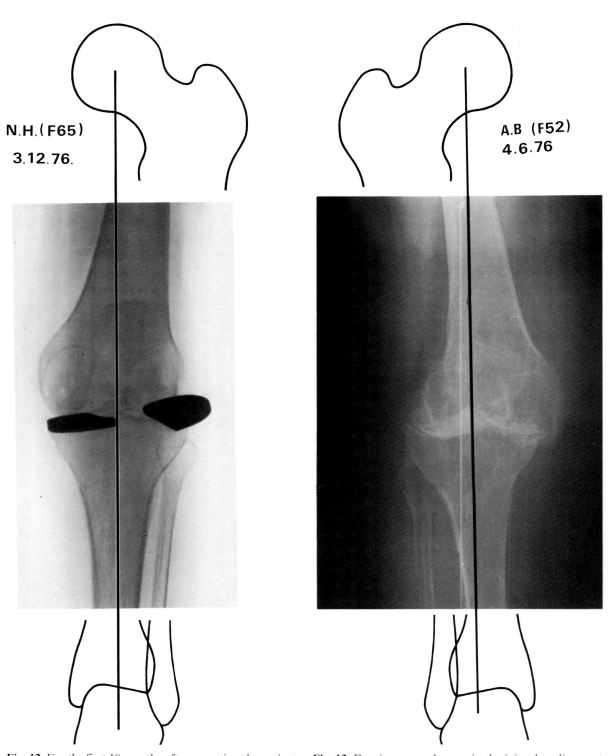

N.H.(F65)
3.12.76.

A.B (F52)
4.6.76

Fig. 12. For the first 18 months after operation the patient complained of discomfort in the knee. Following a sudden painful episode and the appearance of a small lump on the outer side of the joint, the knee became more comfortable. This was because normal leg alignment was restored

Fig. 13. Despite severe changes in the joint, leg alignment remained normal. Although movement was painful, no significant discomfort occurred on weight bearing

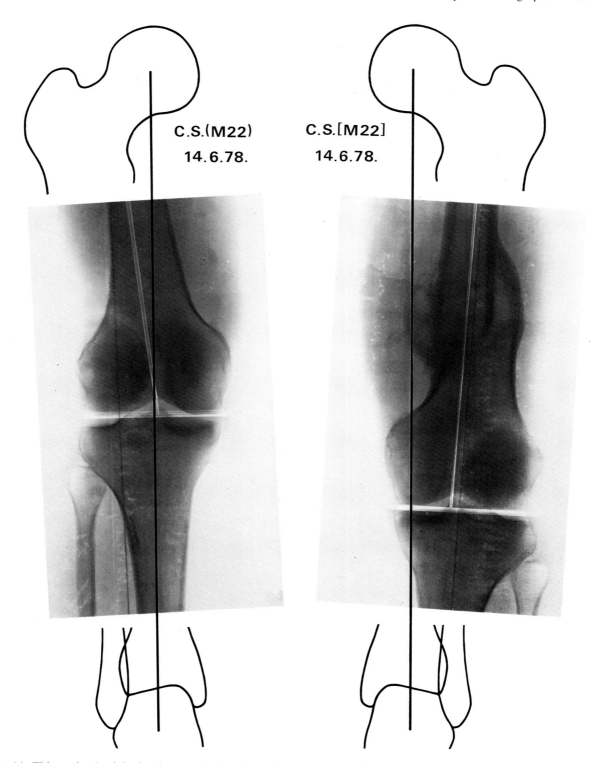

Fig. 14. This patient's right leg is normal. On the left a supracondylar fracture has occurred. This has resulted in malunion, which is confirmed by the leg alignment radiograph. Serious consideration should be given to prophylactic surgery to correct this deformity before damage to the medial compartment occurs

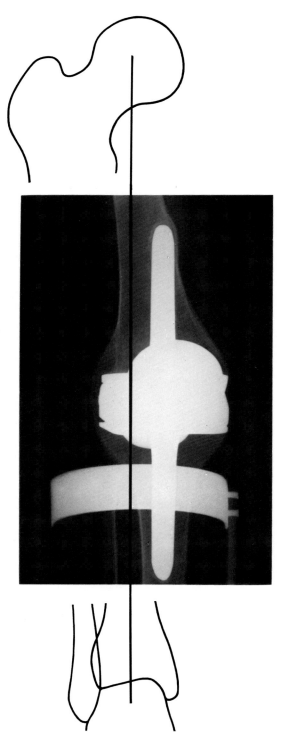

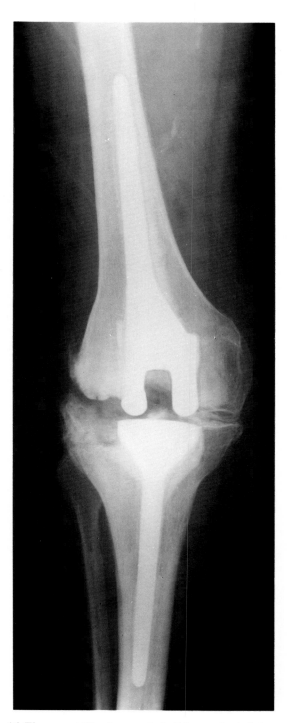

Fig. 15. This prosthesis has been inserted correctly but its design does not allow for the normal 7° valgus angle. This has resulted in pressure exerted by the femoral stem. This is causing painful remodelling of the surrounding bone

Fig. 16. The pre-set 7° valgus angle in this prosthesis helps to ensure satisfactory leg alignment

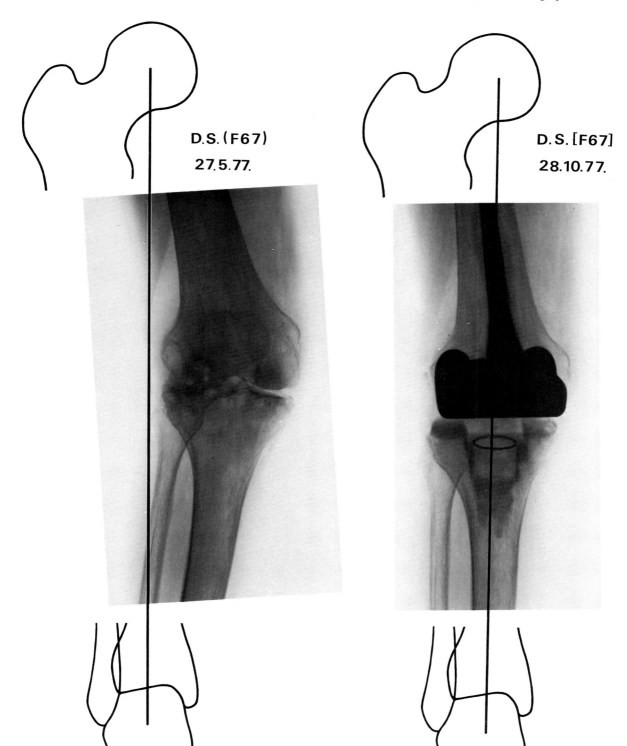

D.S.(F67)
27.5.77.

D.S.[F67]
28.10.77.

Fig. 17. The pre-operative deformity of 27.5.77 has been corrected by this prosthesis whose femoral component has a 7° valgus stem. A removable guide transfixed the tibial component, ensuring correct alignment at a right angle to the bone

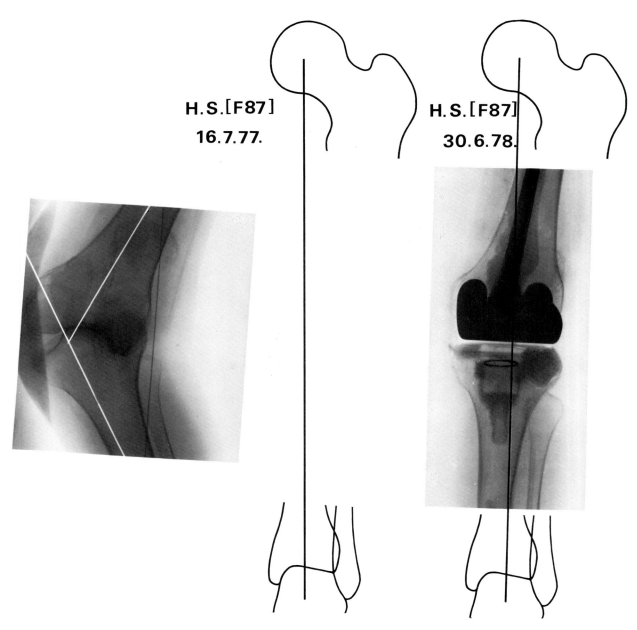

Fig. 18. The leg alignment radiograph taken on 16.7.77 shows a very severe deformity, resulting mainly from destruction of the lateral tibial condyle. Both femoral and tibial components have been aligned correctly. The valgus stem holds the femoral component at the desired angle. The tibial plateau has been inserted at right angles to the shaft, and the lateral condyle has been built up with cement

while the whole leg is rotated. The plane of flexion must be in line with the direction from which the X-rays are coming. With fixed external rotation in the knee, or scoliosis or serious pathology in the hip or peritalar joints, force transmission in the knee is affected and the value of leg alignment radiographs is decreased (Fig. 20).

Even with considerable pre-operative care, the correct estimation of angles and wedges in osteotomy or replacement is difficult. It is essential to

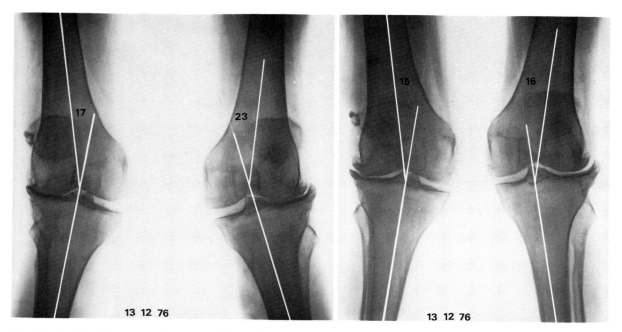

Fig. 19. On the left, the patient is standing with the knees slightly apart and a true picture is obtained. On the right, the knees are pressed together, tending to support each other, and the valgus deformity is diminished

reassess the angle a few months after operation by means of full length, weight-bearing, leg alignment radiographs (Figs. 21 and 22).

Line of Body Weight

Knowledge of the value and direction of the forces which act about the knee joint is essential to the scientific design of a total knee prosthesis and the conduct of osteotomies. The magnitude of these forces must be found either by the direct implantation of strain gauges (which is unacceptable to modern medicine) or by calculations made on the basis of the "line of body weight" radiograph (DENHAM and BISHOP, 1978). When the patient is standing still, this line runs vertically downwards from the centre of gravity of the body to the ground within the boundaries of the feet. The length of the feet from toe to heel helps to prevent overbalancing forwards or backwards, whilst by standing with the feet apart the subject stabilises himself in the lateral plane (Fig. 23).

The importance of the line of body weight radiograph lies in the display of the line of action of the centre of gravity of the body in relation to the bones of the knee joint. In a subject who is standing balanced upon a narrow bar of trapezoidal cross-section, the centre of gravity of the whole body must be directly above the support (Fig. 24). Thus if a radiopaque plumbline intersects the long axis of the bar, the shadow of the plumbline will indicate the distance at which body weight exerts its rotational effect upon the joint. This distance can be measured and calculations of static force transmission made in the antero-posterior or in the lateral plane (Fig. 25).

Although these line of body weight radiographs are essential for calculations of static force transmission, there are practical problems in obtaining accurate pictures in disabled patients who find it difficult to stand on one leg and sometimes find it impossible to balance upon a narrow wedge. There is much to be said for reserving them for research purposes, for obtaining a satisfactory result takes a lot of time and effort. Alternatively, leg alignment pictures are easy to obtain and of great practical value in the planning of treatment and in the assessment of results in surgery, even though they are of no value in calculations of static force transmission in the living subject (Figs. 26–29).

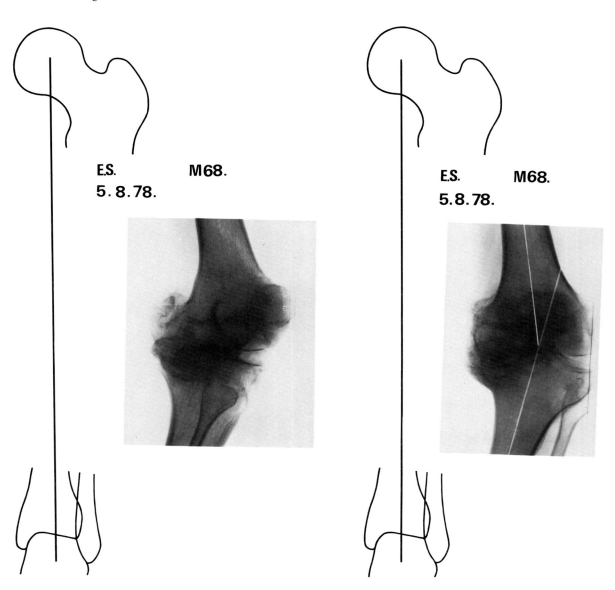

Fig. 20. In the leg alignment radiograph on the right the deformity of 28° (21° plus 7°) of varus is shown. In the radiograph on the left the patient has been asked to rotate the whole leg externally. The fact that he also has 10° of fixed flexion, exaggerates the apparent varus position

Technique

For the AP view of the knee the patient must stand upon the leg to be examined, wearing his shoe, balanced upon the narrow top surface of a 40-cm bar of trapezoidal cross-section (approximately $2 \times 5 \times 7 \times 5$ cm). This bar is firmly attached to a strong raised platform. The X-ray tube is positioned so that it projects along the length of the bar to a cassette fixed behind it. The shadow of the knee must appear on the film. A radiopaque plumbline intersects the upper surface of the trapezium and also casts its shadow upon the 35×40 cm film. The tube–film distance should be approximately 120 cm. At first, the patient stands on the platform with the feet on either side of the bar. The central axis of one foot is then placed upon the bar and the doctor, suitably protected,

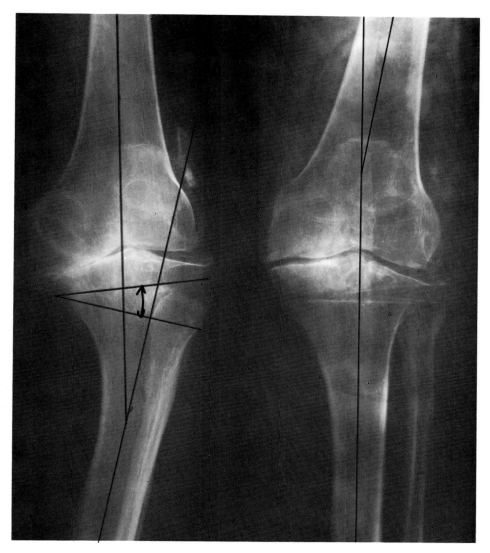

Fig. 21. Measurement of the pre-operative radiograph showed a 20° error in alignment. A wedge osteotomy was performed. The surgeon had not taken ligament laxity into account, and severe overcorrection was obtained. He had to reinsert a 10° wedge to restore correct alignment!

holds the tips of the patient's index fingers. When the radiographer is ready to take the picture, the subject is asked to stand on the one leg on the narrow surface of the bar. It may take the patient a few seconds to balance, but when the doctor feels through the tips of his fingers that the patient is steady, the radiograph is taken. The time of the exposure should not be more than 0.1 s. The problem of balancing an elderly osteoarthritic patient upon a narrow surface is considerable. With a severe deformity this test is not practical, but in patients who have reasonably good coordination and fair muscles the pictures are remarkably consistent (Fig. 30).

The line of body weight radiograph in the lateral plane is taken in much the same way as the antero-posterior picture, but in this case the subject should stand with equal weight on both legs. The cassette is held between the knees and a number of films taken in different degrees of crouching with the patient's body as upright as possible. In this way a series of radiographs can be obtained, from

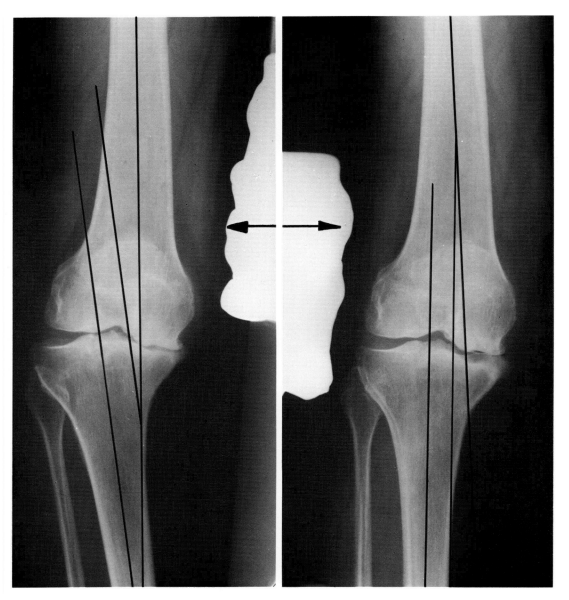

Fig. 22. Stress radiographs with the patient supine and relaxed show considerable ligament laxity. The protected hand of the examiner has forced the knee first into varus and then into valgus

which values of static force transmission can be calculated. In patients who have a lesion in one knee it is necessary to divide the trapezoidal bar and fix the two pieces in line with each other upon two simple bathroom scales. At the moment the radiograph is taken the reaction at each foot is recorded and these readings are used in the subsequent calculations.

Patello-femoral Joint

Special attention must be paid to the patello-femoral joint. Although degenerative change in this area is frequent, the function of the patella and its action within the extensor mechanism are often misunderstood or ignored. Not only does the patella increase the mechanical advantage of the extensor

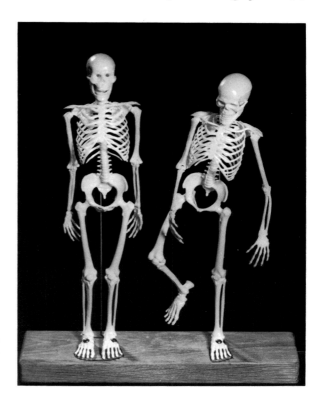

Fig. 23. If the patient is to remain standing his centre of gravity must be directly above a point within the boundaries of the feet (or foot)

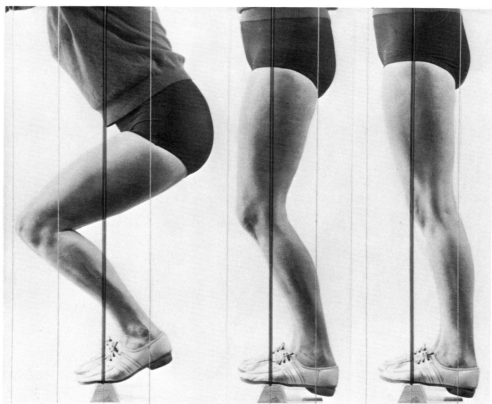

Fig. 24. When the patient is balanced, the centre of gravity must be directly above the supporting surface

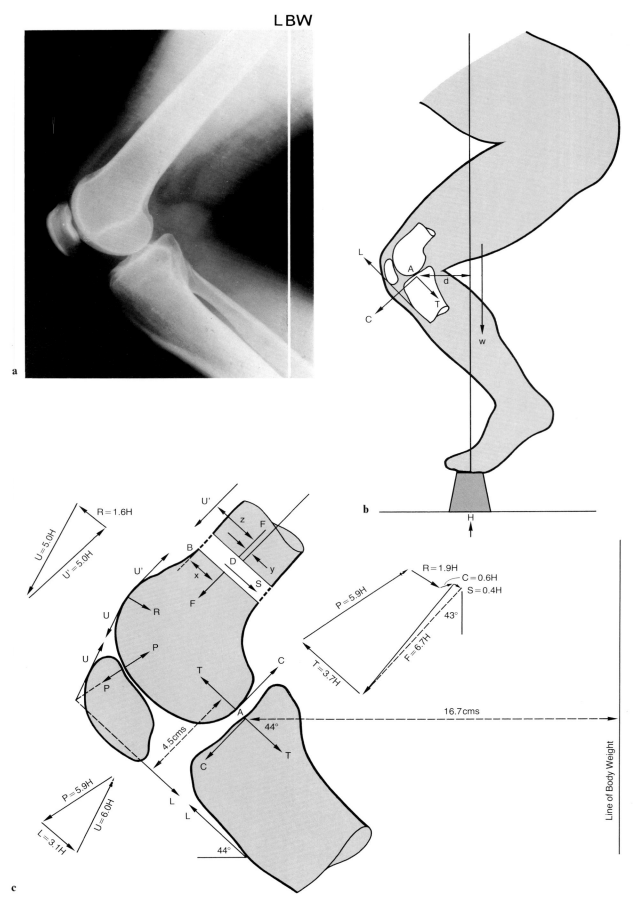

Fig. 25. From the line of body weight radiograph, calculations of static force transmission in the knee can be made

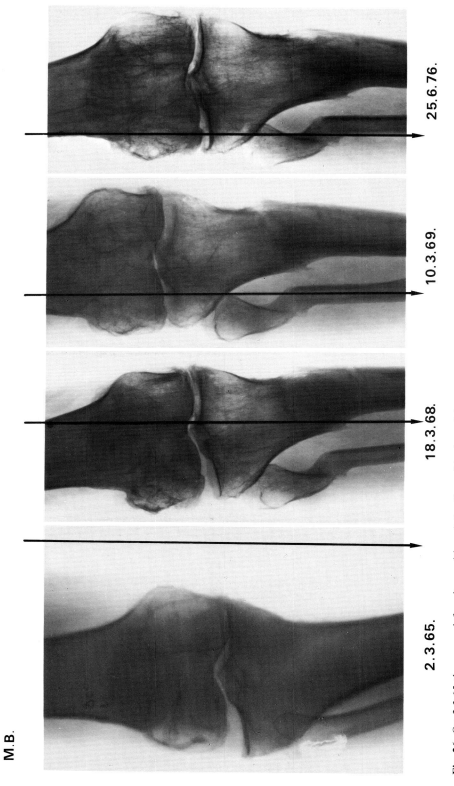

Fig. 26. On 2.3.65 the varus deformity positioned the line of body weight well to the medial side of the knee. A tibial osteotomy succeeded in bringing the line to the centre of the joint. Subsequent degenerative change in the lateral compartment is illustrated by progressive movement of the line of body weight to the lateral side

G.B.(M56)

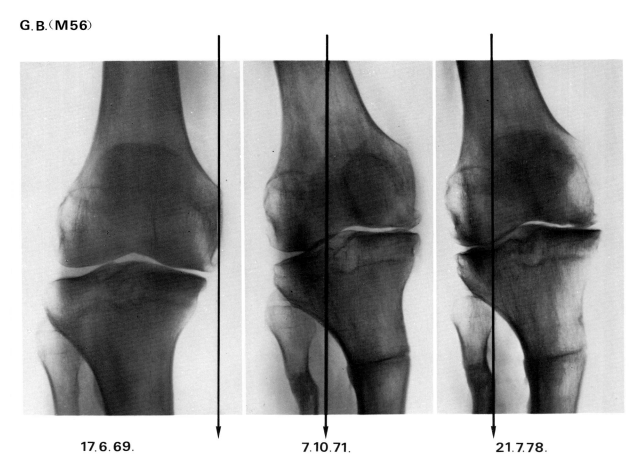

17.6.69.   7.10.71.   21.7.78.

Fig. 27. On 17.6.69 the line of body weight passed to the medial side of the knee. Tibial osteotomy was performed soon after. For 8 years the result has been most satisfactory

mechanism by displacing the quadriceps further from the tibio-femoral joint, but the patella itself has a great influence upon the direction of patello-femoral thrust.

It is important to understand that tension in the quadriceps tendon above the patella can be significantly greater than tension in the patellar ligament, that the direction of the patello-femoral reaction is not half the angle subtended by the two parts of the extensor mechanism above and below the knee cap, and that after about 25° of crouching, the patello-femoral force is greater than the tibio-femoral reaction (Fig. 31). Furthermore, the biomechanical engineer who relates force transmission to the degree of knee bend in a graph which analyses knee function makes a fundamental error. Force transmission must be related to θ, the angle the femur makes with the vertical (Fig. 32).

If force transmission in this joint is to approach anything like its normal value it must be distributed over a wide area or the bones will be damaged. The shape of the contact surface presented to the extensor mechanism changes greatly during movement of the knee. This can only be matched by the patella if the remarkably thick cartilaginous pad on its posterior surface is intact (Fig. 33).

The orthopaedic surgeon should get into the habit of recording the findings in the patello-femoral joint under a separate subheading in the notes immediately after the details of the two tibio-femoral joints. In this way he will become more aware of the problems in this most important joint.

Technique

Lateral pictures taken in full extension and in 90° of flexion are needed, and also skyline views in

M.H.[F56]

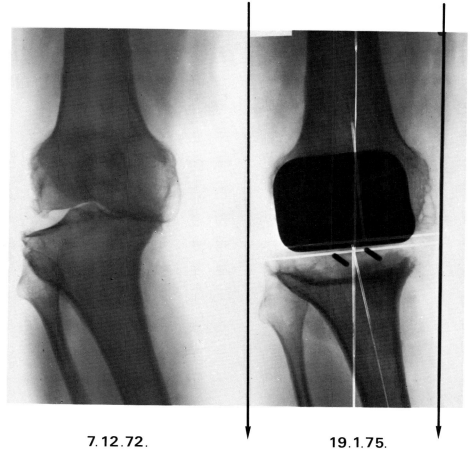

7.12.72.   **19.1.75.**

Fig. 28. The pre-operative radiograph shows a severe deformity with a badly displaced line of body weight. Total joint replacement has not succeeded in correcting the varus. This accounts for the poor clinical result

30°, 60°, and 90° of flexion. These reveal the state of the condylar pathway and the depth of articular cartilage that is available to adapt to the changing bony contour during movement.

The lateral radiograph with the knee in 90° of flexion is of value as a check on the position of the patella within the extensor mechanism. In the normal knee, the patella should be located between the lines drawn along the anterior and posterior margins of the femoral shaft (Figs. 34 and 35). This sesamoid bone has a great influence upon the extent and direction of force transmission. It must be in its normal position if it is to work efficiently.

To exert its best influence upon joint function the patella should be in the midline of the knee. It must not be allowed to sublux laterally over

the femoral condyle or the new femoral component. In joint replacement, efforts should be made to correct an abnormal position. Skyline radiographs are needed after operation.

Figures 36–45 show some of the problems encountered in the patello-femoral joint before and after surgery.

Arthroscopy in Degenerative Arthritis

With more efficient apparatus and with greater clinical experience, arthroscopy has become an important aid to the diagnosis of complicated prob-

A.S.(F79)

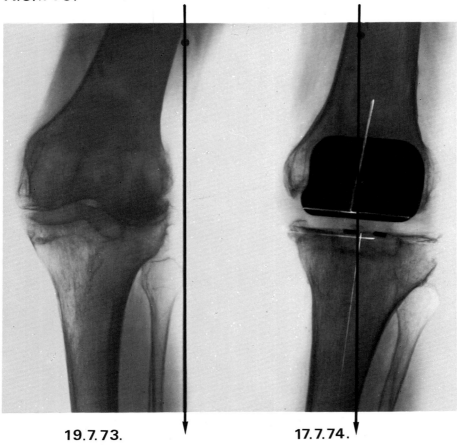

19.7.73. **17.7.74.**

Fig. 29. The lateral tibio-femoral joint is transmitting the sum of body weight and the tensile forces in the ligament and muscles on the medial side of the knee.

After joint replacement the line of body weight is correctly located

P.T.(F49)

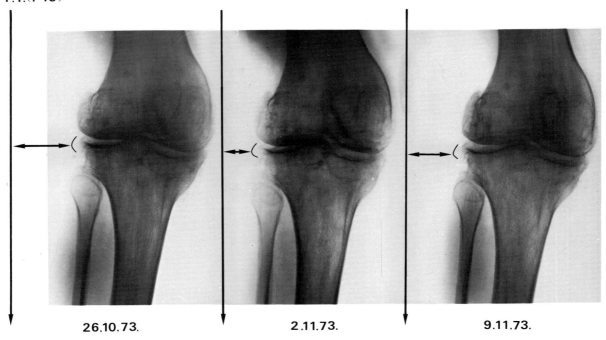

26.10.73. **2.11.73.** **9.11.73.**

Fig. 30. Difficulty in balancing on the narrow wedge produces small variations in the position of the line of body weight. Radiographs taken at weekly intervals illustrate this point

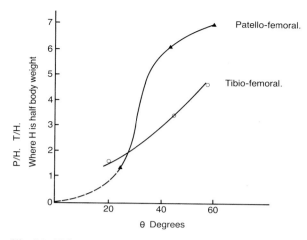

Fig. 31. This graph compares tibio-femoral with patello-femoral reaction. When the angle that the thigh makes with the vertical (θ) is more than about 25°, patello-femoral exceeds tibio-femoral force. For further comment see Denham and Bishop (1978)

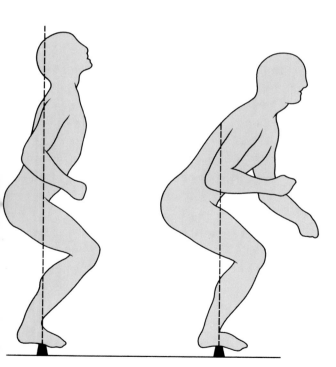

Fig. 32. With knee bend the same, there are wide variations in quadriceps tension as the subject leans backwards or forwards. These changes cause substantial alterations in force transmission in the knee

lems in the knee. In some patients, injury to the menisci, the ligaments, or the articular surface may be difficult to diagnose. The localisation of radiotranslucent loose bodies or small tears can be facilitated by arthroscopy. While there is something to be said for direct inspection of the inside of the joint before osteotomy, I am not in favour of this examination before joint replacement. There are two reasons for this. Firstly, the long-term results of knee replacement have been so uncertain that only the most severely disabled patients should be accepted for surgery; in these, the fine details of intra-articular pathology are not important. Secondly, in all joint replacements it has been found that sepsis is less frequent in joints which have not previously been operated on.

Scintigraphy

Pre-operative radiological studies of a joint under consideration for total prosthetic replacement may be supplemented by scintigraphy, usually with the aid of one of the technetium polyphosphates.

This procedure may be of some value in assessing the degree of activity of an arthritic process of the rheumatoid type, since para-articular uptake is greater in the presence of an acute phase of inflammation. Nevertheless, significant uptake is not uncommonly demonstrated in advanced, but generally inactive, degenerative conditions.

In most cases, therefore, sufficient reliance may be placed on orthodox clinical and radiological assessment to obviate the necessity for this supplementary investigation.

Conclusion

In this chapter a large number of different radiographs have been described. The surgeon must ask for those that are appropriate to the physical signs which have been found. *The patient must not be over-irradiated.* In the early stages of conservative treatment only simple AP and lateral radiographs are needed, but patello-femoral views may be requested if physical examination reveals an abnormality. Line of body weight radiographs are required for research into joint function, but usually

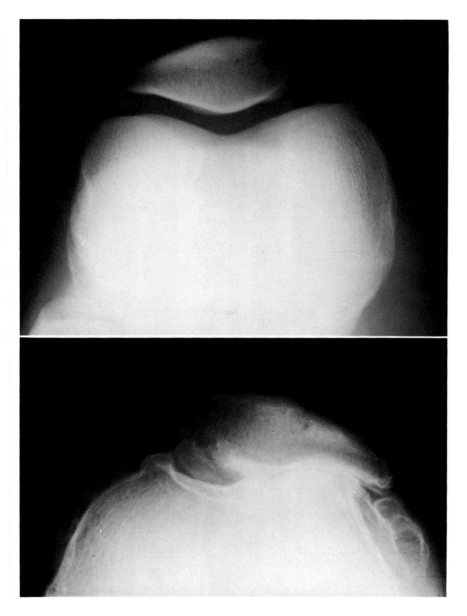

Fig. 33. The normal and the worn patello-femoral joints

they are not necessary for routine treatment. When symptoms and signs become more severe a leg alignment picture may be needed to check the progression of deformity before operation.

If osteotomy or joint replacement is contemplated, long leg alignment radiographs are essential before and after surgery. Until there is general agreement on the 7° valgus angle of the tibia upon the femur smaller films should be avoided. Post-operative skyline views reveal the patello-femoral pathway and indicate degenerative changes in the patella.

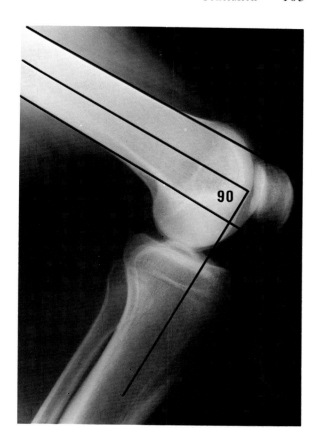

Fig. 34. A radiograph with the knee flexed to 90°. The patella is in the normal position

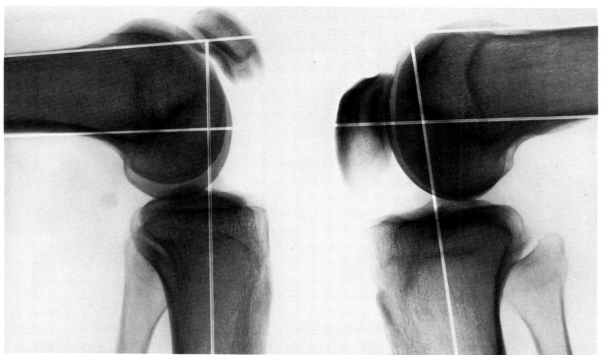

Fig. 35. On the left, patella alta. On the right, the patellar ligament is too short

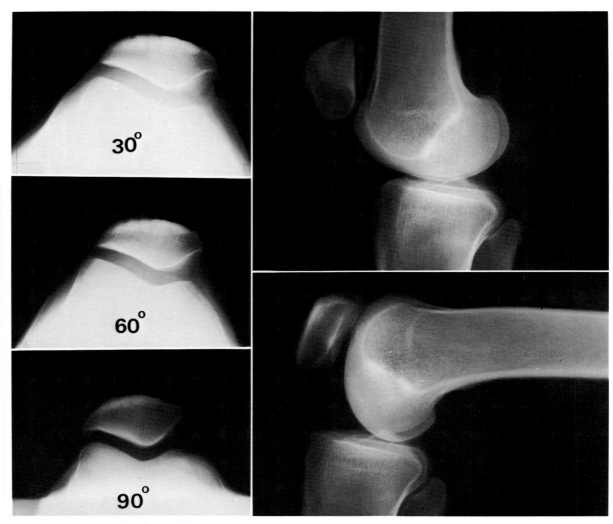

Fig. 36. A normal patello-femoral joint

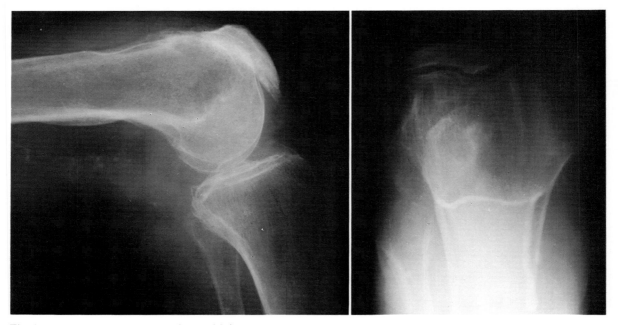

Fig. 37. Severe wear in a patello-femoral joint

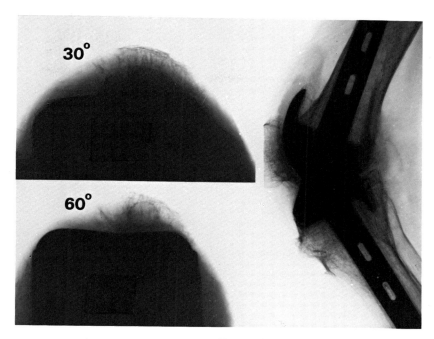

Fig. 38. This prosthesis provides an excellent patello-femoral pathway

D.H.[F42]

15.7.78.

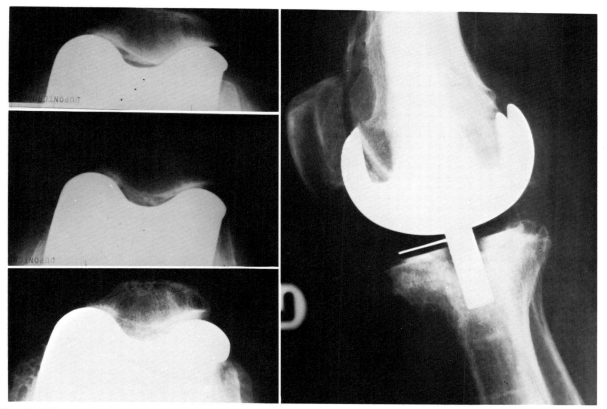

Fig. 39. This prosthesis presents quite a good patello-femoral surface

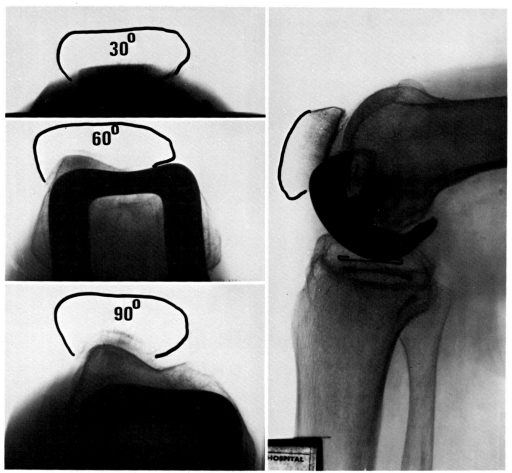

Fig. 40. A *total* knee replacement should include arthroplasty of the three parts of the joint. These radiographs show a prosthesis which does not renovate the patello-femoral articulation

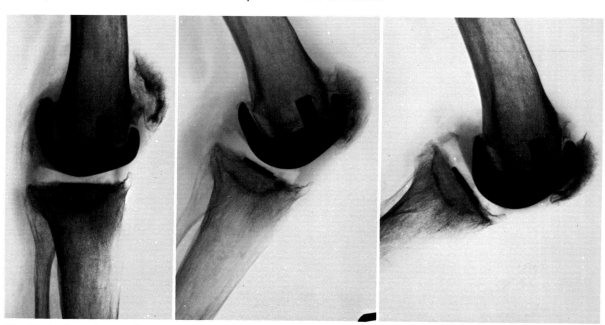

Fig. 41. An irregular patello-femoral pathway can damage the patella

I.W. (F62)

25.8.76.

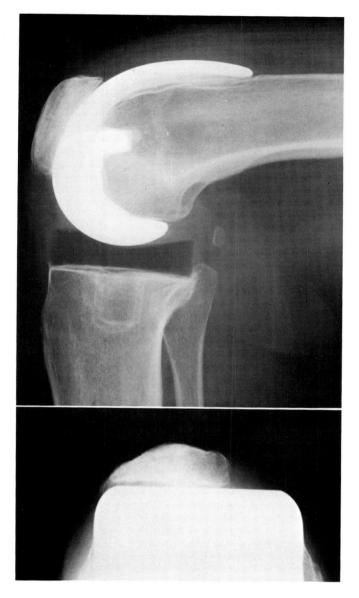

Fig. 42. This prosthesis provides a good patello-femoral
pathway

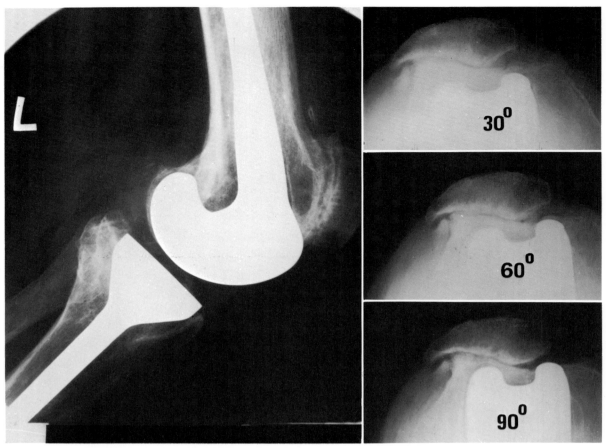

Fig. 43. This prosthesis does not include a patello-femoral arthroplasty

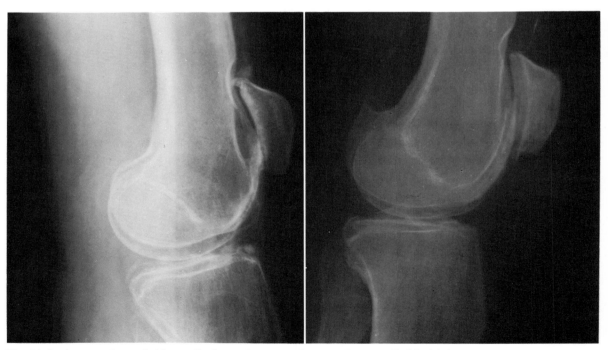

Fig. 44. In degenerative arthritis patello-femoral wear tends to produce a cylindrical joint

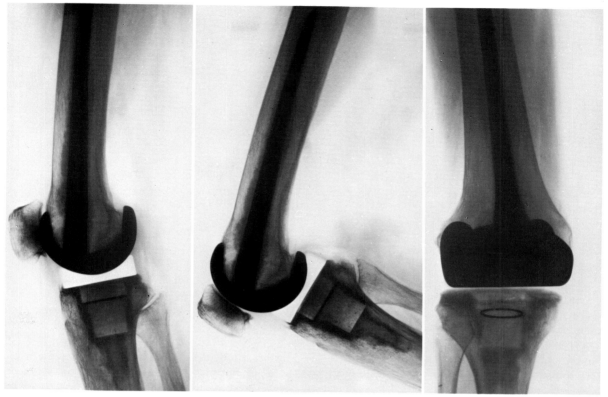

Fig. 45. The patello-femoral surface of this knee replacement is smooth, wide, and cylindrical

D.S.[F68]

20.6.78.

References

DENHAM, R.A., BISHOP, R.D.: Mechanics of the knee and problems in reconstructive surgery. J.B.J.S. **60-B**, 345 (1978)

MAQUET, P.: Biomécanique de la gonarthrose. Acta Orthop. Belg. [Suppl.] **38**, 33–54 (1972)

MURRAY, R.O., JACOBSON, H.G.: Radiology of skeletal disorders, 2nd ed., p. 1851. Edinburgh: Churchill-Livingstone 1977

Chapter 5

Conservative Management

H.L.F. Currey

The London Hospital, London E1 2AD England

The present enthusiasm for developing more effective knee joint replacements is testimony to the fact that current techniques of conservative management are unable to solve the two main medical problems affecting this joint: progressive osteoarthrosis (OA) and rheumatoid arthritis (RA). Nor at this stage do current developments in conservative management appear to open up immediate possibilities for effective control of these diseases as they affect the knee. Nevertheless, conservative management can often slow down the advance of these diseases in the knee joint, can lessen the distress caused to the patient by these processes, and should enable those affected to live fuller lives despite these diseases. Good conservative management is thus the yardstick against which operative treatment of knee arthritis has to be judged, and it should also provide the background of management for patients in whom operative surgical procedures to the knee are performed.

This Chapter attempts to provide a survey of current conservative management as it applies to RA and OA affecting the knee joint. In addition, attention will be drawn to certain aspects of drug treatment that have particular implications for the surgeon operating upon an arthritic patient.

Rheumatoid Arthritis

Damage to one or both knee joints is probably the most important cause of disability in RA. The overall impact of conservative management on the "natural history" of the condition is unknown. However, it is clear that, despite the most conscientious application of currently available techniques of conservative management, some rheumatoid patients continue to progress to a stage of knee joint

Table 1. Treatment of rheumatoid arthritis affecting the knee

A. Systemic drug therapy

B. Local measures:
  (i) Physiotherapy: exercises, splints, etc.
  (ii) Injections: corticosteroids, radioisotopes, chemical ablating agents, and lubricants

C. Aids and appliances: modification of the environment

disability that makes walking either extremely difficult or impossible. Good conservative management can certainly reduce the frequency with which this happens; equally certainly it cannot eliminate it.

Conservative management of the rheumatoid knee cannot be considered in isolation; inevitably one is treating a systemic disease in the patient as a whole and, almost invariably, a disease that is polyarticular. Thus for the rheumatoid patient in whom knee joint disease is the main problem, one can consider conservative management within the framework given in Table 1.

The optimal deployment of these measures usually requires collaboration between hospital services, the general practitioner, and local authority community services. Central to this teamwork is a physician interested in the treatment of RA, working in a hospital with good remedial services (such as physiotherapy), seeing the patient regularly, prepared to accept the load of some psychological dependence on the part of the patient, and (above all) able to win and keep the patient's confidence.

Systemic Drug Therapy

In the absence of any completely effective and safe agent, drug therapy aims to reduce symptoms and delay joint destruction through a combination of analgesic and anti-inflammatory agents and certain "slow-acting" drugs that are believed to retard the disease process in the longer term. Traditionally aspirin was the drug of first choice in RA, but the realisation that 50% of patients cannot tolerate this drug because of gastric irritation has greatly increased the use of newer drugs such as ibuprofen (Brufen) and naproxen (Naprosyn). These are better tolerated, if slightly less potent. However, it seems likely that all these nonsteroidal anti-inflammatory drugs (NSAIDS) achieve their analgesic/anti-inflammatory effects by inhibiting enzymes concerned in prostaglandin synthesis, and this probably also accounts for their gastric irritation, for none is free of this hazard.

The increasing number of drugs appearing on the market complicates the issue of devising a logical plan of drug treatment for RA; but a plan of some sort is necessary if prescribing is not to become an aimless drifting from one preparation to another. The scheme shown in Table 2, although oversimplifying the issue, provides a framework of guidance.

Those who feel that aspirin in full doses is no longer the automatic first choice start the new case on a Group II drug. It may be necessary to try a number of preparations within this group in order to discover which best suits a particular patient. If pain is not relieved, single doses of a Group I drug are added. If morning stiffness is a problem, indomethacin (Indocid) is prescribed as a single dose of up to 100 mg taken on retiring. If symptoms are still not relieved, Group III drugs are introduced, starting with full doses of aspirin. (Phenylbutazone, once so popular, carries a small but definite risk of bone marrow suppression, which may be irreversible.) Again, supplementation with single doses of a Group I drug may be helpful. If the disease continues active, and progressive joint destruction takes place, a Group V drug is introduced. All the drugs in this group have been shown to produce a modest but measurable effect on the disease in the longer term, and to have a definite "steroid-sparing" effect. All Group V drugs are potentially dangerous; their administration requires regular and careful monitoring. The mode of action of the slow-acting drugs is unknown. The antiproliferative agents are described as "immunosuppressive", but there is little proof that actual immunosuppression is necessary to achieve a therapeutic response. What is clear is that these agents increase the risk of neoplasia,

Table 2. Drug treatment of rheumatoid arthritis [a]

Group I

Pure analgesics

Paracetamol (Panadol), codeine, dextropropoxyphene with paracetamol (Distalgesic), and aspirin in small doses (under 2 g daily)

Group II

Analgesics with minor anti-inflammatory properties

Ibuprofen (Brufen), naproxen (Naprosyn), ketoprofen (Orudis), fenoprofen (Fenopron), mefenamic acid (Ponstan), etc.

Group III

Analgesics with major anti-inflammatory properties

Indomethacin (Indocid), phenylbutazone (Butazolidin), aspirin in full doses (at least 3.6 g daily)

Group IV

Pure anti-inflammatory drugs

Corticosteroids and corticotrophin

Group V

Slow-acting drugs

Sodium aurothiomalate (Myocrisin), penicillamine (Distamine), hydroxychloroquine (Plaquenil), immunosuppressives (azathioprine, cyclophosphamide, chlorambucil)

[a] Based on E.C. HUSKISSON, 1974.

particularly lymphoreticular tumours, and this risk is probably in proportion to the total dose administered.

Group IV drugs (corticosteroids) are the only agents that will predictably suppress rheumatoid inflammation. However, this is achieved at such a high cost in undesirable side effects that corticosteroids are used only to reduce an unacceptable level of suffering when this cannot be achieved by other means. Prednisolone is the generally preferred drug and the dose is kept as low as possible. Each milligram of prednisolone over 7.5 mg daily increases the risk of long-term toxicity.

Drug Therapy and Operative Surgery

The surgeon operating on patients suffering from RA will need to have some familiarity with drugs

Table 3. Special precautions necessary in patients taking slow-acting drugs

Drug	Approximate dosage range	Particular hazards	Special precautions [a]
Sodium aurothio-malate (Myocrisin)	50 mg weekly to monthly (IM injection)	Bone marrow suppression, nephritis, dermatitis	Test urine for albumin. Enquire about rash. Full blood count every 2–4 weeks
Hydroxychloroquine (Plaquenil)	200 mg daily	Retinal damage	Specialist eye examination 3-monthly
Penicillamine (Distamine)	250–1 500 mg daily	Bone marrow suppression (especially thrombocytopenia), nephritis, rashes, etc.	Full blood count 2–4 weekly. Test urine for albumin monthly. General enquiry about health
Azathioprine (Imuran)	50–150 mg daily	Bone marrow suppression	Full blood count 2–4 weekly
Cyclophosphamide (Endoxana)	50–100 mg daily	Bone marrow suppression, chemical cystitis	Full blood count 2–4 weekly. Test urine monthly for albumin and blood
Chlorambucil (Leukeran)	2.5–7.5 mg daily	Bone marrow suppression	Full blood count 2–4 weekly
Tetramisole (Levamisole)	50–150 mg daily	Bone marrow suppression (especially thrombocytopenia), oral ulceration, etc.	Full blood count 2–4 weekly. Also general enquiry about health

[a]   Full blood counts should include platelet and differential leucocyte counts.

the patient may be taking. Patients receiving slow-acting drugs, for example, need to be monitored for certain important risks. These are listed in Table 3.

In theory, the immunosuppressive drugs might reduce the patient's resistance to wound infection. In practice these drugs appear not to increase this hazard significantly. There is no particular reason why they should be stopped when operative surgery is contemplated. On the other hand, no harm is done by stopping them for a few days over the immediate operative period.

There are a number of theoretical reasons why corticosteroids might be expected to increase the hazards of infection and lead to delayed healing of surgical wounds. GARNER et al. (1973) studied wound healing in 100 rheumatoid patients and 100 matched non-rheumatoid controls following a variety of orthopaedic operations. Although failure of wound healing by primary intention was somewhat more common amongst the rheumatoid patients (31 as against 16), the overall number of days to wound healing was not significantly different (rheumatoid, 16.6 ± 7.5 days; nonrheumatoid, 15.2 ± 7.9 days). However, amongst the 49 rheumatoid patients receiving corticosteroids (in daily doses ranging from 2.5 to 15 mg prednisolone)

there was a significantly increased incidence of wound infection. Overall there was no significant difference in the time to wound healing between rheumatoid patients receiving and those not receiving corticosteroids; and there was no relationship between the daily dose of corticosteroid and the time to wound healing. However, those 27 patients who had received corticosteroids for more than 3 years showed a definite delay in wound healing (20.3 ± 11 days). Thus in this study corticosteroids did appear to predispose to wound infection, but they delayed healing time only when given for longer than 3 years, irrespective of daily dosage.

In a subsequent study, SCHOM and MOWAT (1977) found that the mean time to wound healing after 42 orthopaedic surgical operations in 21 patients treated with penicillamine was 19.8 (± 13.1) days. Comparing this result with the result of the earlier study, they concluded that this indicated that penicillamine produced a delay in wound healing comparable to that caused by 3 years of corticosteroid therapy. ANSELL et al. (1977), investigating wound healing in patients who had received penicillamine in rather lower doses for a shorter period, found no evidence of any delay attributable to this drug.

A normal response to stress, such as that of a surgical operation, requires normal hypothalamic–pituitary and pituitary–adrenal interactions. Both may become impaired by continued corticosteroid therapy, and may remain impaired for some years after such therapy is stopped. Patients may show no obvious evidence of this defect until the stress of something like a surgical operation produces sudden, sometimes life-threatening, collapse.

Pituitary–adrenal responses may be tested by following the plasma corticol response to an injection of tetracosactrin (Synacthen), while the integrity of the full hypothalamic–pituitary–adrenal sequence may be tested by following the plasma responses to insulin-induced hypoglycaemia. Such tests are somewhat elaborate, and at best provide a warning of which patients are most definitely at risk of collapse. A more practical approach is to assume that anyone who has received more than 1 month of corticosteroid or corticotrophine therapy in the previous year, or 3 months of corticosteroid therapy in the past 2 years, is at risk, and to supplement their endogenous steroids over the operative period.

Intramuscular injections of hydrocortisone hemisuccinate are probably the most reliable form of cover (Myles and Daly, 1974). Doses of 100 mg are given every 8 h, starting with the premedication drugs, and continued for 1, 2, or 3 days, depending on the magnitude of the procedure and the stress to the patient. No "tapering off" of the dose is required, but post-operative patients unable to swallow or absorb must of course have any pre-existing steroid medication continued parenterally. Any collapse that might be due to steroid depletion requires the immediate administration of 100 mg hydrocortisone hemisuccinate IV.

Stress is not the only problem that needs to be remembered when the rheumatoid patient on corticosteroids is admitted for surgery: hypertension, diabetes, hypokalaemia, and pulmonary tuberculosis are all potential hazards.

Local Measures

Physiotherapy

For efficient walking, a knee joint requires to have a free range of movement from full extension to 90° of flexion, to be aligned correctly in a coronal plane, and to be stable. The rheumatoid disease process tends to interfere with all three of these properties, and in the late, neglected knee the combination of flexion and valgus deformities with instability may severely curtail independence. Experience suggests that appropriate physiotherapy can maintain function to a considerable extent despite advancing structural damage. The provision of aids and appliances that supplement physiotherapy is discussed later. For a recent review of physical methods of treatment in RA see Mathews (1978).

Physiotherapy aims to maintain or improve function in the rheumatoid knee by strengthening the power of the muscles acting across the joint, thus improving stability, and by maintaining or increasing the range of movement of the joint. Both objectives are achieved by active muscle exercises; the latter objective may require splinting in addition.

Active rheumatoid disease in the knee produces marked weakness and wasting of the muscles acting across the joint, particularly the quadriceps. This is a major factor in the instability that can so severely interfere with walking and other everyday activities, such as rising from a chair or climbing stairs. Fortunately the weakness can be overcome to a large extent by exercises. These exercises have to be active (neither passive movements executed by the physiotherapist nor electrically induced contractions can strengthen a muscle), but they do not have to involve actual movement of the joint: static exercises that involve tensing of the muscles without moving the joint, as in the familiar "quadriceps drill", are effective. When the range of movement is limited this can be improved by exercises involving active movements against resistance. These are graded according to the initial strength of the muscles and the irritability of the joint. Before intensive physiotherapy is undertaken it is worth considering whether aspirating an effusion and injecting intra-articular corticosteroid may allow the physiotherapy to be more effective.

Splinting also plays an important part in knee physiotherapy. While recent or minor degrees of flexion deformity in the rheumatoid knee can be eliminated by active resistance exercises, the more resistant flexion deformities require splinting. Initially this is likely to involve a "serial splint", i.e., application of a plaster of Paris cast in the position of maximum extension, to be renewed at about weekly intervals, each time taking advantage of any further extension gained. Static exercises are continued throughout inside the cast. In this way quite gross flexion deformities may gradually be eliminated. There is of course a limit to what can be achieved in this way, and a tendency to posterior subluxation of the tibia on the femur is an ominous sign.

The more difficult it has been to eliminate a flexion deformity, the more effort is needed to maintain full extension. Night splints, either plaster of Paris gutter casts or splints made of one of the newer materials such as plastazote, are the most effective means of maintaining extension, supplemented by a daily routine of exercises such as quadriceps drill.

The detailed techniques of exercising and splinting the rheumatoid knee require the expertise of a physiotherapist familiar with the problem, who will also have a psychological role to play in a program that may sorely test the patient's motivation. Some physiotherapists believe that exercises are more easily carried out after applying "counter-irritation" in the form of heat or cold. If this is done it is important that a preoccupation with electrical gadgetry shall not detract from the main issues outlined above.

Judgement is needed about how activity should be graded. Encouraging weight-bearing on knees with flexion deformities and very weak muscles makes the situation worse. Ideally, the patient should be able to extend the knee fully, and raise the leg unaided from a supine position while maintaining full extension before walking is attempted. If this rule is to be broken careful consideration has to be given to the extent of protection that can be provided by crutches or other walking aids; this depends very much on the state of upper limb function.

Until recently no really effective external splint was available to support the unstable rheumatoid knee with a flexion and/or valgus deformity during weight-bearing. Calipers, cages, and reinforced leather braces fitted with padding and straps were often tried, but seldom gave satisfactory results. However, preliminary reports on the new CARS–UBC knee orthosis suggest that the use of a telescopic beam may provide much more effective support, at least for lateral instability (COUSINS and FOORT, 1975; WASSEN et al., 1976).

Injections and Aspiration

Aspiration and injection of the knee joint are very simple procedures that can safely be carried out in the consulting room with the aid of sterile disposable equipment (CURREY and VERNON ROBERTS, 1976).

Apart from diagnostic taps, aspiration is seldom employed alone as a therapeutic measure. If a large effusion is drained to relieve the discomfort of joint distension or to assist a program of physiotherapy (see above), this is usually combined with the injection of a corticosteroid preparation, as otherwise the effusion tends to reaccumulate within days.

Intra-articular injection of drugs has considerable theoretical appeal: it is a means of delivering a drug to the actual inflamed tissue in a concentration that would be difficult or impossible to give safely by systemic administration. Systemic effects are not altogether avoided, however, for some absorption occurs with any drug given by this route.

The most obvious use for the intra-articular route is the administration of corticosteroids to achieve an anti-inflammatory effect. In addition, a variety of different drugs and chemicals has been employed in an attempt to produce a more long-term effect on the rheumatoid synovium. This includes chemical ablating agents, antiproliferative drugs, and radioisotopes. Like the operation of surgical synovectomy, this has the purpose of damping down synovitis and reducing synovial effusions in the longer term. (The intra-articular injection of silicone oil is discussed on p. 117).

Intra-articular Corticosteroids (HOLLANDER, 1972). A variety of insoluble corticosteroid preparations is available for intra-articular injection. Hydrocortisone acetate (50 mg) is still widely used, but there is some evidence that more prolonged relief may be obtained with newer preparations, including:
- Triamcinolone hexacetonide (Lederspan), 20 mg;
- Methylprednisolone acetate (Depo-Medrone), 40 mg;
- Prednisolone tert-butylacetate (Codelcortone-TBA) 30 mg.

It is customary to drain off as much synovial fluid as can easily be obtained before injecting the corticosteroid.

A single intra-articular corticosteroid injection is likely to produce 1–2 weeks of pain relief. The main use of this type of therapy is thus either to damp down a temporary flare in a knee joint (remembering the need to exclude infection by microbiological examination of the synovial fluid) or to facilitate a program of physiotherapy. The very extensive experience of HOLLANDER (1972) suggests that repeated injections may be administered into the same knee joint over many years without any harm. However, most clinicians prefer to employ this treatment as a temporary solution to a local problem and to use it only as an occasional measure in individual patients. In HOLLANDER's series the infection rate was low (18 infections in 250 000 injections) and aseptic necrosis and pictures resembling neuropathic arthropathy were rare. Occasional patients experience an acute flare in the injected joint lasting between a few hours and a few days. The mechanism of this appears to be "crystal synovitis" provoked by the insoluble injected material (McCARTY and HOGAN, 1964), although why only some patients experience this is uncertain. Presumably all these microcrystalline adrenocorticosteroid esters are taken up by macrophages of one sort or another within the joint. These acute flares are usually left to run their course, but the attack may be terminated by aspirating the effusion.

Intra-articular Radioisotopes (GUMPEL, 1974; GUMPEL, 1977). The intra-articular injection of radioisotopes has considerable theoretical appeal. Given a suitable carrier and the right isotope it should be possible to administer a compound that will be taken up by the synovial lining cells and held there while a dose of ionising radiation is delivered to the whole diseased synovium but not to the tissues beyond. Such a "radio-ablation" of the synovium might offer a more precise and less invasive method of achieving the objectives of surgical synovectomy. In fact, while this method of treatment has become popular in a number of centres in continental Europe, its use in Britain has been limited to a very few units. This may be partly explained by problems connected with the treatment: part of the administered dose is absorbed to irradiate the regional lymph nodes and other tissues, while the presence of clots within the joint results in dissipation of radioactivity into the fibrin mass. Also, consideration of radiation hazards means that this treatment should be reserved for patients who have reached the age of 45 years (DOYLE et al., 1977). However, the main reason for the relative neglect of this form of treatment is probably the lack of adequately controlled trials establishing its efficiency.

ANSELL and her colleagues (ANSELL et al., 1963) first showed that colloidal gold-198 (^{198}Au) produced a favourable effect on rheumatoid knee effusions and synovitis. A disadvantage of ^{198}Au is its significant γ emission. For this reason yttrium-90 (^{90}Y), a pure β emitter with a half-life of 2.67 days and a penetration range of 3.6–11.0 mm in soft tissues appears to be more appropriate for the knee (GUMPEL, 1974). Of the various radiopharmaceutical preparations (radiocolloids) of ^{90}Y available, the silicate in a dose of 5 mCi has given satisfactory results in the knee (GUMPEL, 1977). All radiocolloids injected into the knee joint are absorbed to some extent, and deliver radiation, for example, to the regional lymph nodes. Absorption can be reduced to 13% of the injected dose at 5 days by immobilising the joint (leg splintage and bed rest) for 4 days following the injection (GUMPEL et al., 1973). Such rest and immobilisation is probably more important than the choice of radiocolloid in determining how much radiation is delivered to tissues outside the joint (WILLIAMS et al., 1976).

The indications for radioisotope injections into the knee are usually regarded as similar to those for surgical synovectomy, except that patients should have reached the age of 45 years. Knees in which there is evidence of continuing inflammatory activity, with thick synovium and persistent effusion, but with no more than minimal structural damage, are likely to respond best. As with surgical synovectomy, early cases appear to fare better than late. Comparison of the late results of surgical synovectomy and radioisotope injection suggests that the results are similar, except that some loss of range of movement may occur with synovectomy, but not with injection (GUMPEL, 1977). As with surgical synovectomy, a properly conducted long-term controlled trial of intra-articular isotope injection is badly needed.

Intra-articular Chemical Ablating Agents. Apart from radioactive substances, various chemicals have been injected into rheumatoid joints in an attempt to achieve a chemical synovectomy. Most interest has centered round the alkylating agents nitrogen mustard and thio-Tepa, and osmic acid.

The alkylating agents are absorbed from joints following intra-articular injections and, because they are mutagenic and bone marrow suppressants, this places a limit on the total dose that can safely be given into the knee joint. Using 60 mg thio-Tepa injected into the knee joint, GRISTINA et al. (1970) did not show any clear advantage of thio-Tepa over corticosteroid injections. A relatively larger dose of thio-Tepa is permissible in finger joints, but a controlled study in which an average dose of 3.5 mg was injected into rheumatoid finger joints failed to show any advantage of the drug over procaine injections (CURREY, 1965). It appears unlikely that this procedure is much used at present.

Another method of ablating the diseased synovium is to inject osmic acid (BERGLOF, 1964). Injection of 5–10 ml 1% osmium tetroxide solution followed by 40 mg prednisolone produced long-term results that are probably comparable to those claimed for radiocolloid injections. Occasional mild reactions occur, but the procedure appears to be reasonably safe. Vignon and his colleagues (VIGNON et al. 1974) found osmic acid and radiocolloids to be equally effective. Injections of 1% osmic acid into rabbit knee joints inflamed by previous carrageenin injections (AMINI et al., 1971) produced immediate superficial coagulative necrosis followed by delayed death of macrophages deeper in the synovium. After 5 weeks the synovium had returned almost to normal, but electron microscopy revealed changes in chondrocytes, which raised the possibility of some cartilage damage. Like radiocolloid injections, intra-articular osmic acid is a theoretically attractive form of treatment for rheumatoid synovitis of the knee. It has been neglected, probably because of the lack of adequately controlled studies.

Aids and Appliances: Modification of the Environment

Management of the rheumatoid knee is seldom an isolated local problem; more often the knee has to be considered against a background of multiple joint disability. This becomes more relevant as the patient passes from the earlier stages of the disease, in which the therapeutic aim is usually to modify the patient and his joints, to the later stages, in which the objective becomes modification of the environment and provision of aids and appliances to overcome established deformities. Upper limb problems for example, will often preclude the use of axillary crutches or rear wheel-propelled chairs for rheumatoid knee problems. At this stage management requires a team approach, including hospital and community remedial services (NICHOLS, 1976).

Osteoarthrosis

Much of what has been said above regarding the conservative management of the rheumatoid knee

applies also to treatment of the osteoarthrotic joint. The remarks that follow mainly highlight the differences between the approach in dealing with an inflammatory polyarthritis as against a localised degenerative arthropathy.

Systemic Drug Therapy

Much less can be expected from drug therapy in OA than in the inflammatory arthropathies. Indeed, the degree of relief to be expected from the analgesic/anti-inflammatory group of drugs in different types or arthritis is in proportion to the acuteness of the inflammatory change. Thus the acute gouty attack and acute rheumatic fever can be well controlled by systemic drug therapy. OA is at the other end of the scale. The same drugs that are employed in RA (Groups I, II, III; Table 2, p. 111) can be tried, but only partial relief of pain is to be expected. A real danger is that the patient and his doctor, misled by sales promotion claims, may embark on a fruitless round of trying each and every new drug as it appears on the market, convinced that the solution to the problem lies in finding the right drug.

No discussion about the effectiveness of drugs in the treatment of arthritis would be complete without attention having been drawn to the striking "placebo effect" that can be expected when any form of medication is tested (TRAUT and PASSARELL, 1957). Up to 60% of patients will appear to improve on any new treatment offered, and the greater the expectation of patient and doctor, the more marked this effect will be. For this reason it requires the most rigorous double-blind testing against a matched placebo control to detect true drug effects. The same placebo effect of course also complicates the evaluation of physiotherapy and operative surgical procedures; here the problem is usually the lack of adequately matched controls and the near-impossibility of achieving "blindness".

Local Measures

Physiotherapy

The remarks made above regarding physiotherapy in rheumatoid arthritis apply equally to the management of osteoarthrosis of the knee. Active, resisted exercises that improve the power of the muscles acting across the knee can be expected to maintain or increase the range of movement, stabilise the joint in weight-bearing, and reduce pain. Regular periods of exercise, e.g., quadriceps drill, should become a daily routine for anyone with OA of the knee sufficiently severe to produce symptoms.

In seeking to provide symptomatic relief for OA of the knee by physiotherapy it is relevant to consider the mechanism by which pain is produced in this disease. Pain is seldom unchanging day after day; more often pain and swelling appear together and last a few days at a time. Such episodes may be noted to follow minor trauma: moving the joint beyond the usual range, or a lateral strain while weight-bearing. The summation of such episodes may produce an appearance of continuous symptoms, but careful history taking will usually reveal the episodic patterns. If this is the case, then "trauma" in the broadest sense is an important cause of symptoms (and perhaps also of advance of the disease). It follows that physical methods of treatment have an important role to play: improvement of muscle power will reduce instability of the knee, and the provision of correct walking aids and formal training in gait and negotiating stairs, etc., should all help to reduce trauma and strains. The remedial services thus have a key role to play in the conservative management of knee OA.

Injections

Intra-articular injections of radioisotopes and chemical ablating agents are not generally used in OA of the knee, but corticosteroid preparations, used as for RA (p. 114), may be helpful in terminating temporary exacerbations. Soft-tissue injections may also be helpful. When tender areas are detected in the tissues round osteoarthrotic knees, possibly sites of soft tissue "strains" or impingement of soft tissues on marginal osteophytes (KELLGREN, 1965), infiltration of these areas with a mixture of procaine and corticosteroid may relieve symptoms (SHARP, 1969).

Silicone Oil

HELAL and KARADI (1968) tested the effect of injecting silicone oil into joints as an artificial lubricant to facilitate mobilisation. About 10 ml pure silicone oil (200 cSt viscosity) injected into arthritic knees, both rheumatoid and osteoarthrotic, exhibiting dry grating stiffness and "catching" were improved, in that both pain and crepitus were lessened. The silicone appeared to be completely inert and harmless, and was retained in the joint for months (HELAL, 1969). However, WRIGHT and his colleagues (WRIGHT et al., 1971) found that osteoarthrotic joints injected with 300-cSt silicone fared no better than control joints. This technique has not found a place in the routine treatment of arthritic knees.

Aids and Appliances

Little need be added under this heading to what has already been mentioned above in connection with RA. Because OA often affects only one or both knees in isolation, function is usually better maintained than in patients with polyarthritis. Upper limb function will usually permit more effective use of walking aids and, for the unstable knee, calipers are likely to be better tolerated.

References

AMINI, D., DAZIANO, I., GAGNON, J., LAURIN, D.: The use of intra-articular osmic acid to produce chemical synovectomy in rabbits. Clin. Orthop. 79, 164–172 (1971)

ANSELL, B.M., CROOK, A., MALLARD, J.R., BYWATERS, E.G.L.: Evaluation of intra-articular colloidal gold Au-198 in the treatment of persistent knee effusions. Ann. Rheum. Dis. 22, 435–439 (1963)

ANSELL, B.M., MORAN, H., ARDEN, G.P.: Penicillamine and wound healing in rheumatoid arthritis. Proc. R. Soc. Med. 70, 75–76 (1977)

BERGLOF, F.E.: Further studies on the use of osmic acid in the treatment of arthritis. Acta Rheum. Scand. 10, 92 (1964)

COUSINS, S., FOORT, J.: An orthosis for medial or lateral stabilization of arthritic knees. Orthotics Prosthetics 29, 21 (1975)

CURREY, H.L.F.: Intra-articular thiotepa in rheumatoid arthritis. Ann. Rheum. Dis. 24, 382–388 (1965)

CURREY, H.L.F., VERNON-ROBERTS, B.: Examination of synovial fluid. Clin. Rheum. Dis. 2, 149–177 (1976)

DJAFAR, A., DAZIANO, L., GAGNON, J., LAURIN, C.A.: The use of intra-articular osmic acid to produce chemical synovectomy in rabbits. Clin. Orthop. 79, 164 (1971)

DOYLE, D.V., GLASS, J.S., GOW, P.J., DAKEN, M., GRAHAME, R.: A clinical and prospective chromosomal study of yttrium-90 synovectomy. Rheumatol. Rehabil. 16, 217–222 (1977)

GARNER, R.W., MOWAT, A.G., HAZLEMAN, B.L.: Wound healing after operations on patients with rheumatoid arthritis. J. Bone Joint Surg. (Br.) **55**, 134–144 (1973)

GRISTINA, A.G., PACE, N.A., KUNTER, T.G., THOMPSON, W.A.L.: Intra-articular thiotepa compared with depomedrol and procaine in the treatment of arthritis. J. Bone Joint Surg. (Am.) **52**, 1603–1610 (1970)

GUMPEL, J.M.: The role of radiocolloids in the treatment of arthritis. Rheumatol. Rehabil. **13**, 1–9 (1974)

GUMPEL, J.M.: Synoviothèse; surgical or medical. In: Rheumatoid arthritis. GORDON, G.L., HAZLEMAN, B.L. (eds.), pp. 111–116. Amsterdam: Elsevier/North Holland 1977

GUMPEL, J.M., WILLIAMS, E.D., GLASS, H.I.: Use of yttrium 90 in persistent synovitis of the knee. I. Retention in the knee and spread in the body after injection. Ann. Rheum. Dis. **32**, 223–227 (1973)

HELAL, B.: Silicones in orthopaedic surgery. In: Recent advances in orthopaedics. APLEY, A.G. (ed.), Vol. V, pp. 91–99. London: Churchill 1969

HELAL, B., KARADI, B.S.: Artificial lubrication of joints. Use of silicone oil. Ann. Phys. Med. **9**, 334–340 (1968)

HOLLANDER, J.L.: Intrasynovial corticosteroid therapy. In: Arthritis and allied conditions, 8th ed. HOLLANDER, J.L., McCARTY, D.J. (eds.), Vol. XXXII, pp. 517–534. Philadelphia: Lea & Febiger 1972

HUSKISSON, E.C.: Recent drugs and the rheumatic diseases. Reports on Rheumatic Diseases (No. 54). Arthritis and Rheumatism Council, London 1974

KAJANDER, A., RUOTSI, A.: Effect of intra-articular osmic acid on rheumatoid knee joint affections. Ann. Med. Int. Fenniae **57**, 87–91 (1967) [Abstracted in Ann. Rheum. Dis. **27**, 497 (1968)].

KELLGREN, T.H.: Osteoarthrosis. Arthritis Rheum. **8**, 568–572 (1965)

McCARTY, D.J., HOGAN, J.M.: Inflammatory reaction after intrasynovial injection of microcrystalline adreno-corticosteroid esters. Arthritis Rheum. **7**, 359–367 (1964)

MATHEWS, J.A.: Physical treatment of rheumatoid arthritis. In: Compeman's textbook of the rheumatic diseases, 5th ed. SCOTT, J.T. (ed.), Vol. XVII, p. 447. Edinburgh: Churchill, Livingstone 1978

MYLES, A.B., DALY, J.R.: Corticosteroid and ACTH treatment, pp. 162–167. London: Edward Arnold 1974

NICHOLS, P.J.R.: Rheumatoid arthritis. In: Rehabilitation medicine. The management of physical disabilities. NICHOLS, P.J.R. (ed.), pp. 63–98. London: Butterworths 1976

SCHOM, D., MOWAT, A.G.: Penicillamine in rheumatoid arthritis: wound healing, skin thickness and osteoporosis. Rheumatol. Rehabil. **16**, 223–230 (1977)

SHARP, J.: Osteo-arthrosis. In: Textbook of the rheumatic diseases, 4th ed. COPEMAN, W.S.C. (ed.), p. 414. Edinburgh: Livingstone 1969

TRAUT, E.F., PASSARELL, E.W.: Placebos in the treatment of rheumatoid arthritis and other rheumatic conditions. Ann. Rheum. Dis. **16**, 18 (1957)

VIGNON, G., COLCOMBET, B., LAHNÈCHE, B., BIED, J.-C., MEUNIER, P.: Comparaison des synoviorthèses osmiques et isotopiques dans la polyarthritic rhumatoide. Nouv. Presse. Med. **3**, 2712–2714 (1974)

WASSEN, R., HANNAH, R., FOORT, J., COUSINS, S.: Fabrication and fitting of the CARS-UBC knee orthosis. Orthotics Prosthetics **30**, 3–11 (1976)

WILLIAMS, E.D., CAUGHEY, D.E., HUXLEY, P.J., JOHN, M.B.: Distribution of yttrium 90 ferric hydroxide colloid and gold 198 colloid after injection into knee. Ann. Rheum. Dis. **35**, 516–520 (1976)

WRIGHT, V., HASLOCK, D.I., DOWSON, D., SELLER, P.C., REEVES, B.: Evaluation of silicone as an artificial lubricant in osteoarthrotic joints. Br. Med. J. **1977** ii, 370–373

Chapter 6

Soft-Tissue Operations

J.-F. Goldie

Department of Orthopaedic Surgery, University of Göteborg, Göteborg, Sweden

Various surgical procedures have been suggested over the years to deal with both degenerative and inflammatory disease of the knee joint. In this chapter the relevant soft-tissue operations will be described as they have been used in the past and are practised at present.

The operations are:
Synovectomy
Removal of Baker's cyst
Soft-tissue releases (lateral release and posterior capsulotomy, resection of the anterior cruciate ligament)
Nerve resection
Meniscectomy
Débridement (the "spring clean" procedure)
Patellectomy.

Synovectomy

Rheumatoid Arthritis

The synovial membrane readily becomes a target organ for the initiating agent in rheumatoid disease. The resulting inflammatory response calls for active therapeutic measures, of which synovectomy has been said to be one of the most advantageous (CHAPCHAL, 1967; GSCHWEND, 1977). Synovectomy can be a successful procedure if it is performed for the right indications, at the right time and in the right patient (GEENS, 1969), but before an unprejudiced evaluation of the use of synovectomy in rheumatoid disease can be carried out it is necessary to consider (1) what the biological rationale behind synovectomy is; (2) what point in the course of the disease is the time of choice for synovectomy; (3) what the long-term results are; and (4) the nature of the indications and contra-indications.

Historical Aspects

The original indication for synovectomy was arthritis, which could be tuberculous, septic, chronic degenerative, or rheumatoid. With time the procedure became limited to rheumatoid disease only, since the results in other conditions were unsatisfactory. Of late, however, and in Japan especially, synovectomy has been used for articular pathology of various kinds (T. KODAMA, personal communication, 1970; HIROHATA, 1973).

The first surgeon known to have performed a synovectomy of the knee joint was VOLKMANN, who in 1877 carried out the procedure in a case of tuberculosis. The idea of removing inflamed synovial tissue of the knee joint kindled the imagination of a number of surgeons during the late 1800s and early 1900s. Commencing in 1887 with SCHÜLLER, who reported good results in four patients with RA in whom complete synovectomy had been carried out, a number of reports were published presenting satisfactory results with short post-operative observations in groups of patients numbering between five and ten (TUBY, 1870; MÜLLER, 1894; GOLDTHWAIT, 1900; MURPHY, 1916; SPEED, 1924; SWETT, 1926).

In due course, synovectomy acquired a good reputation and became a widely used procedure. However, the disadvantages accompanying its popularisation soon became apparent: as the indications grew wider the results became so variable that by the 1940s synovectomy had come into disrepute. For some 20 years surgical activity subsided, but in the mid-1960s a more optimistic and enthusiastic approach emerged among orthopaedic surgeons all over the world, and some of the long-term results now appearing do seem to provide

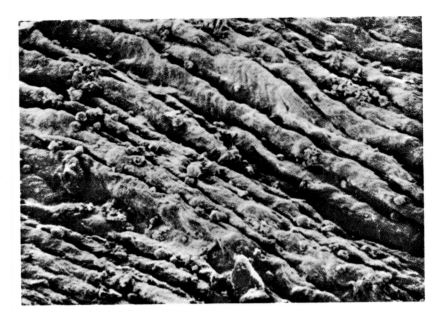

Fig. 1. Scanning electron micrograph of furrowed synovial tissue with some villi from normal knee joint (from REDLER and ZIMMY, cited in I. GOLDIE, Semin. Arthritis Rheum. **3**, 219, 1974). ×1250

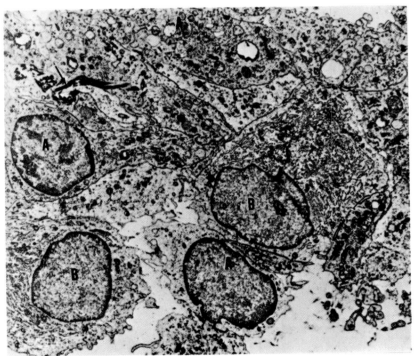

Fig. 2. Synovial tissue with A cells: filopodia, Golgi's complex, fibrils, and vacuoles; and with B cells: vacuoles, mitochondria, and ergastoplasm. (BARLAND et al., 1962; cited in I. GOLDIE, Semin. Arthritis Rheum. **3**, 219, 1974). ×7600

grounds for recommending the procedure (GSCHWEND, 1977).

Synovial Morbid Anatomy

The appearance of the synovial tissues in RA has been described by numerous authors (see for example GARDNER, 1972). For the purposes of this Chapter the essential points that emerge from these descriptions are that the synovial membrane is the first tissue in a joint to be affected and that it is reasonable to think that damage to others is secondary to events in the membrane. Figures 1–5 illustrate aspects of normal and rheumatoid knee joints.

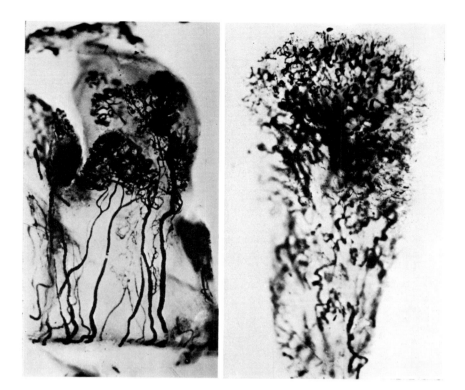

Fig. 3. *Left*, normal vascular architecture of synovial villus; *right*, rheumatoid synovial villus with distorted vessels, diapedesis, oedema, and congested vessels. Intravital freezing technique, × 60

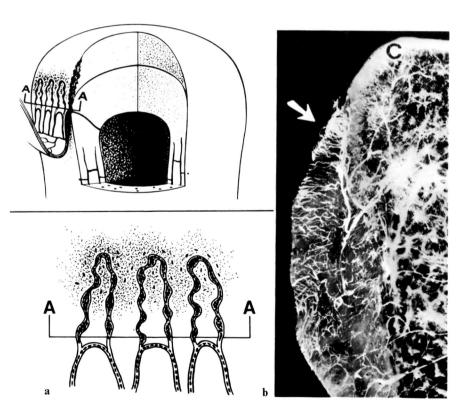

Fig. 4. a Schematic presentation of bone cartilage zone with synovial vessels forming an arcade-like design and connecting with the marrow space. *Intersection* at A shows shunt mechanism above which the circulation in the vascular loops becomes stagnated and diapedesis develops. **b** Microangiogram of vascular connection (*arrow*) between synovial tissue and bone marrow. C, cartilage.

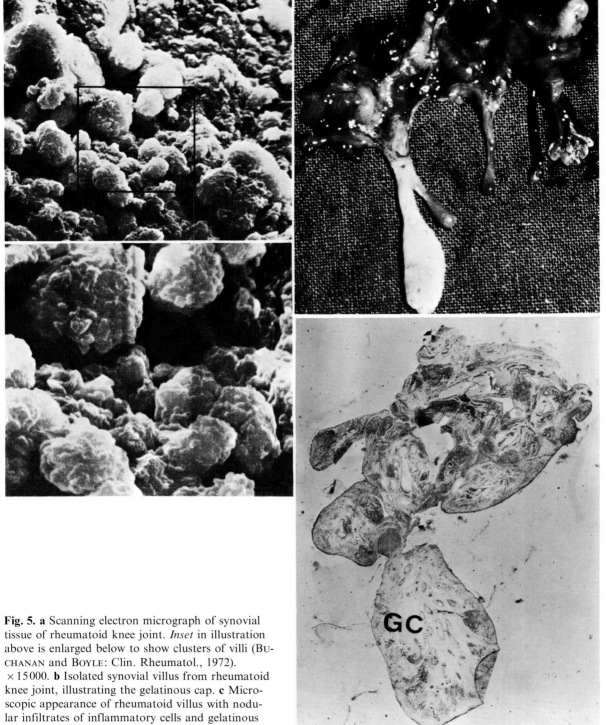

Fig. 5. a Scanning electron micrograph of synovial tissue of rheumatoid knee joint. *Inset* in illustration above is enlarged below to show clusters of villi (Bu-CHANAN and BOYLE: Clin. Rheumatol., 1972). × 15000. **b** Isolated synovial villus from rheumatoid knee joint, illustrating the gelatinous cap. **c** Microscopic appearance of rheumatoid villus with nodular infiltrates of inflammatory cells and gelatinous cap (GC) with some vessels. H and E stain. × 11.5

It has been shown (GOLDIE, 1974) that in RA two macroscopic types of synovial tissue are encountered, hypertrophic and hypotrophic. It seems likely that synovectomy is indicated, only for the former.

The hypertrophic variety is seen in joints that clinically exhibit synovial swelling and an effusion (Fig. 6a–c). The synovial tissue is congested and has a glossy surface covered by a fibrin layer. Microscopically, the synovial tissue appears to be oedematous, although this is difficult to confirm in histologic sections, for technical reasons. There is a heavy infiltration of inflammatory cells, predominantly lymphocytes, that occur as irregularly scattered infiltrates aggregated to resemble lymphoid nodules or as concentrations around vessels. Plasma cells are common but neutrophils scanty. Small scattered areas of fibrinoid necrosis are seen. In some samples tufts resembling granulation tissue invade the bone. The synovium is highly vascular.

The hypotrophic variety occurs in joints that would clinically be referred to as "dry". The synovial tissue appears as a white, almost leathery membrane without oedema or hypervascularity. Microscopically, the cellular infiltration qualitatively resembles that of the hypertrophic variety, although it is much more sparse. The predominant features are hyalinisation and fibrosis. Focal necrotic areas also occur.

The activity of the inflamed synovial tissue — especially of the hypertrophic variety — seems to be such that inflammatory fibrous tissue grows over the joint cartilage and destroys it. At the junction of the bone and the cartilage outgrowths of this tissue invade the bone, giving the radiological appearance of erosions.

Synovial Regeneration

Clinical experience has shown that the activity of synovial tissue can be reduced considerably by drug administration. The results of surgical synovectomy indicate that the removal of pathological tissue has a comparable effect. The rationale for synovectomy is based upon the thought that further destruction of cartilage will be arrested most efficiently by a surgical procedure. This cannot remain unchallenged, however, as there is now radiological evidence that a definite retardation of cartilage and bone destruction occurs once active conservative therapy has been instituted (MC-EWEN, 1977).

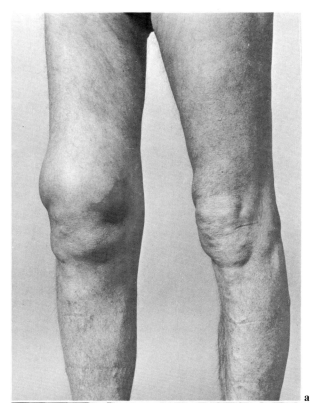

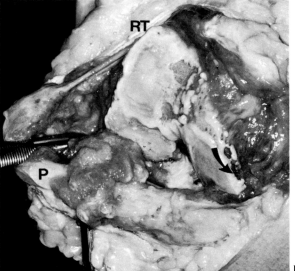

Fig. 6. a Legs of 55-year-old man with RA. Right knee joint is swollen, particularly in the suprapatellar pouch, which was partly closed off by a membrane. Quadriceps wasting. **b** Same knee joint as shown in Fig. 6a, at operation. The incision is medial to the patella and high up in the rectus tendon (RT), thus giving good access to the joint. Patella (P) is well everted. Synovial tissue is congested and femoral cartilage is destroyed. Erosions with invading granulation tufts are seen (*arrow*)

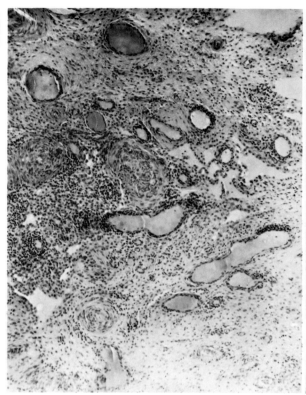
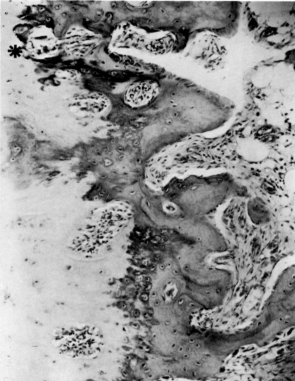

Fig. 6c. Left, histologic section from rheumatoid synovial tissue of knee joint seen in Fig. 6b. Infiltration of cells, which are lymphocytes and plasma cells. A number of dilated thin-walled venules are seen. H and E stain. × 100.

Right, histologic section of bone–cartilage zone at *arrow* in Fig. 6b. Breakthrough of invasive soft tissues at *asterisk*. H and E stain. × 160

Experimentally, synovial tissue regenerates: new synovial tissue is formed by metaplasia of the underlying connective tissue (KEY, 1925). According to MARMOR (1967) and PRESTON (1968), this occurs in man, so that after synovectomy for RA normal synovium is redeveloped. This view has been substantiated by MITCHELL and SHEPHERD (1972), who found that the subsynovial inflammatory infiltrations characteristic of rheumatoid disease disappeared and that the morphology of the chondrocytes gradually improved after synovectomy.

On the other hand, it has been shown (GOLDIE, 1974) that the regenerated synovial tissue has features identical to those present in the original rheumatoid synovium (Fig. 7). These observations were made on tissues obtained at arthrotomy and needle biopsy in 26 knee joints 1–3 years after synovectomy. Of the regeneration of synovial tissues, FASS-BENDER (1975) says: "However, if fibrosis is not a prominent feature, then a new loosely textured and vascular synovial layer arises, which is likely to become the setting for renewed synovitis. Such a tissue cannot readily be distinguished from the original inflamed tissue." GSCHWEND (1977) also studied cases 2¹/₂ years after synovectomy, and found that the microscopic appearance of regenerated tissue resembled that of the original. („Die Histologie ergab eindeutig eine Wiedererkrankung der Synovialis an cP".)

Morphologically, it thus appears that the regenerated synovial tissue remains the target organ for the inflammatory reaction in rheumatoid disease. If this is the case, is synovectomy useful? The answer to this question depends in part upon the function of the new tissue.

Function of Regenerated Synovial Tissue

Five methods, described below, have been used to evaluate the function of regenerated synovial tissue after synovectomy.

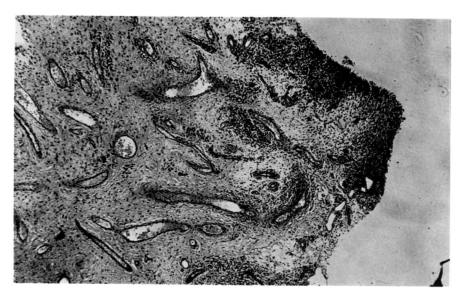

Fig. 7. Regenerated synovial tissue from rheumatoid knee joint synovectomised 1 year before biopsy. Conglomeration of plasma cells and lymphocytes. Thin-walled dilated venules. H and E stain. ×100

Direct Measurement of the Temperature of the Joint. On the assumption that a connection might exist between the activity of the disease and temperature, intra-articular temperatures have been studied (BRANEMARK et al., 1963; GOLDIE, 1974). The intra-articular temperatures were measured 1–7 days before, and 3–6 months after, synovectomy in ten patients with RA. As a control, the intra-articular temperature was measured in ten volunteers. As compared with the normal joints, the rheumatoid joints reacted inversely to stimulation by heat and cold in all cases: on stimulation with heat the intra-articular temperature of the arthritic joints decreased, whereas with cold the intra-articular temperature rose (Fig. 8). After synovectomy, temperature recordings revealed a normal reaction pattern in all patients, suggesting that synovectomy had had a beneficial effect.

Indirect Measurement of the Temperature of the Joint. It has been demonstrated by thermography that following synovectomy the temperature of the pre-operatively inflamed joint decreases (GOLDIE, 1974). In 27 knee joints, repeated post-operative thermograms showed that in all patients a decrease in heat emission followed synovectomy (Fig. 9). This was interpreted as amelioration of the inflammatory state of the joint. Clinically, improvement paralleled the decreased heat emission.

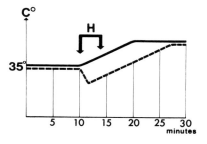

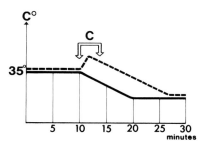

Fig. 8. Reaction of intra-articular temperatures in normal and rheumatoid knee joints after stimulation by heat (H) and cold (C.) *Unbroken line* shows normal reaction. *Broken line* is rheumatoid reaction *Top* heat (approx. 50° C) is applied for 3 min. *Bottom* reactions after cold stimulation; 6 months after synovectomy reaction is normal

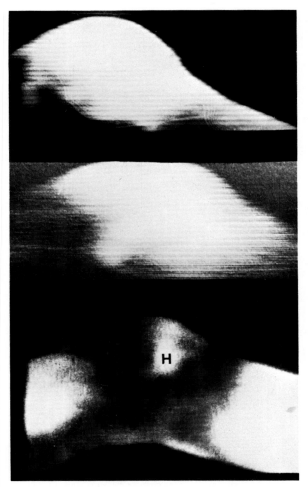

Fig. 9. Thermographic recording of heat emission from right rheumatoid knee joint. *Top,* before synovectomy: increased heat emission. *Middle,* 6 months after synovectomy: increased heat emission, interpreted as an indication of active healing processes. *Bottom,* 1 year after synovectomy: normal emission with increase at Hoffa's fat pad (H)

Table 1. pH values in synovial fluid from normal and rheumatoid knees and rheumatoid synovectomised knees

	Normal knees	Rheumatoid knees	Rheumatoid synovectomised knees
Mean	7.30	6.61	6.79
SD^2	0.033	0.214	0.098
T statistics		[+]diff=4.42	[+]diff=0.95
		[+]diff=4.01	

Determination of Rheumatoid Factor in the Synovial Fluid. In adults with RA the synovial fluid has been shown to contain rheumatoid factor. This persists — like many other immune complexes — after synovectomy, but in a decreased concentration (CRACCHIOLO and BARNETT, 1969). Thus synovectomy may affect the immunological reactions of the diseased joint for the better.

Radiological Appearance of the Joint. It has been a matter of concern that synovectomy might have a deleterious effect upon the cartilage and bone of the joint. Radiologically it appears, however, that surgical synovectomy does not destroy an intact joint, that no sudden increase in already existing destruction occurs following synovectomy, and that no untoward reaction that might subsequently destroy the articular cartilage is initiated by the surgical procedure.

Possible Influence of Synovectomy in One Joint on the Rheumatoid Disease in the Patient as a Whole

Two lines of thought suggest that synovectomy might improve the patient's general condition. First, the diseased joint may contain a local, self-perpetuating tissue injury mechanism of the local autoimmune reaction type, and as the joint is a part of the body that is connected to the general circulation, factors circulating in the blood might influence the synovium in other joints. Second, although the early regenerating synovium can vary in its structural appearance, its function appears to be normal or nearly so. Therefore synovectomy might be expected not only to improve the joint temporarily, but also, by reducing the amount of diseased tissue, to decrease the general activity of the disease. The present author's experience ap-

Measurement of the pH of the Synovial Fluid. An intravital method was used to measure the hydrogen ion concentration in synovial fluids of normal, rheumatoid, and synovectomised rheumatoid knee joints (GOLDIE and NACHEMSON, 1969; GOLDIE, 1974). Normal knee joints had an average pH of 7.3, rheumatoid joints a pH value of 6.6, and rheumatoid joints at varying times after synovectomy a pH of 6.8, with a statistically significant difference only between the first and the two last groups (Table 1). Thus as measured by this yardstick, synovectomy hardly produces a more normal environment in the joint.

Table 2. Reported results of synovectomy

Author	No. of knees	Im-proved	Poor	Follow-up
JONES (1923)	2	2	0	6 months to 1 year
SPEED (1924)	3	2	1	
SWETT (1926)	32	25	7	
ALLISON et al. (1929)	19	14	5	1–5 years
BOON-ITT (1930)	41	25	16	3 years
BERNSTEIN (1933)	25	22	3	
INGE (1938)	26	16	10	
GHORMLEY and CAMERON (1941)	47	26	21	
LONDON (1955)	32	22	10	
LELIK (1961)	27	23	4	
AIDEM et al. (1964)	26	24	2	4 years
TORPPI and HEIKKINEN (1965)	24	22	2	
JAKUBOWSKY (1965)	40	30	10	
GARIÉPY et al. (1966)	56	44	12	2 years
MARMOR (1966)	34	34	0	3 months to 3 years (11 months avg.)
STEVENS and WHITEFIELD (1966)	100	91	9	3 months to 2 years
CONATY et al. (1967)	38	31	7	
PLATT (1967)	42	38	4	3–29 months
FREILINGER (1967)	9	6	3	3–21 months
ARDEN (1967)	29	19	10	2.7 years
BARNES and MASON (1967)	53	40	13	17.6 months (2–48 months)
GEENS (1969)	28	22	6	23 (7–49) months
PARADIES (1969)	48	40	8	18 months
DRABLÖS (1972)	120	94 (6 not recorded)	20	2 years (6 months to 7 years)

Table 2 (continued)

Author	No. of knees	Im-proved	Poor	Follow-up
RANAWAT et al. (1972)	60	44	26	1–8 years
TILLMAN (1972)	82	72	10	6 months to 3 years
MARMOR (1973)	175	93	82	49.4 months
MOHING (1973)	140	133	7	1–7 years
LANVIN et al. (1974)	66	55	11	7.5 years
GSCHWEND (1977)	100	71	29	6.5 years

pears to substantiate these possibilities, since an improvement can often be observed in the individual's general condition following synovectomy, even if it is limited in time. This observation, however, is a matter of controversy.

Timing of Surgical Synovectomy

Since synovectomy does not appear to cause recognisable damage to the joint, and as rheumatoid granulation tissue can rapidly destroy the articular surfaces, an argument can be made out for performing synovectomy as early as possible in the disease, especially during the phase when there is evidence that the synovial tissue is of the active, hypertrophic type. Such a joint is one with palpable synovial thickening and effusion. On this basis it might therefore be suggested that synovectomy should be carried out about 6 months after the first appearance of symptoms in the knee joint, provided that conservative therapy has not proved successful in controlling the synovitis. There may also be a place for synovectomy even if a decrease in symptoms has been observed with conservative treatment, since the object of the removal of synovial tissue is to save the joint from further destruction.

Clinical Experience of Synovectomy of the Rheumatoid Knee Joint

Reported results of synovectomy are presented in Table 2. The results observed at follow-up deserve special comment. BARNES and MASON (1967) found that flexion deteriorated in 50% of the patients. This was related to the length of follow-up, but the patients did not regard the loss of flexion as important. Full extension improved in 50% and deteriorated in 15%. Pre-operative flexion contracture up to 20° was not necessarily followed by a poor result. Stability of the knee joint was unchanged by synovectomy. Continued deterioration in radiographic appearance occurred in 18 of 49 knees. The radiographic deterioration in 23 of 41 knees, however, was less than would have been anticipated had the operation not been performed. There was no correlation between the pre-operative duration of the disease and the result of the operation.

There was some evidence in Barnes' study that the patients' assessment of the result of the operation worsened with the length of follow-up. The same observation has been made by GARIÉPY et al. (1966) and PARADIES (1969).

Long-term clinical studies indicate that following synovectomy the regenerated synovium will eventually become diseased and symptoms will recur if the patient's systemic disease remains active (LONDON, 1955). GARIÉPY et al. (1966) have stated that they observed no systemic exacerbation of disease in 127 cases of synovectomy, but in 56 knees there was a 6% recurrence rate after an average follow-up of 6.5 years. The reported frequency of recurrence varies from zero (MARMOR, 1966; but in a later study in 1973 Marmor reported 82 failures in 175 synovectomies) to 54%. This wide variation may be due to the fact that the reports are based on patients with different disease activity, e.g., monarticular involvement and the classic, severe form of RA. Moreover, there is some divergence in the concept of recurrence: the presence of an effusion only and of an effusion with pain and swollen articular tissues are variously thought to constitute recurrence.

Earlier in this Chapter it was suggested that synovectomy should be carried out early in rheumatoid disease. To some extent this is substantiated by clinical experience; many failures are believed to be the result of the operation being performed at a late stage of the disease and to the duration of the disease and of joint involvement. Thus GARIÉPY et al. (1966) stated that poor results were due to patients being operated on late in the course of their disease and that little benefit could be provided by the operation if it was perfomed at later stages of arthritis, when the disease had already progressed beyond the synovial tissue. GEENS (1969), however, reached quite the opposite conclusion, which is worth quoting: "85% of the procedures in adults were performed in late stages of destruction. All adult patients had classic rheumatoid arthritis with multiple joint involvement. 79% of the knees were rated improved by the patient as compared to 65% rated improved by the examiner. In 46.5% definite or probable recurrence was found."

Present Author's Experience

During 1965–1966, synovectomy of one or both knees was performed in 44 patients. In seven patients the operation was performed on both knees, thus providing a total of 51 knees. The patients fulfilled the criteria of the American Rheumatism Association for classic or definite RA. The material is presented in Table 3.

Pain was graded according to a numerical system: 0 = none, 1 = occasional, 2 = mild, 3 = moderate, 4 = severe. The range of motion was determined in all knees with 0° as full extension and 90° flexion regarded as normal. Radiology was graded according to the scale described in the Atlas of Standard Radiographs of Arthritis, Manchester Royal Infirmary, 1960: 0 = none, 1 = doubtful, 2 = mild, 3 = moderate, 4 = severe.

Table 3. The pre-operative state of 51 knees synovectomised for rheumatoid arthritis in 1965 and 1966

	Stage			
	I	II	III	IV
Women	3	14	8	3
Men	4	4	8	0
Total knees	7	21	20	3
Mean age (years)	47.5	59	61.2	65.6
Duration of rheumatic disease (years)	5.3	11.5	14.7	8
Duration of joint affection (years)	3.1	5	5.9	4.3
Grade of pain	2.3	2.8	3.4	3.3
Extension defect (degrees)	5	10	15	20
Flexion defect (degrees)	0	5	10	31.6
Stability	yes	yes	no	no
Radiological changes	1	2	3.1	4

Table 4. Observations noted over a 12-year follow-up in patients subjected to synovectomy of the knee joint for rheumatoid arthritis

Year	Stage				Knees/ Patients
	I	II	III	IV	
1965	7	21	20	3	51/44
1965 ↓ Lost 1973	0	8 { 2 dead / 2 arthrodesis / 2 ankylosis / 2 arthroplasty	10 { 2 dead / 2 arthrodesis / 2 ankylosis / 4 arthroplasty	1 arthrodesis	19/15
1973 ↓ Lost 1977	0	4 arthroplasty	6 arthroplasty	0	10/10
Total remaining in 1977	7	9	4	2	22/19

Table 5. Pain[a] reported during a 12-year follow-up period by patients subjected to synovectomy of the knee joints for rheumatoid arthritis

Year	Stage			
	I	II	III	IV
1965 (pre-op.)	2.3	2.8	3.4	3.3
1973	0	1.5	1.2	1.5
1977	1	2	2	2

[a] 0, no pain; 1, sporadic; 2, slight; 3, moderate; 4, severe.

Table 7. Stability of knees over a 12-year follow-up period in patients subjected to synovectomy of the knee joint for rheumatoid arthritis

Year	Stage			
	I	II	III	IV
1965 (pre-op.)	+	+	−	−
1973	+	+	−	−
1977	+	+	−	−

Table 6. Flexion contracture during a 12-year follow-up period in patients subjected to synovectomy of the knee joint for rheumatoid arthritis

Year	Stage			
	I	II	III	IV
1965 (pre-op.)	5°	10°	15°	20°
1973	5°	5°	15°	15°
1977	5°	5°	15°	15°

Table 8. Patients' opinion of synovectomy of the knee joint 12 years after surgery

Could you recommend synovectomy?

Yes: 15 ($^1/_3$ of the original population)
No: 4

The patients were reviewed in 1968, 1970, 1973, and 1977. The longest interval from operation to follow-up was 12 years and the shortest, 11.5 years. Four patients had died due to intercurrent disease, thus leaving 40 patients or 47 knees for review.

Of these, however, later failures and progression of disease demanded further surgery in 25 knees (Table 4). Tables 5–8 give a summary of pain, flexion contracture, stability, and the patient's opinions.

In three knees infection developed, which was successfully treated within 1 month with antibiotics. Neither clinical thrombosis nor thrombophlebitis was diagnosed. No deaths attributable to the operation occurred. One patient had a second synovectomy within 1 year of the first procedure because of excruciating pain; it was completely relieved.

Controlled Studies

Although synovectomy has been reported to yield acceptable long-term results (for examples see GSCHWEND, 1977; present author's experience in Tables 5–8), these reports are based mainly on observations after operation without any matched controls.

In Britain and the United States such controlled studies have been carried out. In 1977 MCEWEN presented the preliminary results of a 5-year study carried out as a multicentre evaluation of synovectomy in the treatment of RA under the sponsorship of the U.S. Public Service and Arthritis Foundation. Sixteen hospital centres throughout the USA participated. A total of 70 patients entered the study, of whom nine died before completion of the period of review and four others were lost. Fifty-seven patients were followed for the full 5 years. The synovectomised and control joints were analysed clinically with regard to pain, tenderness, soft-tissue swelling, effusion, local heat, erythema, and active and passive range of motion.

During the course of the study it became evident that synovectomised joints were clinically slightly superior to control joints with respect to a number of these features at the end of 1 year, but that by the end of 3 years only soft-tissue swelling was less in the synovectomised knees than in the controls. After 5 years this difference had also disappeared. The range of active motion was slightly better in the synovectomised knees, but passive motion was better in the controls.

Radiographs were read by two observers without knowledge of the dates when films were taken. The features analysed were: soft-tissue swelling, osteoporosis, evidence of cartilage thinning, marginal and subchondral bone erosions, cyst formation, and deformity. In none of these features was there a statistically significant difference between the synovectomised and control knee joints after 3 and 5 years.

The only striking difference observed over the 5 years was that recurrent rheumatoid inflammation occurred less frequently in the synovectomised knees than in the controls.

In summary therefore, this controlled study of synovectomy showed that the operation produced no benefit over a 5-year period. There was, however, some short-term gain.

Indications and Contra-indications

Surgical synovectomy can be recommended as an acceptable procedure in the rheumatoid knee joint only if conservative treatment has failed and a good result in the short term is desired. The disadvantages of surgery, such as infection and the formation of adhesions, should be balanced against the possible disadvantages of prolonged conservative therapy, which may not arrest the disease in the single joint that is responsible for the patient's disability.

The following indications and contra-indications may be suggested. The indications (assuming adequate conservative treatment to have been tried and to have failed) are

1) Active disease in the joint
2) Disease duration of less than 3 years
3) Slight or mild radiological change
4) Significant pain in the joint prior to operation
5) Effusion
6) Palpable synovial thickening
7) Persistent involvement of short duration in one knee when there is advanced joint destruction of the opposite side.

Synovectomy is contra-indicated in the following circumstances:

1) Disease duration of more than 3 years
2) Severe pre-operative radiological changes
3) Absence of pain
4) Severe instability and loss of articular cartilage
5) Absence of effusion and synovitis.

Operative Technique

The approach to the joint is via a medial parapatellar incision. Figures 6b and 10 show the surgical approach.

As much synovium as possible should be removed. According to TILLMAN (1977), synovectomy should be performed through a medial and a posterior incision, as the amount of tissue removed is much larger and in his experience the results are better. MARMOR (1973) leaves the suprapatellar pouch intact to facilitate knee mobility

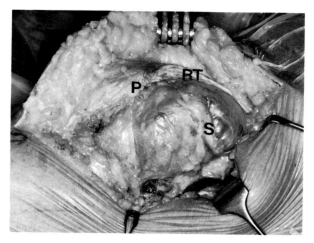

Fig. 10. Approach via medial parapatellar incision to right knee joint. S, bulging synovial tissue; P, patella; RT, rectus tendon. For further approach compare Fig. 6b

and to counteract the formation of adhesions that would impair function.

Degenerated menisci should be removed. The cruciate ligaments remain surprisingly uninvolved but they are often covered by granulation tissue, which should be removed.

Post-operatively, the knee is immediately mobilised.

Osteoarthrosis

In 1899 MIGNON presented his result of synovectomy in one patient with chronic traumatic OA of the knee. There was apparently complete restoration of function in 6 months, but the long-term result was not reported.

During the early 1900s the surgical treatment of OA of the knee was dominated by synovectomy (JONES, 1923; INGE, 1938; STEINDLER, 1955). The studies presented were small, however, and the follow-up periods short. In the later literature it was recommended that synovectomy be combined with more extensive surgery, such as the removal of menisci and excision of osteophytes and destroyed cartilage (see "Débridement", below).

In 1965, MEAD stated that synovectomy is "the most effective way of dealing with the persistent chronically inflamed grossly thickened synovial lining when the anatomy of the joint is otherwise compatible with function." In Japan, HIROHATA (1973) reported on an 85% improvement following synovectomy in OA of the knee joint with a follow-up time of no less than 13 years.

Present Author's Experience

In the spring of 1972 synovectomy was carried out as the only procedure in ten knee joints affected by OA. A follow-up was carried out in the spring of 1973, and in no instance was there any improvement. All the patients have subsequently been re-operated upon, eight undergoing arthroplasty and two, arthrodesis.

Comment

With the advent of more sophisticated methods, i.e., arthroplasty, for the surgical management of OA of the knee joint, it now appears that synovectomy no longer has any place.

Removal of Baker's Cyst

In 1877, BAKER reported on the formation of synovial cysts in the leg in connection with diseases of the knee joint. He described eight patients in whom the cysts appeared to be tuberculous in origin. In one case there was a question of RA. The cysts generally have a direct connection with the joint, and according to TAYLOR and RANA (1972), popliteal cysts appear in 40% of patients with RA affecting the knee joint. The cysts can vary in size and the occasional cyst can extend through the calf to the tendo Achilles.

The cysts form a bulging mass in the popliteal region and are obvious on inspection. The cyst may rupture due to increased pressure in the knee joint, decreased resistance of the capsule, or a sudden increase of the load on the knee joint.

Rheumatoid Arthritis

The cyst should be removed in its entirety. There is a risk of recurrence but this is diminished if synovectomy is carried out through an anterior incision at the same time as the cyst is removed. The best approach is a curved incision commencing at the lower medial aspect of the popliteal fossa and carried transversely to the lateral margin. The incision will then follow Langer's lines.

Present Author's Experience

In the material previously presented on synovectomy in this Chapter, a popliteal cyst was encountered in ten cases. They were all removed at the time of synovectomy and there has been no recurrence.

Osteoarthrosis

A popliteal cyst is a rare occurrence and should be treated by removal if this is symptomatically warranted. Aspiration can be considered as an alternative, but this only yields temporary relief since the cyst rapidly re-fills. (It should be pointed out that a pre-operative arthrogram is of value as it has happened in the author's experience that the "cyst" has proved to be a soft-tissue tumor.)

Comment

In RA a Baker's cyst should be removed if it is the patients' chief complaint. A simultaneous synovectomy is recommended as the chance of recurrence then decreases considerably.

In OA removal of a popliteal cyst is a matter of choice and is indicated only if sufficient symptoms are present. It should be borne in mind that a popliteal cyst can mimic a soft-tissue tumor.

Soft-Tissue Release Procedures

Rheumatoid Arthritis

In a knee with a flexion contracture, the pull of the hamstrings causes posterior subluxation and external rotation of the tibia. Lack of extension causes a loss of stability of the knee. The limitation of movement will cause a constant loading within a small, restricted area of the joint surface. According to PERRY (1967), the load on the knee with a fixed flexion deformity of 20° is 1.2 times the body weight and at 40°, 2.6 times the body weight. The aim of soft-tissue release procedures is to prevent fixed deformities such as these.

In 1921, PUTTI described posterior capsulotomy and division of the gastrocnemius by which correction of more than 15° of fixed flexion could be obtained. PRESTON (1968) combined extra-articular procedures such as posterior capsulotomy and tendon resections with intra-articular procedures such as the excision of menisci, division of the posterior cruciate ligament, and patelloplasty. Good results were obtained in 82% of 13 operated knees 6–24 months after operation. RUSZCYNSKA and JAKUBOWSKY (1970) and JAKUBOWSKY and DUBINSKA (1974) have reported good results in 60% and satisfactory results in 33% of knees with a lateral release procedure that also involved the severance of the lateral collateral ligament.

Present Author's Experience

Twenty-six patients, 19 women and 7 men, representing 39 knees, have been operated upon. All patients had classic RA according to the ARA classification. Their ages varied from 20 to 80 years. The pre-operative flexion contractures are listed in Table 9: the majority had fixed flexion deformities between 20° and 30°, and correction of these was the main indication for a release procedure. In all knees further flexion from the position of deformity was not less than 50°, i.e., all knees could flex to or beyond 90°.

The duration of disease varied from a maximum of 23 years to a minimum of 4 years, with a mean of 12 years, and as a rule the joint operated on had become involved at the time of onset of disease.

In all patients a valgus deformity varying between 10° and 20° was present, and prior to surgery all patients had been subjected to physiotherapy in varying forms.

Table 9. Pre-operative fixed flexion deformity assessed radiologically in 39 rheumatoid knees treated by soft-tissue release

Pre-operative extension deficit (degrees)	No. of knees		
	Men	Women	Total
15–20	1	4	5
21–25	2	8	10
26–30	5	12	17
31–35	2	3	5
36–40		2	2
	10	29	39

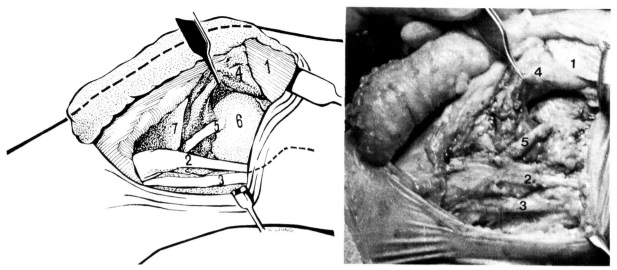

Fig. 11. *Left*, lateral release procedure (schematic) in left knee-joint in RA. 1, ilio-tibial band; 2, biceps tendon; 3, peroneal nerve; 4, synovial membrane; 5, lateral collateral ligament; 6, lateral femoral condyle; 7, lateral tibial condyle. *Right*, operative field of structures to be considered at lateral release

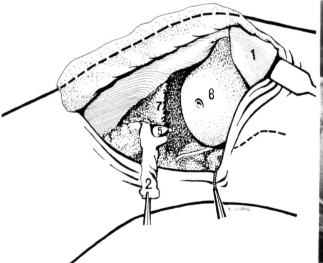

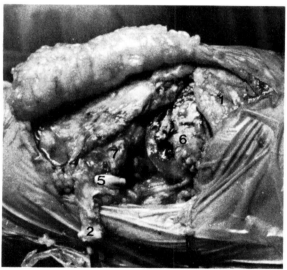

Fig. 12. *Left*, schematic description of completed lateral release in left knee joint. Relevant structures have been severed. Figures denote same structures as in Fig. 11.

Right, operative field at completion of lateral release procedure

Ten patients (14 knees) had previously undergone synovectomy. The indications for surgery in these patients were:

1) Certified diagnosis of RA (by the ARA criteria)
2) Fixed flexion in excess of 15°
3) Flexion of at least 50°
4) Failure of conservative measures
5) No radiological signs of deep excavation in the tibial plateaus

6) A co-operative attitude in the patient, to make post-operative physiotherapy practicable.

Operative Technique

The iliotibial band is completely transected (Fig. 11). The biceps tendon is incised with a Z-shaped incision. The lateral collateral ligament is divided. The joint capsule is opened and a lateral synovectomy is carried out, including excision of the suprapatellar bursa (Fig. 12). The lateral head of the gastrocnemius and the popliteus tendon are divided. The posterior capsule is incised. Extension of the knee is now tested. If it is not satisfactory, the posterior capsulotomy is extended medially and the medial head of the gastrocnemius is released from its attachment to the femur. The biceps tendon is sutured without tension and only the skin is closed (thus leaving all other severed structures unsutured).

Post-operative Course

A plaster cast is applied from groin to ankle for 10 days. The wound is then inspected and further knee extension is carried out if necessary. A new plaster is applied for 4 weeks. Active physiotherapy is carried out with intensive quadriceps and walking exercises, with full weight-bearing on the operated leg. After removal of the plaster, active knee extension is practised.

Results

Reviews were carried out 6 months, $1^1/_2$ years, and 5 years after surgery and the results are presented in Table 10. The most striking observation was that between 8 and 12 weeks after the operation there was almost complete stability of the knee joint, despite the cutting of all the structures mentioned above. At 6 months all patients had to use walking aids. Most of the patients could walk 100 m without rest, and climbing stairs had

become possible for 12 patients. At $1^1/_2$ years further improvement was noticed, and the walking distance had now been increased to 200 m without rest. There was slight pain on weight-bearing, but this did not decrease the patients' general activity. Finally, there was no instability in any knee joints. Stabilising braces were used by nine patients, however. At this time no knee exhibited any valgus deformity.

At 5 years there was no change in the observations as compared with the $1^1/_2$-year follow-up.

The results with regard to flexion deformity and the range of movement are set out in Tables 10 and 11. It will be seen that full extension was

Table 11. Range of motion (ROM) before and 5 years after soft-tissue release (ALR) in 30 rheumatoid knees with different degrees of pre-operative fixed flexion deformity

Pre-operative extension deficit (degrees)	n	ROM			
		Pre-operative		ALR	
		60–80	81–100	81–100	101–110
15–20	5	3	2	2	3
21–25	7	5	2	3	4
26–30	12	7	5	10	2
31–35	4	4		4	
36–40	2	2		2	

Table 10. Post-operative assessment of soft-tissue release for fixed flexion in the rheumatoid knee joint

Pre-operative extension deficit (degrees)	Post-operative extension deficit (degrees)														
	6 months					$1^1/_2$ years					5 years				
	0↓10	11↓20	21↓25	26↓30	31↓35	0↓10	11↓20	21↓25	26↓30	31↓35	0↓10	11↓20	21↓25	26↓30	31↓35
15–20	5					5					5				
21–25	7	3				10					7				
26–30	10	7				13	1				10	2			
31–35	2	3				4	1				3	1			
36–40			2			1	1						2		
Total	24	13	2 = 39			33	3 = 36				25	3	2 = 30		
Comments						3 patients deceased (3 treated knees)					6 patients deceased (9 treated knees)				

well maintained and that movement was preserved.

Of 30 patients, 25 were so satisfied with the results that they felt they could strongly recommend the procedure to other patients. The remaining five, who had very slight residual fixed flexion and no deformity, were unhappy for reasons that were difficult for the investigator to analyse in detail, as they were part of a more general complaint.

Complications. There were four cases of early complications with sloughing of the wound, but eventual healing occurred. No further early or late complications were observed.

Osteoarthrosis

There seems to be no place for an isolated soft-tissue release procedure in OA.

Comment

In view of the introduction of total arthroplasty of the knee, isolated soft-tissue release may become out-dated. On the other hand, it might still be an acceptable introductory procedure to minimise skeletal resection at the time of arthroplasty. In the author's investigation quoted above, lateral release was not carried out with future replacement surgery in mind. Up to 1975 none of the knees had been subjected to replacement procedures, but during the last 2 years five of the patients have been subjected to total arthroplasty. Soft-tissue release procedures now of course form an integral part of some replacement procedures (see, for example, Chap. 13).

Resection of the Anterior Cruciate Ligament

In 1960 SOMERVILLE reported good results after division of the anterior cruciate ligament in eight patients with flexion contracture due to RA. Judging from the literature the method has not gained wide acceptance, and the author has no experience of this procedure.

Nerve Resection

In 1947, KESTLER reported that nerve resection can be of some value in treating intractable pain of the knee in the aged and also in RA. The operation consisted of dissection and then resection of the sensory nerves supplying the posterior capsule of the knee. A curvilinear skin incision was used to expose the posterior tibial, common peroneal, and recurrent anterior tibial nerves. The branches reaching the capsule were excised. Eight or ten days later, with the patient in the supine position, the branches of the obturator nerve and the femoral nerve that supply the anterior knee capsule were excised. KESTLER stated that the results were encouraging but that the follow-up was too short to allow a final conclusion.

Comment

The author has no experience of this procedure and so far as he is aware the operation is no longer carried out.

Meniscectomy

Rheumatoid Arthritis

When at synovectomy the menisci appear to have degenerated, they should be removed. In those instances where no degeneration is present it is worthwhile inspecting the space inferior to the menisci, as quite often granulation tissue grows between the tibial plateau and the rim of the meniscus. This granulation tissue should be removed. If the menisci are not degenerate, they should be left in place, since the menisci carry much of the body weight — for example, the medial meniscus takes some 50% of the load that falls on the medial tibio-femoral articulation and the lateral meniscus takes some 70% of the load in the lateral tibio-femoral articulation. (In this context, it should be remembered, however, that the medial tibial condyle takes about 10 times more load than the lateral [KETTELCAMP et al., 1970; WALKER and ERCHMAN, 1975].)

Osteoarthrosis

According to SMILLIE (1974), "The return of function coupled with the relief of symptoms is exceptionally rapid following the excision of a meniscus, the site of a horizontal cleavage lesion, from the medial compartment, even when osteoarthrotic change is in an advanced state. This statement has occasioned surprise bordering on disbelief. It is factual and was acquired in the hard school of experience." The excision of a meniscus in OA removes an obstruction to motion, particularly in final extension when the joint is "screwed home". Without giving any figures, SMILLIE makes the statement that the resulting benefit is dramatic in effect.

Comment

The author has limited experience of this procedure, but it does occasionally happen that in patients with osteoarthrosic change in the knee joint, the clinical picture is suggestive of a torn meniscus. At operation the meniscus — usually medial — is thin and degenerate and small ruptures can be seen within it. The large horizontal cleavage mentioned by SMILLIE has never been observed by the author. The improvement, if not dramatic, is sometimes considerable, but in contrast to what is experienced after meniscectomy in young people, the post-operative period is long and demands intensive physiotherapy, with special attention to the quadriceps mechanism. Similar observations have been made by APPEL (1970). Meniscectomy therefore cannot readily be recommended as a single procedure for operative treatment of the osteoarthrosic knee, but rather as part of a procedure whose aim is to "refashion" the articular surfaces as described below (see "Débridement"). On the other hand, it should be remembered that locking phenomena in the osteoarthrosic knee can be due to a ruptured meniscus, which should then be removed.

Débridement (the Spring-clean Procedure)

Early in the last century, Napoleon's surgeon, Baron LARREY, conceived the idea that pain and

spasm in infected war wounds were caused by the bands that bridged their interior. LARREY introduced the term débridement into the surgical literature to signify the act of releasing tight bands deep in wounds, not removing the debris. Used in its correct sense, débridement had a place in the treatment of chronic arthritis: where intra-articular adhesions were tough and unyielding a scalpel could be slipped into the joint and swept up and down, severing all the tight bands that offered resistance (KELIKIAN, 1949). With time, however, the term débridement came to refer not only to the cutting of adhesions but also to synovectomy, the excision of osteophytes, the removal of destroyed cartilage, and often the drilling of denuded bone.

Rheumatoid Arthritis

As débridement involves synovectomy and the excision of osteophytes and degenerate cartilage, it can be regarded as part of the synovectomy procedure for RA. Débridement should therefore almost always be carried out in the rheumatoid knee joint when synovectomy is done.

Osteoarthrosis

In the treatment of OA of the knee joint débridement was popularised by MAGNUSSON, who reported on more than 100 débridements in 1946. To quote MAGNUSSON "...many of these patients have left the hospital walking without a limp in less than 3 weeks. If cases for this operation are properly selected and operative technique and after-treatment are carefully adhered to, the results of débridement for traumatic or hypertrophic arthritis of the knee and hip are among the most satisfactory in any form of joint surgery." MAGNUSSON presents the symptoms, tests for joint function, operative description, and post-operative care. However the follow-up of the 100 patients is more a personal account than a systematic analysis.

The work of MAGNUSSON has had a number of followers, of whom HAGGART of the United States and PRIDIE of Bristol, England were the foremost. The work of PRIDIE was summarised and presented by INSALL in 1967, who described 62 operations in 60 knees with a follow-up of 6.5 years. Forty-six patients thought the operation was a success and 14 were dissatisfied. The reviewer found the result to be good in 40 knees (no limp, full extension, no extension lag, flexion to 90°, no pain on movement), fair in 11 knees (9 limps, 1 flexion to 15°, 1 instability), and poor in 11 knees (5 arthrodeses, 2 limps, 2 stiff, 2 extension lags). Pain was markedly relieved in 40 patients, unchanged in 16, and worse in 4. Prior to operation 36 knees were unstable and 33 of these became stable post-operatively. There was a general improvement in the range of motion, and pain on movement was considerably decreased. There was a definite impression that surgery tended to improve the radiological appearance.

Other series (HAGGART, 1947; ISSERLIN, 1950) show results of the same kind.

Operative Technique

The aim of the operation is to remove synovial tissue, osteophytes, softened fibrillated cartilage, torn or degenerated menisci, and loose bodies and to drill holes into denuded bone (COONSE and ADAMS, 1943; MAGNUSSON, 1946; HAGGART, 1947).

Present Author's Experience

In 1970, débridement as described by MAGNUSSON (1946) was carried out in 15 patients (15 knees). There were nine women and six men. The average age was 56 years, with ten patients over 60 years and five under 50.

A review was carried out in 1975 and the patients' assessment was success in ten and dissatisfaction in five. On objective examination the results were good in six (no pain, no limp, full extension, full stability); fair in three (occasional weight-bearing pain, occasional limp, full extension, acceptable stability); and poor in six (pain, limp, extension lag, and slight instability). The six patients in whom the results were classified as poor have since been subjected to arthroplasty, with initially good results. Of the three patients with results classified as fair, two used a cane when walking outdoors.

Comment

Once OA of the knee has reached a stage that necessitates an operation and in which a spring-clean procedure becomes an alternative this may be carried out, particularly in view of the good results over a $6^1/_2$-year period reported by INSALL (1967). However, in the wake of successes with total hip replacement the osteoarthrosic knee is now replaceable. Though with a shorter observation time than the $6^1/_2$ years cited above for spring-clean procedures, the current results with total knee replacement are so promising that knees with such advanced changes as to justify any operation should seriously be considered for replacement surgery. There are studies — though perhaps not large enough — with up to 4 years' follow-up yielding 85%–90% good results following replacement (e.g., GSCHWEND, 1977). Another fact in favour of replacement surgery in the severely damaged knee is the possibility this operation offers of decreasing the instability of the knee and correcting pre-operative deformities in varus or valgus. The latter is difficult if not impossible with débridement procedures.

Patellectomy

In 1937 BROOKE stated that: "The patella has been adapted to play a part in the movements of the knee joint, but it was not designed for this purpose; and although theoretically its presence should enhance the power of the quadriceps muscle, in practice there is considerable doubt as to its mechanical value in assisting movements at that joint. Rather is there evidence that it has become imperfectly adapted to the mechanism of the joint and thus has a deterrent action on a machine for which it was never designed."

In contrast to this opinion, BRUCE and WALMSLEY (1942) presented evidence that the patella is an integral part of the quadriceps tendon and that the bone exercises a protective role as regards the patellar surface of the femur. In animal experiments, BRUCE and WALMSLEY (1942) demonstrated that removal of the patella was followed by severe degenerative changes in the articular cartilage of the patellar surface of the femur. On the other hand there was no apparent change in gait or in joint efficiency. Clinical observations also led BRUCE to the conclusion that removal of the patella caused localised OA of the patello-femoral compartment of the knee joint. BRUCE therefore agreed with the general view that the patella forms a pulley that maintains the tendon of the quadriceps in front of the axis of movement of the joint and so increases its effectiveness.

Later studies, particularly those considering patellectomy in relation to fractures of the patella, have shown that following removal of the patella the quadriceps mechanism is weakened, quite often to the point of there being an extension lag.

The pressure between the patella and the femur has attracted some investigative interest. MAQUET (1969) found that if the body weight is applied to a flexed knee the pressure between the patella and the femur amounts to 256 kgf (for a body weight of 60 kg) at 36° of flexion and to 420 kgf at 47°. If the tibial insertion of the patellar ligament is moved anteriorly there is a considerable reduction in the pressure between the patella and the femur, and for this reason MAQUET recommended a ventralisation of the tibial tubercle as a method of treatment of OA of the patello-femoral joint (see Chap. 9)

FÜRMAIER (1953) pointed out that the absence of the patella increases the pressure between the femur and the tibial plateau.

Rheumatoid Arthritis

Patellectomy should never be carried out as a single procedure. A partial patellectomy may, however, be justified as part of synovectomy, débridement, or arthroplasty.

Osteoarthrosis

Removal of the patella in chronic arthritis was first suggested by LUDLOFF in 1926 (cited in BRUCE and WALMSLEY, 1942). WATSON-JONES (1939) also recommended patellectomy as the treatment of choice for OA confined to the patello-femoral compartment of the knee joint.

After the work of BROOKE (1937), patellectomy became a popular method in the treatment of OA in the patello-femoral joint. In 1939 BERKHEISER, who has been widely cited in the literature on patellectomy for OA, reported good results in eight of eleven patients after patellectomy. He claimed that the range of motion of the knee joint was increased and that the quadriceps muscle became much stronger. His indications were:

Osteoarthrosis of a number of years' standing

Persistence of symptoms in spite of conservative treatment

Fixed flexion of not more than 20°

"Quiescence" of arthritis at the time of surgery.

With an average follow-up of 9 years in 27 patients after patellectomy, GECKELER and QUARANTA (1962) reported excellent results in 14 knees (52%), good in 6 (22%), fair in 4 (15%) and failure in 3 (11%). The failures were found in patients who were thought to have been wrongly selected for the procedure. In the remaining patients there was no progress of the degenerative change in the knee.

During 1950–1954 HALIBURTON and SULLIVAN (1958) carried out 154 patellectomies in 136 patients. The cause of the OA was trauma in 45 patients, recurrent dislocation of the patella in 20, and obesity in 10. In the remaining 51 patients a variety of conditions preceded OA, such as genu valgum, genu varum, osteochondromatosis, and osteochondritis. There was an overall improvement in 87%, absence of pain in 61%, full extension in 96%, and 90° flexion in 92%. The conclusion of these authors was that patellectomy for degenerative joint disease gave subjective improvement in a high proportion of patients, particularly in those with advanced disease.

Operative Technique

The usual technique for patellectomy is that suggested by BOYD and HAWKINS (1948) (Fig. 13).

Comment

In spite of the favourable results described above, opinion has now swung away from patellectomy in OA. It is the author's opinion that patellectomy in OA leads to little if any reliable short-term improvement and that it prejudices later toal knee replacement.

Summary

In the author's opinion, synovectomy combined with a débridement procedure may have a part to play in the treatment of appropriately selected early cases of RA. Meniscectomy is occasionally indicated in OA. None of the other procedures discussed in this Chapter is any longer indicated for either disease.

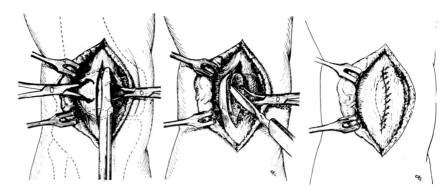

Fig. 13. Patellectomy as described by H.B. Boyd and B.L. Hawkins: Surg. Gynecol. Obstet. **86**, 357 (1948). The patella is sawn into two halves (*left*) and enucleated (*middle*), and finally the capsule is imbricated (*right*)

References

Aidem, H.P., Baker, L.D.: Synovectomy of the knee joint in rheumatoid arthritis. JAMA **187**, 4–6 (1964)

Allison, N., Coonse, G.K.: Synovectomy in chronic arthritis. Arch. Surg. **18**, 824 (1929)

Appel, H.: Late results after meniscectomy in the knee joint. Acta Orthop. Scand. Suppl. 133 (1970)

Arden, G.P.: The results of synovectomy in rheumatoid arthritis. Synovectomy and arthroplasty in rheumatoid arthritis. Stuttgart: Thieme 1967

Baker, N.M.: The formation of synovial cysts in the leg in connection with diseases of the knee joint. St. Bartholomew's Hospital Report **21**, 177 (1877)

Barnes, C.G., Mason, R.M.: Synovectomy of the knee joint in rheumatoid arthritis. Ann. Phys. Med. **9**, 83–102 (1967)

Berkheiser, E.J.: Excision of the patella in arthritis of the knee. J. Am. Med. Assoc. **113**, 2303 (1939)

Bernstein, M.A.: Synovectomy of the knee joint in chronic arthritis. Ann. Surg. **98**, 1096 (1933)

Boon-Itt: A study of the end results of synovectomy of the knee. J. Bone Joint Surg. (Am.) **12**, 853 (1930)

Boyd, H.B., Hawkins, B.L.: Patellectomy. A simplified technique. Surg. Gynecol. Obstet. **86**, 357 (1948)

Branemark, P.I., Lindström, J., Hansson, B.: Intra-articular temperature in man. Under normal and pathological conditions. Fifth european congress of rheumatoid diseases 1963

Brooke, R.: The treatment of fractured patella by excision. A study of morphology and function. Br. J. Surg. **24**, 733 (1937)

Bruce, J., Walmsley, R.: Excision of the patella. Some experimental and anatomical observations. J. Bone Joint Surg. (Br.) **23**, 311 (1942)

Chapchal, G.: Synovectomy and arthroplasty in rheumatoid arthritis. Suttgart: Thieme 1967

Conaty, J.B., Garrett, A.L., McWister, W.: Synovectomy and salvage procedures in rheumatoid arthritis. J. Bone Joint Surg. (Am.) **49**, 193 (1967)

Coonse, K., Adams, J.D.: A new operative approach to the knee joint. Surg. Gynecol. Obstet. **77**, 344 (1943)

Cooper, N.S.: Pathology of rheumatoid arthritis. Med. Clin. North Am. **52**, 607 (1968)

Cracchiolo, A., Barnett, E.W.: Immunologic changes in synovial fluid following synovectomy. J. Bone Joint Surg. (Am.) **51**, 475–486 (1969)

Cruickshank, B.: Interpretation of multiple biopsies of synovial tissues in rheumatic dieseases. Ann. Rheum. Dis. **11**, 137 (1952)

Drablös, P.A.: Synovectomy of the knee in rheumatoid arthritis and air-laid conditions. Scand. J. Rheumatol. **1**, 49 (1972)

Fassbender, H.G.: Pathology of rheumatic diseases. Berlin-Heidelberg: Springer 1975

Freilinger, G.: Is synovectomy in the late stage of rheumatoid arthritis still of some use? Synovectomy and arthoplasty in rheumatoid arthritis, p. 36. Stuttgart: Thieme 1967

Fürmaier, A.: Beitrag zur Mechanik der Patella und des Gesamtkniegelenkes. Arch. Orthop. Unfallchir. **46**, 78 (1953)

Gardner, D.L.: The pathology of rheumatoid arthritis. London: Arnold 1972

Gariepy, R., Demers, R., Laurin, C.A.: The prophylactic effect of synovectomy of the knee in rheumatoid arthritis. Can. Med. Assoc. J. **94**, 1349 (1966)

Geens, S.: Synovectomy and debridement of the knee in rheumatoid arthritis. J. Bone Joint Surg. (Am.) **51**, 617 (1969)

Geckeler, E., Quaranta, A.: Patellectomy for degenerative arthritis of the knee. Late results. J. Bone Joint Surg. (Am.) **44**, 1109 (1962)

Ghormley, R.K., Cameron, D.M.: End results of synovectomy of the knee joint. Am. J. Surg. **53**, 455 (1941)

Goldie, I.: Synovectomy in rheumatoid arthritis. A general review and an eight-year follow-up of synovectomy in 51 rheumatoid knee joints. Semin. Arthritis Rheum. **3**, 219 (1974)

Goldie, I., Nachemson, A.: Synovial pH in rheumatoid knee joints. Acta Orthop. Scand. **40**, 634–641 (1969)

GOLDTHWAIT, I.E.: Knee joint surgery for non-tubercular conditions. Boston Med. Surg. J. **143**, 286 (1900)

GSCHWEND, N.: Die operative Behandlung der chronischen Polyarthritis. Stuttgart: Thieme 1977

HAGGART, G.E.: Surgical treatment of degenerative arthritis of the knee joint. N. Engl. J. Med. **236**, 971 (1947)

HALIBURTON, R., SULLIVAN, C.: The patella in degenerative joint disease. A clinico-pathologic study. Arch. Surg. **7**, 677 (1958)

HIROHATA, H.: Synovectomy in arthritis of the knee joint. International congress of rheumatology, Kyoto Japan 1973

INGE, G.A.L.: Eighty-six cases of chronic synovitis of knee joint treated by synovectomy. J. Am. Med. Assoc. **111**, 2451 (1938)

INSALL, J.N.: Intra-articular surgery for degenerative arthritis of the knee. A report of the work of the late K.H. Pridie. J. Bone Joint Surg. (Br.) **49**, 211 (1967)

ISSERLIN, B.: Joint debridement for osteoarthritis of the knee. J. Bone Joint Surg. (Br.) **32** 302 (1950)

JABUKOWSKY, S.: Frühzeitige Synovektomie der Kniegelenke bei primär chronischer Polyarthritis. Beitr. Orthop. Traumatol. **12**, 680–682 (1965)

JAKUBOWSKI, S., DUBINSKA, A.: The treatment of flexion contracture in knee joint with posterior capsulotomy in RA patients. Acta Orthop. Scand. **45**, 235 (1974)

JONES, E.: Synovectomy of the knee joint in chronic arthritis. J. Am. Med. Assoc. **81**, 1586 (1923)

KELIKIAN, H.: Surgery in the treatment of chronic arthritis. Surg. Clin. North Am. **29**, 87 (1949)

KESTLER, O.C.: Surgical treatment of the aged arthritic. Geriatrics **2**, 283 (1947)

KETTELKAMP, D.B., CHAO, E.I.: A method for quantitative analyses of medial and lateral compression forces at the knee during standing. Clin. Orthop. **83**, 202 (1972)

KETTELKAMP, D.B., JOHNSON, R.J., SMIDT, G.L., CHAO, E.Y.S., WALKER, M.: An electrogoniometric study of knee motion in normal gait. J. Bone Joint Surg. (Am.) **52**, 775–790 (1970)

KEY, J.A.: The reformation of synovial membrane in the knee of rabbits after synovectomy. J. Bone Joint Surg. (Am.) **7**, 793 (1925)

KULKA, P.: Vascular derangement in rheumatoid arthritis. Modern trends in rheumatology. HILL, A.D. (ed.). London: Butterworth 1966.

LANVIN, C.A., DESMARCHAIS, J., DAZIANO, L., GARIEPY, R., DEROME, A.: Long-term results of synovectomy of the knee in rheumatoid patients. J. Bone Joint Surg. (Am.) **56**, 521 (1974)

LELIK, F.: Unsere Erfahrungen über die operative Heilbehandlung der Synovitiden verschiedenen Ursprungs. Z. Orthop. **95**, 182 (1961)

LONDON, P.: Synovectomy of the knee in rheumatoid arthritis. An essay and surgical treatment. J. Bone Joint Surg. (Br.) **37**, 392 (1955)

LUDLOFF, M.: Die Verkleinerung der Patella als funktionsverbessernde Maßnahme bei bestimmten Knieaffektionen. Zentralbl. Chir. **52**, 786 (1925)

McEWEN, C.: A multicentre evaluation of synovectomy in the treatment of rheumatoid arthritis. Results after five years. XIV international congress on rheumatology, San Francisco 1977

MAGNUSSON, P.B.: Technique of debridement of the knee joint for arthritis. Surg. Clin. North Am. **26**, 249 (1946)

MAQUET, B.: Biomécanique du genou et gonarthrose. Rev. Med. Liege **24**, 170 (1969)

MARMOR, L.: Synovectomy of the rheumatoid knee. Clin. Orthop. **44**, 151–162 (1966)

MARMOR, L.: Surgery of rheumatoid arthritis. Philadelphia: Lea and Febiger 1967

MARMOR, L.: Surgery of the rheumatoid knee. Synovectomy and débridement. J. Bone Joint Surg. (Am.) **55**, 535 (1973)

MEAD, N.C.: Surgery in arthritis of the lower extremity. Surg. Clin. North Am. **45**, 201 (1965)

MIGNON, A.: Synovectomie du genou. Bull. Mem. Soc. Chir. Paris **26**, 1113 (1900)

MITCHELL, N.S., SHEPHERD, N.: The effect of synovectomy on synovium and cartilage in early rheumatoid synovitis. Clin. Orthop. **89**, 178 (1972)

MOHING, W.: Die Synovektomie des Kniegelenks. Orthopäde **2**, 75 (1973)

MÜLLER, W.: Zur Frage der operativen Behandlung der artritis deformans und des chronischen Gelenkrheumatismus. Arch. Klin. Chir. **47**, 1 (1894)

MURPHY, J.B.: Hypertrophic villous synovitis of the knee joint. Surg. Clin. Chicago, **5**, 155 (1916)

PARADIES, L.H.: Synovectomy of the knee. Early synovectomy in rheumatoid arthritis. New York: Excerpta medica 1969

PERRY, J.: Structural insufficiency. Pathomechanics. Principals of lower extremity bracing. Am. Phys. Ther. Assoc. **81**, 172–176 (1967)

PLATT, G.: Synovectomy in rheumatoid arthritis. In: Synovectomy and arthroplasty in rheumatoid arthritis, p. 31. Stuttgart: Thieme 1967

PRESTON, R.L.: The surgical management of rheumatoid arthritis, p. 69. Philadelphia: Saunders 1968

PUTTI, V.: Popliteal capsulotomy in the treatment of flexor retractions of the knee. Chir. Organi Mov. **5**, 11 (1921)

RANAVAT, C.S., ECKER, M.L., STRAUB, L.R.: Synovectomy and debridements of the knee in rheumatoid arthritis (a study of 60 knees). Arthritis Rheum. **15**, 571 (1972)

RUSZCZYNSKA, J., JAKUBOWSKI, S.: Prophylactic significance of lateral tenotomy of the knee in juvenile rheumatoid arthritis. Rheumatologia **8**, 129 (1970)

SCHÜLLER, M.: Chirurgische Mitteilungen über die chronisch-rheumatischen Gelenkentzündungen. Arch. klin. Chir. **45**, 153 (1893)

SMILLIE, I.S.: Diseases of the knee joint. Edinburgh, London: Churchill Livingstone 1974

SOMERVILLE, E.W.: Flexion contractures of the knee. J. Bone Joint Surg. (Br.) **42**, 730 (1960)

SOKOLOFF, L.: Pathology of rheumatoid arthritis. Arthritis

and air-laid diseases, p. 187. Philadelphia: Lea & Febiger 1966

SPEED, J.S.: Synovectomy of the knee joint. J. Am. Med. Assoc. **83**, 1814 (1924)

STEINDLER, A.: Synovectomy and fat pad removal in knee joint. J. Bone Joint Surg. (Br.) **37**, 392 (1955)

STEVENS, J., WHITEFIELD, G.A.: Synovectomy of the knee in rheumatoid arthritis. Ann. Rheum. Dis. **25**, 214 (1966)

SWETT, P.P.: Synovectomy in chronic infectious arthritis. Ann. Joint Surg. **40**, 49 (1926)

Symposium: Early synovectomy in rheumatoid arthritis. Amsterdam, New York: Excerpta medica 1969

TAYLOR, A.R., RANA, N.A.: Popliteal and calf cyst. J. Bone Joint Surg. (Br.) **54**, 172 (1972)

TAYLOR, A.R., HARDISON, J.S., PEPPLER, C.: Synovectomy of the knee in rheumatoid arthritis. Ann. Rheum. Dis. **31**, 159 (1972)

TILLMAN, K.: Die Indikationsstellung zur Synovektomie der Kniegelenke bei chronischer Polyarthritis. Z. Rheumaforsch. [Suppl.] **31** (2), 278 (1972)

TILLMAN, K.: Vergleich von Langzeitergebnissen nach partieller und subtotaler Synovektomie der Kniegelenke bei chronischer Polyartritis. (In press) (1977)

TORPPI, P., HEIKKINEN, E.: Partial synovectomy as a therapeutic method for rheumatoid and non-specific synovitis of the knee. Ann. Chir. Gynaecol. Fenniae **54**, 29 (1965)

TUBY, A.H.: Arthritis deformans with a notice of its surgical treatment. Lancet **II**, 1528 (1870)

VOLKMANN, N.: Zur Synovectomie des tuberkulosen Kniegelenkes. Dtsch. Z. Chir. **6**, 39 (1877)

WALKER, P., BAIN, A.: Total knee replacement, Mechanical engineering publications limited for the institution of mechanical engineers 1974

WALKER, P.F., ERCHMAN, M.J.: The role of the menisci in forced transmission across the knee. In: Total knee replacement. London, New York: Mechanical Engineering Publications for the Institution of Mechanical Engineers 1975

WATSON-JONES, R.: Fractures and other bone and joint injuries. Edinburgh: Livingstone 1939

Chapter 7

Arthrodesis

M.A.R. FREEMAN
The London Hospital, London E1 2AD England

J. CHARNLEY
Wrightington Hospital, Near Wigan, Lancashire, WN6 9EP England

Preface

(J. CHARNLEY)

It is probably difficult for young orthopaedic surgeons to imagine why we were enthusiastic about knee fusion in the treatment of serious arthritic conditions of the knee 20 years ago. The fact was that all the knee arthroplasties at that time were very poor and a primary knee fusion by means of a compression technique was the quickest of all the major orthopaedic operations to achieve its result. Bony fusion strong enough to permit unsupported weight-bearing could be achieved in a total period of 8 weeks and with a remarkably small failure rate.

In a difficult problem, as after a failed total knee replacement, a perfect combination is required of (1) three or more points of contact between the cortical bone of the hollow but large-diameter bone ends; (2) rigid external fixation; and (3) continuously acting, spring-loaded compression. Provided this combination is maintained for about 3 months, and provided that sepsis is not gross, there is a good chance of achieving osseous union. The problem is how to achieve these three factors simultaneously and maintain them for an adequate period. One of the best ways is to suspend the lower extremity in balanced traction, the limb being immobilised in an external fixation apparatus, and withhold weight-bearing until clinical union has started.

Historical Background

(M.A.R. FREEMAN)

Arthrodesis was originally devised for the treatment of the infected, particularly the tuberculous, knee. When first used for the arthritic knee, the acceptability of fusion as a method of treatment was severely limited not only by the disadvantage of stiffness, but also by the difficulty of achieving fusion with the techniques originally employed. Adequate immobilisation cannot be secured by external splintage alone unless a hip spica is employed for as long as 3 months. Clearly for any patient this is a formidable undertaking, but for a patient with a nonfatal disease involving joints other than the knee, which are likely to be made worse by such prolonged immobilisation, it is quite inappropriate.

The disadvantage of prolonged, general immobilisation was eliminated by the use of compression applied across the knee for a period of approximately 4 weeks. This technique, although originally described by KEY in 1932, was developed to such an extent by the work of CHARNLEY (1948) (who refers to KEY in his publications) that the technique is now rightly associated with his name. CHARNLEY (1953) listed the following factors as being responsible for the efficacy of compression:

A) Mechanical
   1) Enhancement of fixation
   2) Persistence of intimate contact
   3) Prevention of repeated shearing and flexural movements at the arthrodesis site
B) Biological
   1) Osteoclasis
   2) Osteogenesis.

It is the present view of one of the authors (JC) that the biological role of compression is unproven but that the mechanical role cannot be in dispute.

Using compression (applied through Steinmann pins, one in the femur and one in the tibia, by a screw mechanism joining the pins with a relatively flexible linkage) CHARNLEY and LOWE (1958) reported an average time for walking free of plaster of 8.5 weeks after operation in osteoarthrosis (OA) and 9.0 weeks after operation in rheumatoid arthritis (RA). There were no major complications causing longterm disability, and union occurred in 98.8% of cases. Now, when a patient is advised to have the knee replaced rather than arthrodesed, the surgeon must first be sure that an acceptable result can be achieved with sufficient reliability to off-set the disadvantages of a stiff knee, given that compression arthrodesis will produce permanent pain relief in virtually 100% of knees after 2 months.

Disadvantage of Stiffness at the Knee

For cultural reasons, a stiff knee is more acceptable in some countries (for example the United Kingdom) than others. Nevertheless, in any country a single stiff knee represents a serious disability. In particular, the patient limps; stairs and inclines cannot be negotiated normally; rising from and sitting in a chair are interfered with; sitting in a confined space, such as in a theatre or bus, is at best awkward; the foot usually cannot be reached for toilet and dressing; driving, entering, and sitting in a car are difficult; and getting up from the floor if one has fallen may be impossible. All these impediments are made very much worse if the remaining joints in the legs and arms are less than perfect. On the other hand they are materially mitigated by even a little movement: although a fully controlled painless arc of about 100° is required for a virtually normal nonathletic life, an arc from 0° to only 30° will usually improve the walking gait, improve stair and incline ascent and descent, render sitting in a confined space less difficult and ugly, and make the foot more accessible. Over and above this, many patients — especially those with arthritis — cherish movement for emotional, almost symbolic reasons out of proportion to its objective functional significance.

If one knee is stiff the swing phase of gait is prejudiced, since the heel tends to catch on the floor. This can be off-set by the slight true shortening (about 2 cm) produced by the bone excision required to arthrodese the knee. There is therefore no reason on this basis to add apparent shortening by fusing the knee in flexion. In the stance phase of gait a flexion deformity in excess of 10° is disabling, since ankle dorsiflexion and hip flexion must then be maintained against gravity to hold an upright posture. Although other aspects of the disability listed above are diminished by fusing the knee in more than 10° of flexion, such gains are minimal and do not outweigh the functional loss encountered in walking. If the object of arthrodesis is to allow the patient to walk, the knee should therefore be stiffened at 0°–10°. Cosmetically 10° is perhaps preferable to 0°, especially for women.

Bilateral arthrodesis of the knee was discussed by CHARNLEY (1953), who pointed out that the disability, although obviously much greater than after unilateral fusion, was not overwhelming. Interestingly, the shorter the legs are, the less severe is the disability. Having said this, the disability is sufficiently severe to make two stiff knees a result to be avoided if at all possible.

Indications for Primary Arthrodesis of the Knee in 1977

The results of replacement are now sufficiently good in any knee, regardless of how severely it is damaged, for primary arthrodesis to be rarely indicated now. Nevertheless it should be considered for an elderly patient who has had little or no movement in the knee for many years and in whom pain and/or deformity are intolerable, or for a young patient with a knee that is already stiff and in whom the prospect of a successful replacement is negligible (Fig. 1). In the author's experience, whilst useful movement can be gained in such a completely stiff knee by replacement, this cannot be guaranteed and becomes less likely the longer stiffness has been present. Most young patients with a stiff knee prefer the hope of movement following replacement to the certainty of stiffness following arthrodesis, and for them nothing is lost by attempting replacement provided this is of a kind that does not prejudice subsequent fusion. For an elderly patient, however, the possibility of two operative procedures may be unacceptable, and hence primary arthrodesis may be preferred: the author (MF) has carried out only two such procedures in the last 5 years.

Arthrodesis as a Revision Procedure

It is in this context that arthrodesis has a modern role. Obviously many failed procedures can be

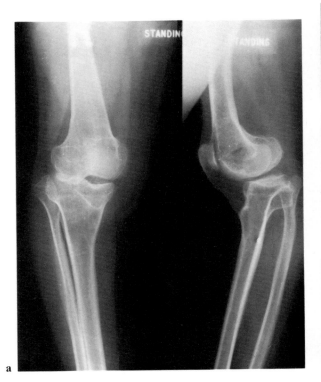

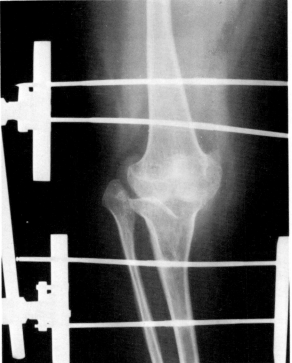

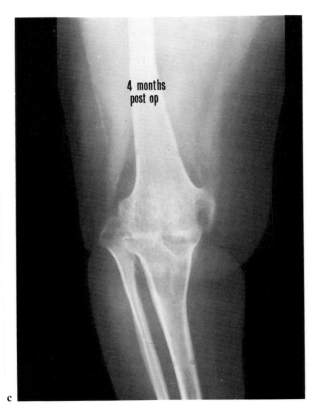

Fig. 1. a Pre-operative radiographs of the knee of a patient with achondroplastic dwarfism. This patient had previously had a high tibial osteotomy, which had been unsuccessful in relieving pain. The knee was too small for a conventional prosthesis, was painful and unstable, and had only 30° of movement. The patient wished for only one further operative procedure. It was decided to carry out a primary arthrodesis rather than to attempt what would almost certainly have been an unsuccessful joint replacement. Arthrodesis was particularly indicated for this patient, since her legs were short. **b** The same knee 3 weeks after operation, to show the frame illustrated in Fig. 3 in place. The tibia and femur were deliberately placed in straight alignment so that the arthrodesed knee would be similar in appearance to the other knee. **c** Bony union 4 months post-operatively

salvaged by total replacement, but the results of such repeated operations became less and less satisfactory as bone is lost, the skin is repeatedly scarred, and the tissues damaged and exposed to infection. Thus the point at which it is wiser to proceed to a virtually certain arthrodesis rather than to risk prejudicing eventual arthrodesis by a further revision procedure is a matter of surgical judgement, about which no general statement can be made.

Requirements for Successful Arthrodesis

Two factors severely reduce the chance of obtaining successful arthrodesis at the knee: the absence of cancellous bone and the presence of infection.

Union occurs more rapidly in cancellous than in cortical bone — probably because the number of cells with osteogenic potential in any cross-section of the bone is much greater in cancellous bone. Similarly the blood supply is better and the area over which accurate coaptation can be achieved is greater. Mechanically, arthrodesis of the knee suffers the disadvantage that fusion is being attempted between two long levers: the bending moments at the fusion site are therefore potentially large. These can best be countered by achieving fixation and bony union as far as possible from the neutral axis of the section being bent, i.e., by achieving fusion between the expanded cancellous bone ends rather than between the narrower tubular shafts. Implants for the total replacement of the knee should therefore be designed and implanted in such a way that they preserve the cancellous bone through which a primary arthrodesis normally occurs. Of this bone, that of the condyles is of more use than that of the midline: in the tibia the midline cancellous bone is relatively porotic and in part lies opposite the intercondylar notch of the femur. Intramedullary stems may not themselves therefore damage bone of crucial importance. If, however, they are connected to the bearing by a conical section, implantation of which requires the removal of cancellous bone from the condyles, their use is less attractive. Equally, of course, the use of cement remote from the bone surfaces raises the danger that the bones will have to be seriously damaged in the course of removing it.

Thus, ideally the implantation of a prosthesis should not result in damage to, nor even invasion of, the bone beyond arthrodesis surfaces. In practice this ideal cannot easily be achieved. It is, however, possible virtually to confine implant material to the surfaces themselves or to the midline of the bones within a short distance from the surface.

Having said this, satisfactory fusions have been achieved following the failure of a variety of implants, some of which transgress these ideals to varying extents. Specifically, fusion has been achieved with acceptable shortening after ICLH, Total Condylar, Geomedic, Polycentric, and Sheehan arthroplasty, to mention only some of those discussed in this volume.

Sepsis interferes with bone union. Therefore arthrodesis may fail as a revision procedure for an infected prosthesis unless the infection can be eradicated. This requires the removal of all dead and foreign material without thereby creating a dead space in the knee that cannot be obliterated and is difficult to drain. Dependent drainage is impossible to achieve in the knee if the patient is in bed, and suction drainage can only be maintained for a short period. Therefore the retention of cancellous bone when a prosthesis is implanted is of double significance: not only does its retention provide the tissue through which union will most readily occur, but it also allows the implant to be removed without thereby creating a surgically unmanageable intra-osseous dead space. Furthermore, speaking generally, infection in cancellous bone is more easily eradicated than infection in cortical bone: thus it is preferable to have cancellous rather than cortical bone at the interface with the prosthesis. Arthrodesis can be secured in the situation shown in Fig. 2 but it is not easy.

Techniques of Fusion Useful in the Revision of Failed Arthroplasty

Fixation and compression can best be secured by the use of four, rather than two, pins (Denham pins, which are threaded, being preferable to Steinmann pins) connected to a modern, rigid frame (Fig. 3). Such apparatus can be used satisfactorily in the presence of infection and is preferable to the original Charnley apparatus since it provides more secure fixation especially in bending about a medio-lateral axis (i.e., in the flexion–extension

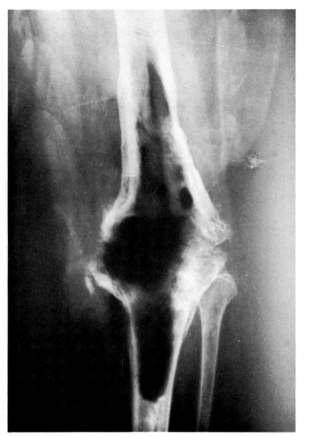

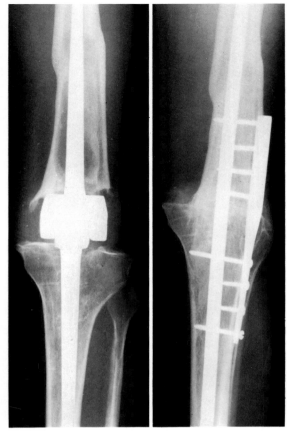

Fig. 2. The knee after the removal of an infected prosthesis, the implantation of which required the removal of substantial quantities of cancellous bone. Arthrodesis can be achieved in this situation, but it is not easy

Fig. 4a and b. Arthrodesis of the knee after Shiers arthroplasty, using an intramedullary nail and an onlay plate. **a** The pre-operative state; **b** bony union

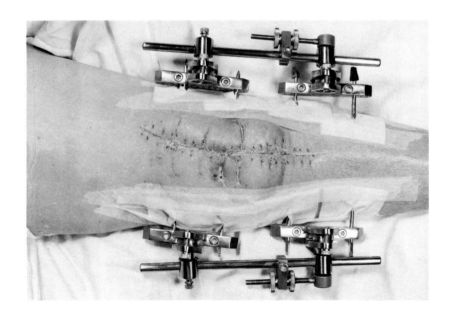

Fig. 3. The ICLH (Day) frame used to provide rigid external fixation and compression in arthrodesis of the knee following failed joint replacement. This frame is shown merely as an example of one of a number of modern devices capable of providing adequate fixation and compression

direction). If a prosthesis with an intramedullary stem has been employed and if cortical bone has then become infected, a frame either cannot be used at all or can only be used with difficulty since the pins cannot be placed in infected bone. For such a knee revision by arthrodesis may be impossible.

Even in the absence of infection, arthodesis may be difficult after the use of some implants because of the loss of cancellous bone through which union occurs. For such knees arthrodesis over an intramedullary nail passed down the femur into the tibia combined with an onlay plate to control rotation can be employed (Fig. 4). This technique has the added advantage of providing an immediately comfortable knee upon which the patient can bear weight.

allows the knee to be fully extended when the patient lies supine at night and to be slightly flexed in a chair by day. If the implantation of the original prosthesis has required the removal of more than 2 cm of bone from the long axis of the limb, the resultant ankylosis may be unacceptably unstable.

Simple removal of the prosthesis, without any subsequent attempt at fusion, should therefore be considered as a primary salvage procedure for a patient whose other disabilities make a chairbound existence inevitable, and may be considered as a possibly acceptable outcome for a knee in which infection prevents arthrodesis.

The only alternatives are amputation or a full débridement followed by re-implantation of a prosthesis with the aid of antibiotic-impregnated cement, both procedures that fall outside the scope of this Chapter.

Excision Arthroplasty as a Salvage Procedure

Excision of the knee can lead to a comfortable fibrous ankylosis that is acceptable to a patient who is in any event chairbound. Pain is relieved and with the use of a removable polypropylene splint sufficient stability can be achieved to allow weight-bearing during transfer activities. At the same time the small degree of movement permitted with a short fibrous ankylosis may be worthwhile if it

References

CHARNLEY, J.: Positive pressure in arthrodesis of the knee joint. J. Bone Joint Surg. (Br.) **30**, 478 (1948)

CHARNLEY, J.: Compression arthrodesis. Edinburgh, London: Livingstone 1953

CHARNLEY, T., LOWE, H.G.: A study of the end results of compression arthrodesis of the knee. J. Bone Joint Surg. (Br.) **40**, 633 (1958)

KEY, J.A.: Positive pressure in arthrodesis or tuberculosis of the knee joint. South. Med. J. **25**, 909 (1932)

Chapter 8

Osteotomy

P.G.J. MAQUET

25, Thier Bosset, B-4070 Aywaille, Belgium

Osteotomy about the knee has been used for many years to correct deformity of the limb, the aim being to straighten a varus, a valgus, or even a flexed or hyperextended knee. A wedge osteotomy of the distal end of the femur and a V-shaped osteotomy of the proximal end of the tibia have been described by LANGE (1951) ("Pendelosteotomie"). JACKSON and WAUGH (1961, 1969, 1970, 1974) proposed a cylindrical osteotomy through cancellous bone at the level of the tibial tubercle, "in order to realign an osteoarthritic knee joint having significant lateral angulation." COVENTRY (1965, 1970, 1973) resects a wedge proximal to the tibial tuberosity and fixes the fragments with staples and a plaster cast. HERBERT (1967) cuts the upper tibia obliquely, impacts the fragments and screws these to the proximal extremity of the fibula. RAMADIER (HERBERT et al., 1967; RAMADIER, 1965) also impacts the fragments, which are immobilized by two staples. DUPARC (HERBERT et al., 1967) inserts a graft between the osteotomy surfaces that are separated. GARIÉPY (HERBERT et al., 1967) fixes the fragments of an oblique osteotomy of the upper end of the tibia with compression clamps, as does MACINTOSH (1970). BLAIMONT (1970) proposed the same fixation after a curved osteotomy proximal to the tibial tuberosity and a rotation of the convexity of the distal fragment inside the concavity of the proximal. More recently, IZADPANAH and KEÖNCH-FRAKNÓY (1977a and b) advocated a transverse displacement osteotomy proximal to the femoral condyles as a treatment for osteoarthritis (OA) with a varus deformity. NITSCH and YANSEN (1976) use a supracondylar osteotomy of the femur to correct any deformity, either varus or valgus.

All these procedures, except that of BLAIMONT (1970), are designed to restore the normal anatomy by correcting a deformity. However, none of them takes the patello-femoral joint into account. American, English, French and German reports (BOUILLET and VAN GAVER, 1961; COVENTRY, 1965, 1970, 1973; DEBEYRE and ARTIGOU, 1973; HARDING, 1976; INSALL et al., 1974; IZADPANAH and KEÖNCH-FRAKNÓY, 1977a and b; JACKSON and WAUGH, 1961, 1970, 1974; KLEMS, 1976; MACINTOSH, 1970) all lack accurate measurements of the deformity and of its correction. Most authors plan their surgery on X-rays showing only the lower end of the femur and the upper end of the tibia, neglecting full-length views. In the French literature (HERBERT et al., 1967; RAMADIER, 1967) an accurate measurement of the deformity on whole-limb X-rays is mentioned but the number of knees under- or overcorrected after surgery reveals a lack of accuracy in the operative procedures (DEBEYRE and ARTIGOU, 1973; HERBERT et al., 1967; and MASSE, 1976).

"Tibial osteotomy frequently is done in order to transfer the load from the worn to the comparatively normal compartment" (MACINTOSH and WELSH, 1977). However, if this is really achieved, the stress in the "comparatively normal compartment" must obviously become much higher than the physiological stress, because it is confined to this one compartment. This in turn might be expected to accelerate the onset of degenerative changes in the comparatively normal compartment.

Several authors confine the indication for a tibial osteotomy to knees with a varus deformity smaller than 15° or 20°, without significant collateral laxity (COVENTRY, 1973; INSALL et al., 1974; MACINTOSH and WELSH, 1977).

With a different objective in mind, BENJAMIN (1969) carried out a double osteotomy, dividing the lower end of the femur and the upper end of the tibia in cases of rheumatoid arthritis (RA) and OA. This double osteotomy was aimed at "the mere surgical division of various structures, such as blood vessels, nerves and bone." The prerequisites were "the absence of gross deformity" and "a range of movement of 90 degrees."

Pathogenesis of Osteoarthritis of the Knee

Since osteotomy is designed, at least in part, to arrest the progression of degenerative changes in the knee, the pathogenesis of these changes must be understood if an osteotomy is to be planned rationally. Osteoarthritis appears as the result of a disturbance of the equilibrium that normally exists between the biological resistance of the tissues and their mechanical stressing (MÜLLER, 1929; PAUWELS, 1973; RADIN et al., 1972) when the joint can no longer withstand its mechanical environment. Treatment must reduce the articular stresses sufficiently to make them tolerable. This aim usually cannot be achieved simply by restoring the anatomy to normal (MAQUET, 1969a and b, 1970, 1976).

The mass of the body minus that of the supporting lower leg and foot eccentrically exerts a force P on the knee of the stance leg by its weight and accelerations. Force P must be balanced by active muscular forces L and by passive ligamentous forces. Force R is the resultant or the vectorial sum of all these forces (MAQUET, 1969a and b; 1970, 1972; MAQUET et al., 1975a and b). Its line of action must be perpendicular to the articular surfaces of the femoro-tibial joint, since there is equilibrium and the coefficient of friction of a joint is negligible (RADIN and PAUL, 1970; RADIN et al., 1970) (Fig. 1). Force R is transmitted from the femur to the tibia through articular surfaces that vary during movement of the joint. From extension to flexion they decrease in size and move posteriorly on the tibial plateaux (Fig. 2a). The menisci take part in transmitting the femoro-tibial force. They represent approximately 50% of the weight-bearing surfaces (MAQUET et al., 1975a and b). These surfaces are thus reduced by meniscectomy (Fig. 2b), an operation that often precedes OA.

Force R creates compressive stresses in the joint. According to PAUWELS' law (PAUWELS, 1965, 1973b; KUMMER, 1959, 1972), the quantity and structure of osseous tissue depend on the magnitude of the stresses applied to it. The symmetrical, subchondral dense bone, of even thickness throughout, that underlies the tibial plateaux of a normal knee thus betokens an even distribution of the articular compressive stresses. Hence, the overall load R supported by the knee must act through the centre of gravity of the weight-bearing surfaces of the joint (MAQUET, 1970, 1976) (Figs. 3 and 5a).

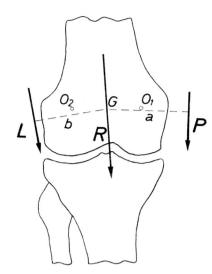

Fig. 1. Loaded knee projected on the coronal plane. P, force exerted by the part of the body supported by the knee; L, lateral muscular stay; a, lever arm of P; b, lever arm of L; R, resultant of P and L; O_1, centre of curvature of the medial condyle; O_2, centre of curvature of the lateral condyle; G, central point on the axis of flexion of the knee

Force R can be displaced medially by a weakening of the muscles L, by an increase of force P, by a varus deformity, or by a displacement of the centre of gravity of the body in a horizontal transverse direction away from the loaded knee (MAQUET, 1970, 1976). The medial displacement of the line of action of resultant R alters the distribution and magnitude of the stresses in the joint and soon decreases its effective weight-bearing surfaces (Fig. 4). Between certain physiological limits, increased stresses provoke apposition of bone and decreased stresses, resorption. Consequently, the shape of the subchondral sclerosis in a joint corresponds to that of the stress diagram or load distribution within it (PAUWELS, 1973a and b). Medial displacement of R will thus appear on the X-ray: the subchondral sclerosis underneath the medial plateau increases and becomes triangular in shape (Fig. 5b). The trabeculae of the cancellous bone become more apparent under the medial joint space, and less so under the lateral. The normal lateral subchondral sclerosis fades away. At a later stage, the medial joint space disappears, reflecting destruction of the articular cartilage, the lateral joint space widens, and the medial subchondral sclerotic triangle increases (Fig. 5c). Finally, the tolerance of the bone to mechanical stress is

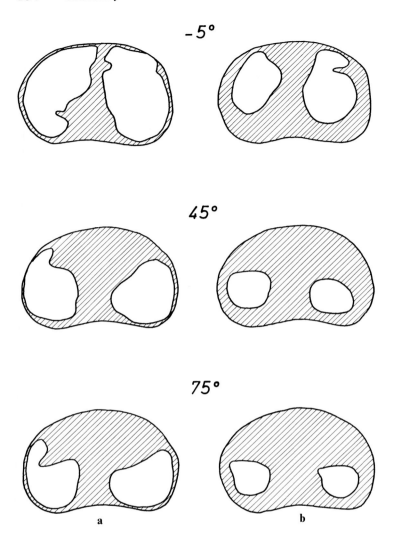

−5°

45°

75°

a   b

Fig. 2a and b. Tracings of the load-transmitting areas of the femoro-tibial joint at 5° hyperextension, 45° flexion, and 75° flexion. **a** knee with menisci; **b** knee without menisci

overwhelmed so that bone destruction occurs. This causes or aggravates the varus deformity and leads to or accentuates ligamentous laxity laterally, with eventual subluxation of the femur on the tibia (Fig. 5d).

In a varus deformity of the knee (Fig. 7), the femur, and hence the lateral muscles L, are less inclined to the line of action of force P than in a normal knee (Fig. 6). But overstressing due to the medial displacement of the resultant force R finally erodes the medial border of the plateau, which is usually somewhat enlarged by osteophytes. Because of this change in shape, the plateau remains perpendicular to the line of action of resultant R (Fig. 7). Equilibrium is maintained and the knee is stable as long as R does not act further medially than the medial border of the joint (Fig. 8). If

there were to be no flattening of the articular surfaces, equilibrium would be disrupted as soon as R acts medially to the centre of curvature of the medial condyle.

Thickening of the sclerotic area under the lateral plateau constitutes the first sign of OA in the lateral compartment of the knee (Fig. 9a). Later, this sclerosis increases further, while that under the medial plateau tends to fade away and the structure of the cancellous bone under the medial plateau becomes less apparent (Fig. 9b). The lateral joint space is narrowed and the femur subluxates on the tibia. Destruction of the cartilage and resorption of bone in the lateral part of the knee provoke or accentuate the valgus deformity (Fig. 9c). The pathological distribution of the stresses visible on X-rays betokens a lateral displacement of the force

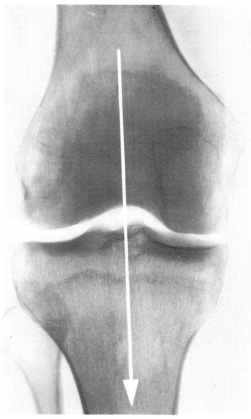

Fig. 3. The outline of the dense subchondral bone underlying the tibial plateaux corresponds to the stress diagram

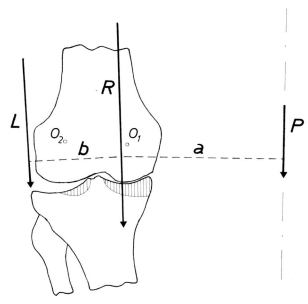

Fig. 4. Increased stresses in the medial compartment of the knee resulting from a medial displacement of resultant R. P, force exerted by the mass of the body supported by the knee; L, lateral muscular stay; R, resultant of P and L; O_1, centre of curvature of the medial condyle; O_2, centre of curvature of the lateral condyle; a, lever arm of P; b, lever arm of L

R, which soon leads to a reduction of the effective weight-bearing surfaces of the joint. Force R can be displaced laterally by an increase of the muscular force L, by a valgus deformity of the leg, or by a transverse horizontal shift of the centre of gravity of the body towards the loaded knee (MA-QUET, 1970, 1976). The muscular force L is produced partly by bi-articular muscles spanning the knee and the hip. An abnormal increase of this force L may be demanded by the conditions of equilibrium at hip level. Laterally displaced, the resultant R increases and concentrates the stresses in the lateral aspect of the joint, where they can attain an enormous magnitude (Fig. 10).

In a valgus deformity, the femur, and hence the lateral muscles L, are more inclined to the line of action of force P than in a normal knee. Therefore, the resultant R is also more oblique. It is perpendicular to the intercondylar eminence in the lateral part of the joint (Fig. 11), and no longer to the transverse plane tangential to both plateaux (Fig. 6). In relation to this plane, the resultant R acts with a perpendicular component N and a tangential component T. The perpendicular component N presses the femur against the tibia and its reaction N′ presses the tibia against the femur. The tangential component T tends to displace the femur medially on the tibia, and its reaction T′ tends to displace the tibia laterally under the femur. These mechanical conditions concentrate and increase the compressive stresses on the lateral plateau towards the intercondylar eminence rather than on the lateral margin of the joint. Erosion permits the femoral condyle to sink into the deepened tibial plateau (Fig. 9c). Here, as soon as the force R acts outside the centre of curvature of the lateral aspect of the joint, the knee holds only thanks to its medial ligaments. Eventually these give way, as does any ligament stretched for long enough. The knee thus becomes

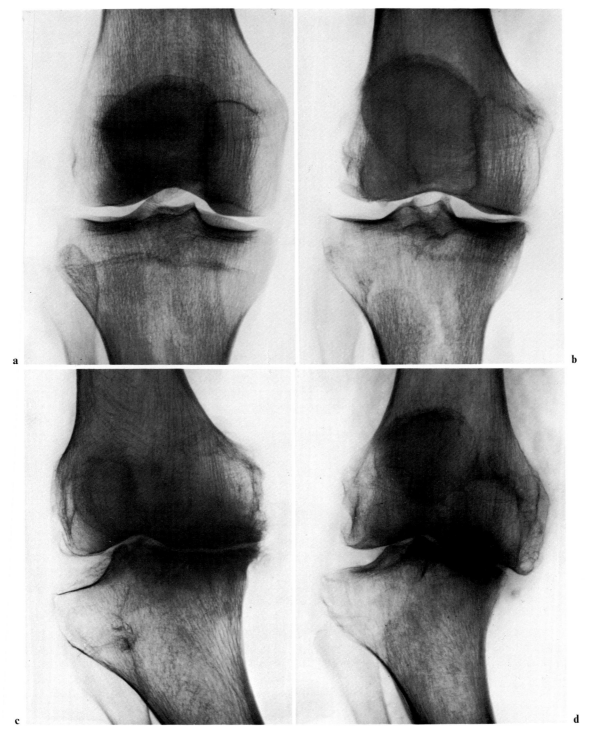

Fig. 5. a Normal knee; **b** dense triangle underlining the medial tibial plateau; **c** larger triangle and narrowing of the joint space; **d** sclerosis under the eroded medial tibial plateau and subluxation of the joint

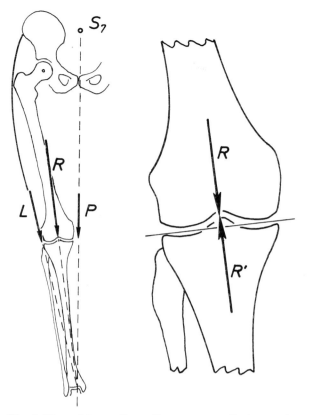

Fig. 6. Normal knee. Force R acts perpendicular to the plane tangential to the tibial plateaux.

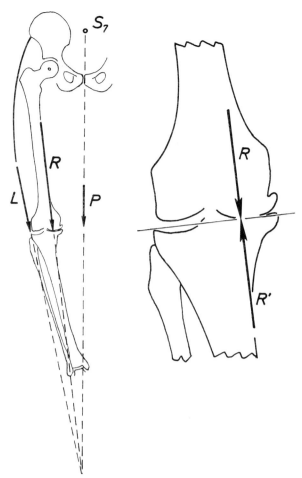

Fig. 7. OA with varus deformity. The resultant force R keeps acting perpendicular to the plane tangential to the tibial plateaux

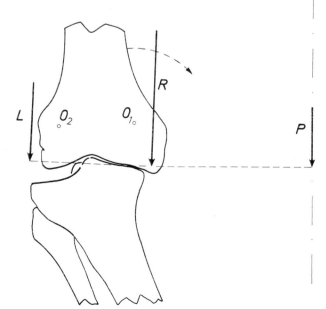

Fig. 8. Unstable varus knee. The line of action of resultant R is medial to the medial border of the tibia

unstable (Fig. 12), sooner than in OA with a varus deformity.

The difference in evolution between medial and lateral OA can be observed on X-ray plates and is crucial in the choice of treatment. A dense triangle of bone, the base of which is medial, underlies the medial plateau in OA with a varus deformity (Fig. 5). In OA with a valgus deformity the pathological subchondral sclerosis is more centrally localized underneath the lateral plateau, extending into the region of the intercondylar eminence (Fig. 9). Lateral OA with valgus deformity can be compared with OA of the hip with protrusio acetabuli, whereas the development of medial OA with varus deformity is more like that of OA of the hip, with progressive lateral subluxation of the femoral head.

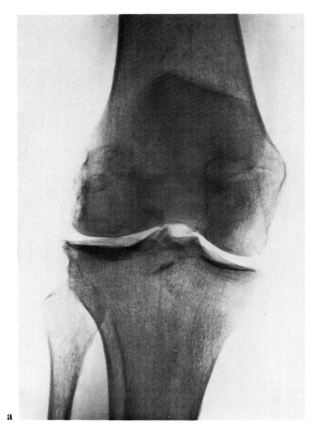

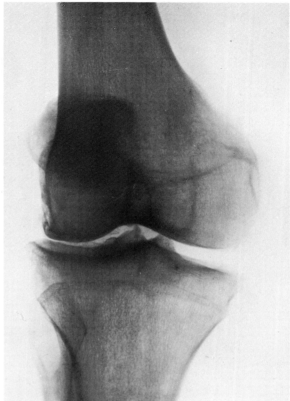

a

b

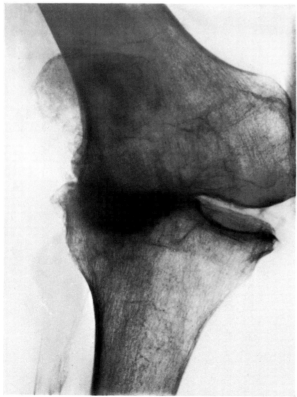

c

Fig. 9a–c. OA with valgus deformity. **a** cup-shaped sclerosis under the lateral tibial plateau; **b** dense triangle underlining the lateral tibial plateau; **c** narrowing of the joint space with impingement of the femur into the tibia

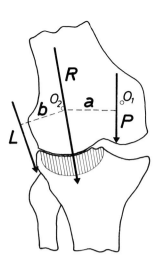

Fig. 10. Increased stresses in the lateral compartment of the knee resulting from the lateral displacement of resultant R. Symbols have same meanings as in Fig. 4

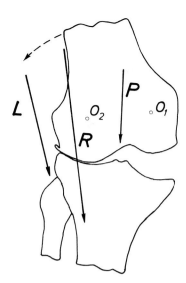

Fig. 12. Unstable valgus knee. The line of action of resultant R is outside the centre of curvatur O_2 of the lateral condyle. Symbols have same meanings as in Fig. 4

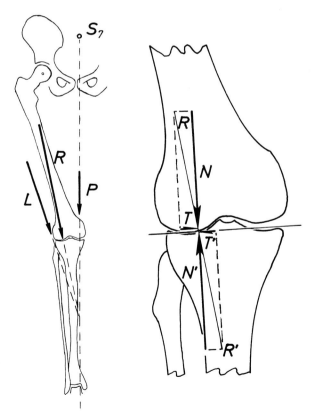

Fig. 11. OA with valgus deformity. Resultant R acts on the tibial plateaux with a perpendicular component N and a tangential component T

The subchondral sclerosis underlying the tibial plateaux in a lateral view of a normal knee demonstrates that the stresses are also evenly distributed in the sagittal plane (Fig. 13 a). The resultant force R must therefore cross the centre of the weight-bearing surfaces when projected on the sagittal plane. Force R must also pass through the axis of flexion of the joint (FICK, 1910; HUSSON, 1973 a and b, 1974; KUMMER, 1962, 1965; MENSCHIK, 1974, 1975).

The dense triangle developing under the posterior part of the osteoarthritic joint indicates an uneven distribution of the stresses and a posterior displacement of the load, with subsequent reduction of the weight-bearing articular surfaces (Fig. 13 b).

The subchondral area of the patella normally presents a thin ribbon of dense bone the shape of which corresponds to the stress distribution in the patello-femoral joint (Fig. 14 a). This sclerosis can increase in thickness and take the form of a dense cup in cases of patello-femoral OA (Fig. 14 b and c). Such an alteration indicates an increase of the force R_5 pressing the patella against the femur (MAQUET et al., 1975 a and b; MAQUET, 1976).

Force R_5 can be increased by an augmentation of the forces Mv, developed in the quadriceps tendon, and Pa, exerted by the patella tendon, or,

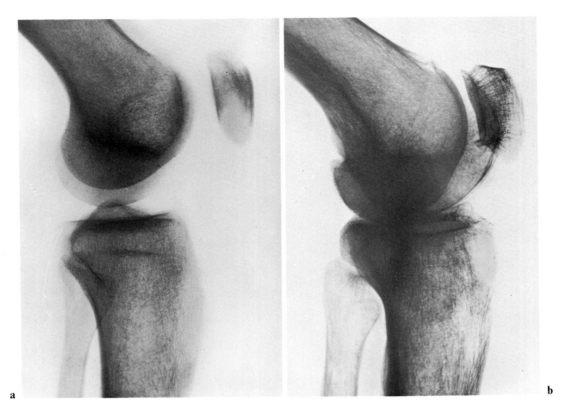

Fig. 13. a Normal knee. A dense strip of even thickness underlies the tibial plateaux. **b** Osteoarthritic knee. A dense triangle indicates the locally increased stresses

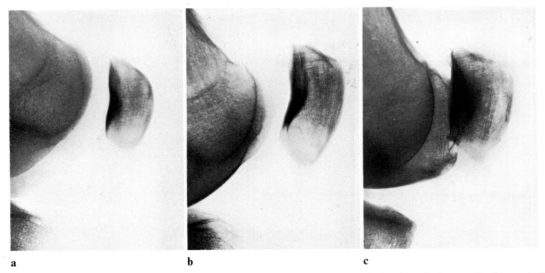

Fig. 14. a Patella of a normal knee. **b** Thickening of the subchondral sclerosis in patello-femoral OA. **c** Thick cup-shaped subchondral sclerosis at a later stage of the condition

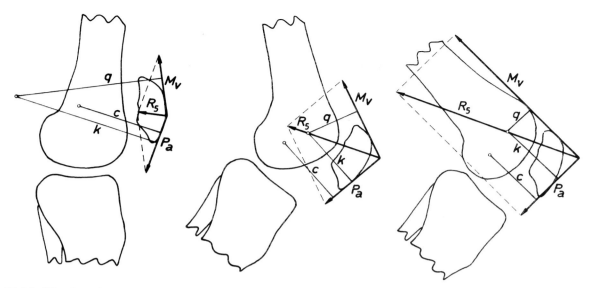

Fig. 15. Modification of the lever arms during movement. Mv, quadriceps muscle; Pa, patella tendon; R_5, resultant of Mv and Pa; q, lever arm of force Mv acting on the patella; k, lever arm of force Pa acting on the patella; c, lever arm of force Pa acting on the femoro-tibial joint

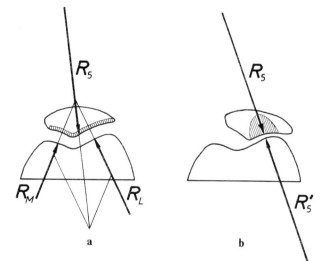

Fig. 16 a and b. Reduced weight-transmitting articular surfaces following lateral displacement of the patella. R_5, force pressing the patella against the femur; R_L, lateral component of R_5; R_M, medial component of R_5; R_5, reaction pressing the femur against the patella

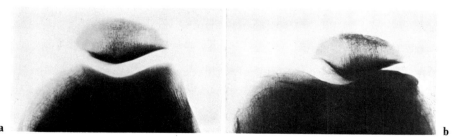

Fig. 17. a In a normal patello-femoral joint, the subchondral sclerosis underlies both articular facets of the patella equally. **b** In a subluxated patella, the sclerosis is much thicker under the lateral facet

above all, by closing the angle formed by the lines of action of these forces Mv and Pa (Fig. 15). The magnitude and distribution of the stresses in the patello-femoral joint depend on the magnitude and situation of force R_5. A lateral displacement of the patella will reduce the weight-transmitting articular surfaces and concentrate and increase the stresses in the joint (Fig. 16). This again can be observed on X-rays. In a normal patello-femoral joint, the subchondral sclerosis underlies both articular aspects of the patella equally (Fig. 17a). The sclerosis is much thicker and concentrated under the lateral aspect of a subluxated patella (Fig. 17b).

Rationale for Surgical Treatment of OA of the Knee

Re-alignment of the leg as advocated by most authors (BOUILLET and VAN GAVER, 1961; DEBEYRE and ARTIGOU, 1973; HARDING, 1976) would restore a normal anatomical shape and thus replace the knee in the very same mechanical situation that caused the pathological condition to appear in the first place. Surgery must aim at reducing and evenly redistributing the stresses over the largest possible articular surface. This can usually be achieved only by overcorrecting the deformity and by creating a somewhat abnormal shape to the skeleton (MAQUET, 1969a and b, 1976).

Choice of a Surgical Procedure

In the author's practice, OA with a varus deformity is generally treated by an osteotomy of the upper end of the tibia, OA with a valgus deformity by a supracondylar osteotomy of the femur, and OA of the patello-femoral joint by an anterior and, if necessary, medial displacement of the tibial tuberosity. In some cases, the condition will heal after the correction of a deformity of the skeleton at a distance from the affected knee (MAQUET, 1970, 1976). Although such a result confirms the mechanical effect of the treatment, the discussion in this Chapter will be limited to osteotomies about the knee and the advancement of the tibial tuberosity.

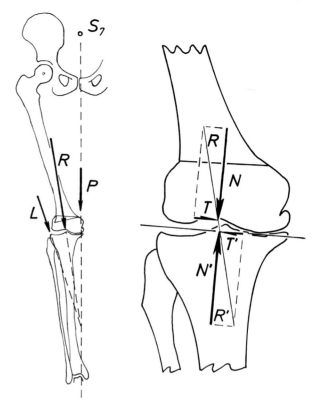

Fig. 18. After an osteotomy of the lower end of the femur, the resultant force R acts on the tibial plateau with a perpendicular component N and a tangential component T

The first question to arise is why, as a rule, an upper tibial osteotomy is chosen for cases of OA with a varus deformity, and a lower femoral osteotomy for those with a valgus deformity. KUMMER (1977) has provided an explanation for the varus deformity. The same reasoning will be applied to the valgus deformity.

As mentioned above, in OA with a varus deformity the line of action of the resultant force R is displaced medially and is less inclined to that of force P than in a normal knee. Because of the erosion of the medial margin of the tibial plateau, R remains perpendicular to the latter (Fig. 7). After a supracondylar osteotomy of the femur overcorrecting the deformity, the femur and the lateral muscles L are re-oriented more obliquely in relation to the line of action of force P (Fig. 18). The intersection of forces L and P is brought closer to the joint. Therefore, the resultant force R turns (counter-clockwise in the drawing). The whole lower leg and the distal fragment of the femur

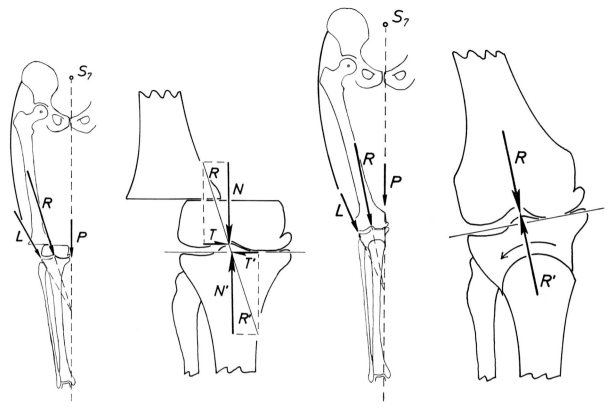

Fig. 19. The amount of correction provided by a displacement supracondylar osteotomy is limited by the width of the femur

Fig. 20. After an appropriate osteotomy of the upper end of the tibia, force R acts perpendicular to the plane tangential to the tibial plateaux

pivot around the heel, which must remain on the line of action of the force developed by the body weight plus the forces of inertia. Because of this rotation of the lower leg (clockwise in the drawing) and the opposite rotation of the resultant R, force R is no longer perpendicular to the plane tangential to the tibial plateau. It acts then with a perpendicular component N, pressing the femur against the tibia, and a tangential component T which tends to displace the femur medially on the tibia. Components N′ and T′ of reaction R′ act inversely on the tibia. Therefore, force R cannot be redistributed evenly over the weight-bearing surfaces of the joint.

A transverse-displacement supracondylar osteotomy of the femur has also been proposed for correcting a varus deformity (IZADPANAH and KEÖNCH-FRAKNÓY, 1977a and b). It is, however, subject to the same criticism as applies to supracondylar osteotomy. Moreover, the amount of correction, not to mention overcorrection, provided

by such an osteotomy is much restricted by the very width of the femur. This is illustrated by the grotesque situation in Fig. 19.

Correction of a varus deformity by an osteotomy of the upper end of the tibia will also open the angle formed by the femur and the lateral muscles L with the line of action of force P (Fig. 20). The resultant force R turns (counter-clockwise in the drawing). But the upper fragment of the tibia pivots in the same direction, i.e., in the opposite direction to the distal fragment, which rotates clockwise around the heel supported by the ground. Therefore, the resultant R remains perpendicular to the plane tangential to the tibial plateaux. If the overcorrection has been sufficient, force R is brought back to the centre of gravity of the weight-bearing surfaces and the stresses are then optimally redistributed over the joint (KUMMER, 1977).

As described above, in OA with a valgus deformity, the line of action of the resultant R is dis-

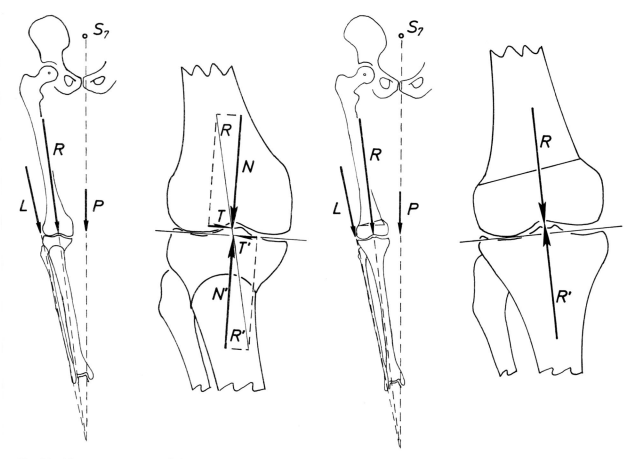

Fig. 21. After an osteotomy of the upper end of the tibia carried out for OA with a valgus deformity, force R remains oblique to the plane tangential to the tibial plateaux

Fig. 22. After an appropriate osteotomy of the lower end of the femur carried out for OA with a valgus deformity, force R acts perpendicular to the plane tangential to the tibial plateaux

placed laterally and is oblique to the plane tangential to the tibial plateaux. (Fig. 11). This follows from the direction of the lateral muscles about a valgus knee and is substantiated by the shape and location of the subchondral sclerosis underlying the lateral aspect of the joint (Fig. 9).

Correcting or overcorrecting the deformity reorientates the femur and the lateral muscles L. The intersection of forces L and P is displaced further away from the knee (Figs. 21 and 22). This reorientation of force L changes the direction of R, which turns (clockwise in the drawing). If the correction is achieved through an osteotomy of the proximal end of the tibia (Fig. 21), the upper fragment of this bone rotates clockwise i.e., in the opposite direction to the lower fragment, which pivots counter-clockwise around the heel. Turning

the upper fragment in the same direction as the resultant force does not allow force R to be made perpendicular to the plane tangential to the tibial plateaux. Force R, oblique to this plane, keeps acting with a tangential component T. This hinders an optimal redistribution of the stresses, which remain concentrated in the area lateral to the intercondylar eminence. Since the operation has lengthened the lever arm of force P, the resultant R is increased and poorly distributed. Aggravation of the symptoms and X-ray signs confirm the predicted mechanical deterioration.

A supracondylar osteotomy of the femur overcorrecting the valgus deformity, in contrast, turns the tibial plateaux counter-clockwise (Fig. 22). This rotation and the clockwise rotation of the resultant R make the latter perpendicular to the plane tangential to the tibial plateaux. Force R then acts as a purely compressive force. If the overcorrection has been sufficient, force R, although somewhat increased, causes reduced compressive stresses, evenly distributed over the largest possible weight-bearing surfaces of the joint.

Tibial or femoral osteotomy can be considered in RA. But since the evolution of the disease is due primarily to a biological rather than a mechanical disorder, its treatment must aim first at correcting this disorder, and lies in the field of internal medicine or rheumatology. Only when the mechanics of the knee are disturbed should an osteotomy be considered during a remission of the disease. We have combined osteotomy with as complete a synovectomy as possible in these circumstances. The osteotomy then follows the same principles as for OA, since it actually deals with the same mechanical disturbance. It is usually carried out through the upper tibia for a varus deformity, or through the lower femur for a valgus deformity. If the joint is grossly destroyed by RA, osteotomy should not be considered.

Femoral or Tibial Osteotomy

Planning a femoral or a tibial osteotomy requires X-rays of good quality. The A P view is taken with full weight bearing on the affected knee, the patella being directed forward. The lateral view is taken in a standard position of flexion, the patient lying on his side. We choose 45° of flexion.

In order better to outline the subchondral sclerosis and the cancellous structure, it is advisable to overexpose and to underdevelop. Contact printing of the X-rays on photographic paper further accentuates the appearance of these structures.

In addition to these X-rays centred on the knee it is necessary to have an AP X-ray showing the whole of the affected limb while the patient is standing and supporting the full body weight (Fig. 23) (DE MARCHIN et al., 1963a and b; RAMADIER, 1967). A line drawn from the centre of the femoral head to the midpoint of the cross-section at the level of the osteotomy defines the axis of the upper part of the limb; another drawn from the midpoint of the cross-section at the level of the osteotomy to the middle of the ankle joint represents the axis of the lower part of the limb. In a normal leg, both axes are in line. The angle (α) they form in abnormal cases measures the varus or the valgus deformity.

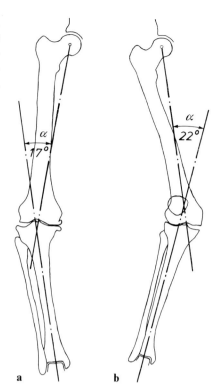

Fig. 23 a and b. From the X-ray of the whole loaded leg the angle α can be determined. Angle α is formed by the so-called mechanical axes of femur and tibia. In a normal knee angle α is zero. **a** Varus deformity; **b** Valgus deformity

Barrel-Vault Osteotomy of the Tibia

Planning. Before performance, a barrel-vault osteotomy is planned graphically on the tracing of a standing AP view of the affected knee (Fig. 24). For an osteotomy of the upper end of the tibia, a transverse line is drawn through the proximal end of the shaft, perpendicular to the tibial axis. Another transverse line is drawn just below the joint space, forming an angle α + 3° to 5°, open laterally, with the first transverse line. The 3°–5° provide the overcorrection. Its exact magnitude varies with each individual: it is less in a young, strong patient, more in an old, obese lady. A curve of 2.5 cm radius is drawn, embracing the tibial tuberosity and concave downward. The distal fragment with its transverse line is then traced onto a second sheet of transparent paper. This sheet is turned on the first until the transverse line through the distal fragment is parallel with that below the joint

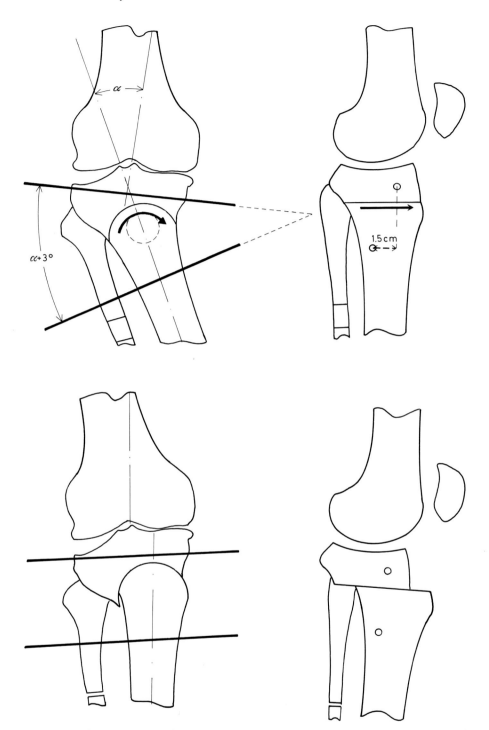

Fig. 24. Surgical procedure of the barrel-vault osteotomy, combining overcorrection of varus deformity and anterior displacement of the patella tendon

space on the first sheet. The proximal fragment with its transverse line and the femur is then traced on the second sheet.

This is a graphical method of planning a barrel-vault osteotomy overcorrecting a varus deformity. In the rare cases in which a tibial osteotomy is used to treat OA with a valgus deformity, overcorrection is usually less and the angle α should be 1°–2° open medially.

Attempts have been made to provide more accuracy for the overcorrection (BLAIMONT et al., 1971; KETTELKAMP and CHAO, 1972), relying for instance on the actual strength of the muscles (BLAIMONT et al., 1971). As yet these have not been successful.

Operative Technique. Surgery is carried out without a tourniquet to reduce the risks of thrombosis and embolism. The technique which we have proposed causes very little bleeding. Third of the fibula is first divided obliquely through its middle third, below the periosteum, great care being taken to avoid the fibular veins. The tibial tubercle is approached anteriorly through a 5-cm longitudinal incision. The patella tendon is dissected free on both sides and the tibia stripped of muscular insertions at this level. Two Steinmann pins are inserted in the transverse plane, corresponding to the transverse lines of the drawing, the upper one being 1.0–1.5 cm more anterior than the lower. The bone is cut above and around the tibial tuberosity with a narrow chisel along a curved line previously marked by holes drilled antero-posteriorly with a Kirschner wire. The fragments are rotated and the distal one displaced anteriorly until the two Steinmann pins are parallel and in the same coronal plane. They are then fixed under compression with two clamps. If there is a tendency for the fragments to tilt, a third Steinmann pin can be inserted parallel to the proximal one, and the pins can then be fixed with the mobile units of the compression clamps, one of which is provided with two holes. This is very rarely necessary. The barrel-vault osteotomy thus achieves a precise overcorrection of the deformity and an anterior displacement of the patella tendon. The two wounds, the lateral and the anterior, are sutured on suction drainage.

To ensure the accuracy of the procedure, two special instruments have been devised. An Osteotomy Guide allows holes to be drilled with a Kirschner wire along a regular curve (Fig. 25). Secondly, a Pin Guide ensures that the Steinmann pins are inserted at the desired angle (Fig. 26).

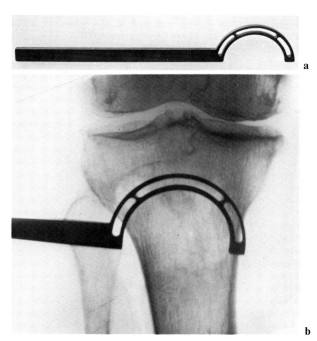

Fig. 25. **a** Osteotomy Guide for the barrel-vault osteotomy. Two sizes are available. **b** X-ray during operation

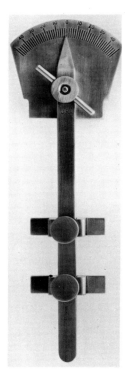

Fig. 26. Pin Guide for proximal tibial and distal femoral osteotomy

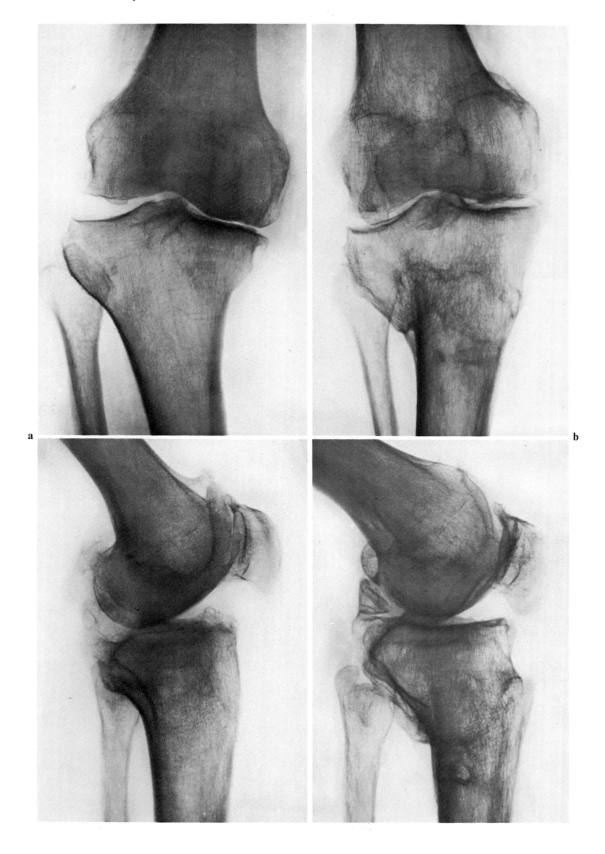

a   b

If an irreducible flexion contracture exists, division of the posterior capsule at the level of the femoral condyles precedes the osteotomy.

The day after surgery, the patient stands and walks with crutches. These are soon discarded. The pins are removed after 2 months.

When the overcorrection has been sufficient to bring back the resultant force R to the centre of gravity of the femoro-tibial joint surfaces, the clinical and radiological evolution demonstrates the redistribution of the articular stresses. On the X-ray, the exaggerated subchondral sclerosis under the medial plateau decreases and the structure of the cancellous bone becomes symmetrical under both plateaux (Fig. 27). Pain disappears, the range of movement improves, and the patient can walk for greater distances.

Indications for the Barrel-Vault Tibial Osteotomy. The indications for a barrel-vault osteotomy are medial OA of the knee, usually with a varus deformity, and lateral OA resulting from an exaggerated overcorrection of a varus deformity. Exceptionally it may be used for lateral OA with a mild valgus deformity.

Several authors (COVENTRY, 1973; INSALL et al., 1974; MACINTOSH and WELSH, 1977) confine their indications for a tibial osteotomy to deformities of less than 20° (MACINTOSH and WELSH, 1977) or even 10° (INSALL et al., 1974) and to knees without significant collateral laxity. MACINTOSH and WELSH (1977) write: "If insufficient cartilage space remained, the patient was not considered as a candidate for the procedure." Others claim that a fixed flexion contracture of more than 20° is a contra-indication for osteotomy (JACKSON et al., 1969).

In our experience, gross deformity or instability in the coronal plane due to laxity of the collateral ligaments and even subluxation of the femur on the tibia do not constitute contra-indications for barrel-vault osteotomy. When the deformity is sufficiently overcorrected by surgery to attain an even distribution of the stresses in the knee, the ligaments tighten spontaneously and the knee again becomes stable (Fig. 28). In such cases the proper degree of overcorrection may be difficult to ascer-

tain. An exaggerated overcorrection seems to accelerate healing and stabilization of the knee, but it may have to be followed by a second osteotomy to restore a more moderate valgus deformity. In proper mechanical conditions, a large joint space develops even in cases in which absolutely none was present before surgery (Fig. 29; MAQUET, 1976). Flexion contracture is corrected by a posterior capsulotomy.

A significant deformity due to partial destruction of the medial plateau does not necessarily contra-indicate treatment by osteotomy (Fig. 30). When stressed again in a tolerable way the living tissues have a considerable capacity for repair and adaptation to the new situation.

It is recommended by several authors (COVENTRY, 1965; and HERBERT et al., 1967) that osteotomy be carried out by taking a wedge from the lateral side of the knee. Osteotomy with resec-

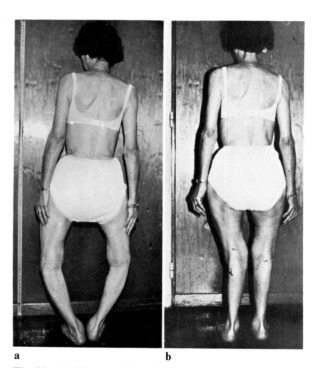

Fig. 28a–d. 69-year-old patient, before (**a**) and 7 years after (**b**) a bilateral proximal tibial osteotomy and anterior displacement of the patella tendon. Standing AP and lateral X-rays before (**c**) and after (**d**) surgery

◄ **Fig. 27 a and b.** Right knee of a 66-year-old patient, before (**a**) and 5 years after (**b**) a barrel-vault osteotomy overcorrecting the varus deformity

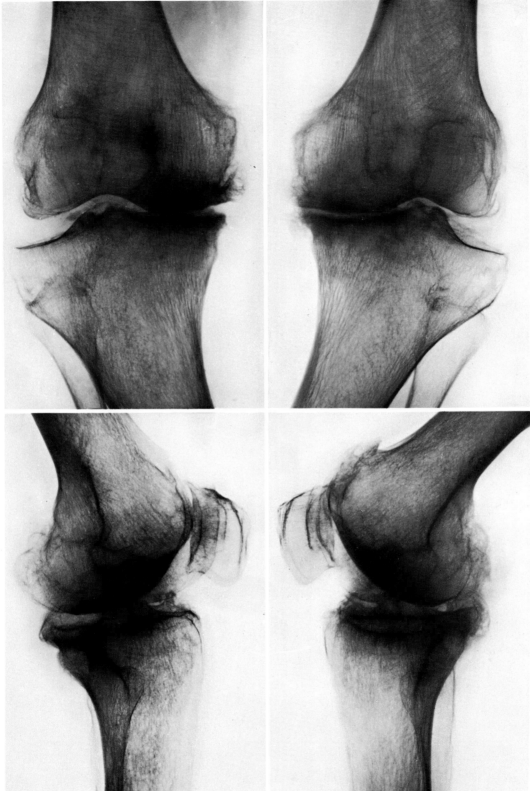

Fig. 28c

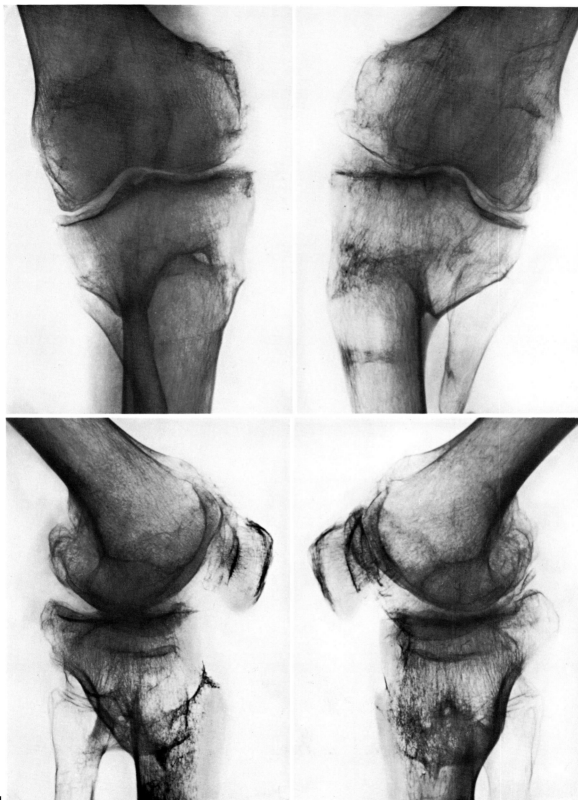

Fig. 28d

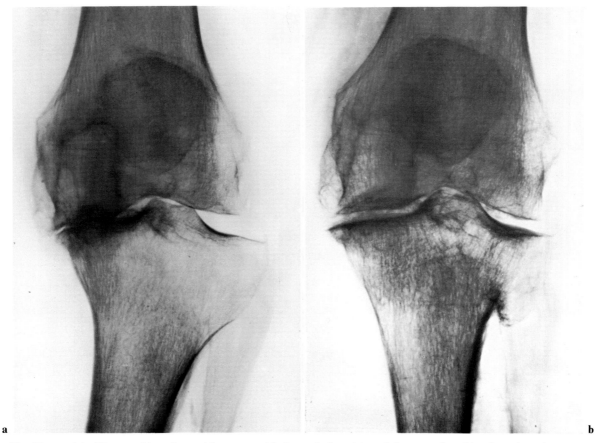

a

b

Fig. 29 a and b. 79-year-old patient with an unstable knee, before (**a**) and 5 years after (**b**) a barrel-vault osteotomy overcorrecting the varus deformity

tion of a lateral wedge between the joint and the insertion of the patella tendon can indeed be carried out relatively accurately. But it cannot be used for the correction of large deformities, because the space between the tibial tuberosity and the joint is seldom large enough to allow excision of a wide wedge. Fixation of the fragments with staples often needs to be supplemented by plaster immobilization, after which flexion of the knee may be limited. If performed below the anterior tuberosity of the tibia, the osteotomy heals much more slowly and does not permit a simultaneous anterior displacement of the patella tendon. It requires longer immobilization or formidable internal fixation.

The barrel-vault osteotomy as described above combines an accurate overcorrection of the varus deformity and an anterior displacement of the patella tendon, without any troublesome bulge below the knee. It does not require plaster immobiliza-

tion and allows immediate weight-bearing. The advantage of a forward displacement of the tibial tuberosity has been explained elsewhere (BANDI, 1972; GUILLAMON et al., 1977; MAQUET, 1963, 1976), and will be restated below.

The purpose of overcorrecting a varus deformity is to compensate for the weakness of the lateral muscles. It has been demonstrated that this weakness represents the most common primary cause of OA with subsequent varus deformity (BLAIMONT, 1970; MAQUET, 1967b).

Supracondylar Osteotomy of the Femur

In most cases of lateral OA with a valgus deformity, a barrel-vault osteotomy of the tibia would entail an unacceptable obliquity of the tibial plateaux in relation to the axis of the tibia and to the line of action of the resultant force R. There-

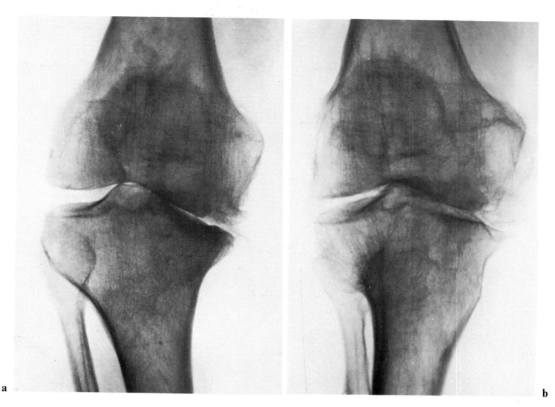

Fig. 30 a and b. 62-year-old patient before (**a**) and 10 years after (**b**) a barrel-vault osteotomy overcorrecting the varus deformity

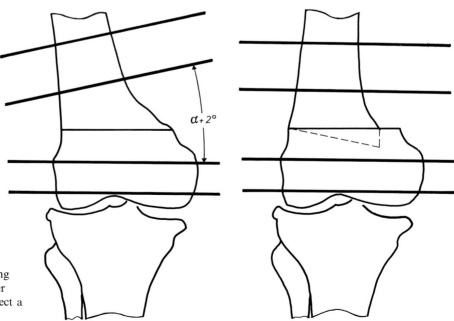

Fig. 31. Pre-operative planning for an osteotomy of the lower end of the femur to overcorrect a valgus deformity

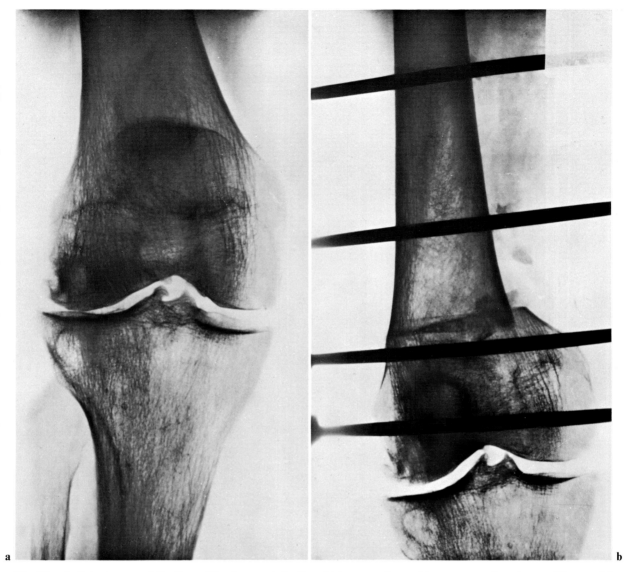

Fig. 32 a–d. Osteotomy and fixation of the fragments by four Steinmann pins and two compression clamps. 74-year-old patient before (**a**) and after (**b**) surgery, 4 months later (**c**) and 3 years later (**d**)

fore, a supracondylar osteotomy of the femur is usually indicated in these cases, as explained above in more detail.

The operation must be planned graphically (Fig. 31). On a tracing of an AP X-ray of the weight-bearing knee, two pairs of transverse lines are drawn, one through the condyles, approximately parallel to the joint space, and the other through the lower end of the shaft of the femur. They form an angle $\alpha + 1°$ to $2°$, open medially. The osteotomy is transverse and supracondylar.

Surgery is carried out through a medial incision. Two Steinmann pins are inserted parallel to the lower lines of the pre-operative diagram and two more parallel to the upper, using the pin guide to ensure accuracy. The four pins are in the same coronal plane. After a transverse osteotomy, sparing part of the lateral cortex, which is used as a hinge, and bevelling the medial corner of the proximal fragment, the fragments are impacted medially until the Steinmann pins are parallel (Fig. 32). The pins are fixed by two compression

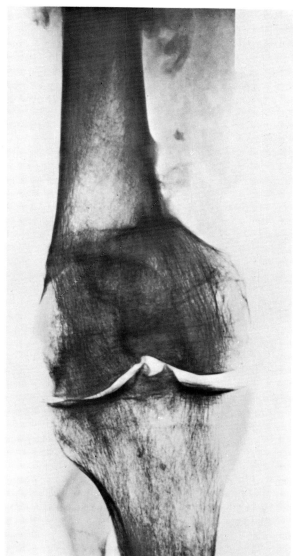
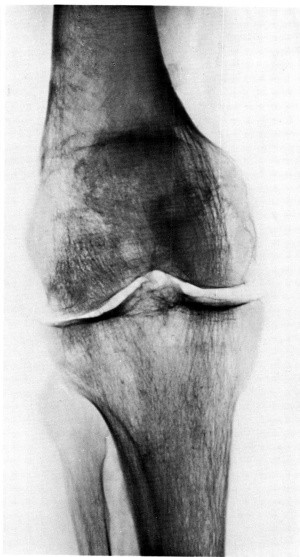

c d

clamps, each equipped with four mobile units. The impaction of the fragments is easy in elderly patients with soft bones. In younger patients a wedge with a medial base may have to be resected.

The patient walks and puts weight on the treated leg from the day after surgery. The pins are removed after 2 months.

In the author's experience, the clinical results and the radiological changes demonstrate a redistribution of the stresses over the largest possible articular surfaces, as long as the overcorrection has been sufficient to bring back the resultant force R to the centre of gravity of the femoro-tibial

articular surfaces. The subchondral scleroses tend to become symmetrical and the structure of the cancellous bone under both tibial plateaux becomes more nearly normal (Fig. 33). Gross laxity in the coronal plane does not influence the end results: when the overcorrection is sufficient, the ligaments tighten spontaneously and the laxity regresses or even disappears. The good results are lasting (Fig. 34).

Distal femoral osteotomy is thus generally indicated in OA with a valgus deformity. However, in some cases a second-stage osteotomy may be required to restore a proper alignment of the leg

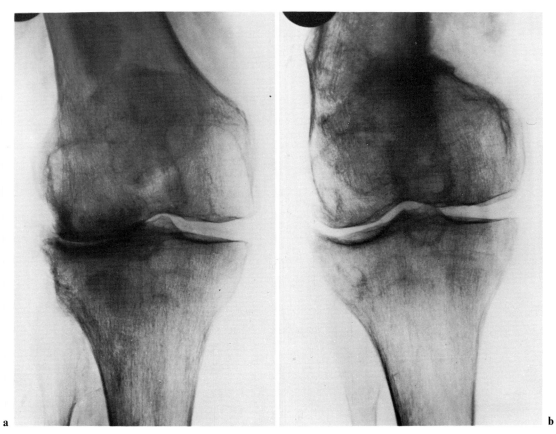

a   b

Fig. 33 a and b. 73-year-old female patient before (**a**) and 1 year after (**b**) an osteotomy of the lower end of the femur overcorrecting the valgus deformity

after the knee has healed following an exaggerated overcorrection of a valgus deformity through a supracondylar osteotomy. Then the realignment (=correction of the varus deformity) must be achieved through a new osteotomy of the lower end of the femur. In such cases the approach is lateral and the angle formed by the Steinmann pins opens laterally.

Patello-femoral OA Treated by Advancement of the Tibial Tuberosity

In the treatment of OA of the patello-femoral joint, the aim of surgery is to diminish and eventually to recentre the force R_5, which compresses the patella against the femur. This aim can be attained by displacing the tibial tuberosity forward and, if necessary, medially (MAQUET, 1963, 1974, 1976a and b).

The incision is medial to the tibial crest, about 15 cm long, through skin and periosteum. It starts from the tibial tuberosity and extends distally. The patella tendon is dissected free from its lateral attachments. The bone is divided parallel to the tibial crest to allow advancement of the crest and of the tuberosity together with the insertion of the patella tendon (Fig. 35). The advancement is maintained by inserting iliac grafts between the tuberosity and the main part of the tibia. The anterior displacement must be sufficient to ensure a significant change in magnitude of the compressive force R_5. The patient walks immediately after surgery.

The anterior displacement of the patella tendon lengthens the lever arm of force Pa somewhat. The force that must be exerted by the patella tendon to achieve a specific extension moment is thus reduced, and so therefore is the compressive force R transmitted from the femur to the tibia. But the procedure acts mainly by opening the angle β formed by the quadriceps tendon Mv and the

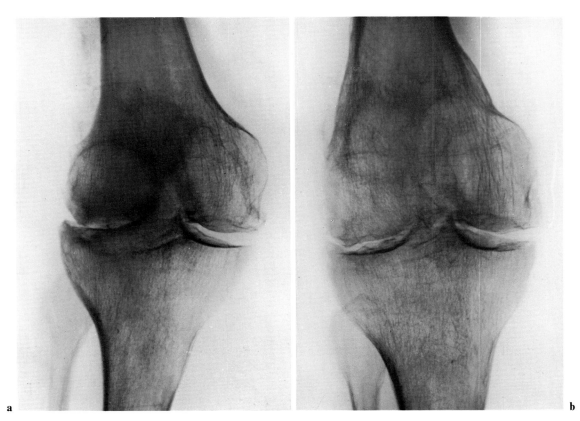

Fig. 34 a and b. 66-year-old female patient before (**a**) and 8 years after (**b**) a distal femoral osteotomy overcorrecting the valgus deformity

patella tendon Pa (Fig. 36). An advancement of 2 cm decreases the force R_5 compressing the patella against the femur by about 50% (Table 1). Beyond 2 cm, medial and lateral relief incisions are sometimes called for to avoid tension in the skin. Even so there is a risk of skin necrosis at the apex of the anterior bulge. When this happens, the skin finally heals, although slowly. This is the most common complication of this procedure.

An anterior displacement of the tibial tuberosity reduces the force R_5 more considerably in extension or near-extension. During the phases of gait when the quadriceps muscle acts, the flexion demanded of the knee is less than 30°. Therefore the effects of an anterior displacement of the patella tendon are exerted at the most favourable phases of gait, when the mechanical stresses are at their greatest and the degree of flexion is small.

Here again, in the author's experience, the postoperative outcome demonstrates the mechanical effect of the procedure: pain disappears and the range of movement is improved. On the X-ray,

Table 1. Decrease of patello-femoral compressive force caused by 2 cm advancement of tibial tuberosity (MAQUET, 1976b)

Phases	Pull of the patella tendon		Patello-femoral compressive force	
	before P_a (kg)	after surgery P_a (kg)	before R_5 (kg)	after surgery R'_5 (kg)
12	283.149	257.408	218.992	102.889
13	146.920	133.564	126.847	64.801
14	157.042	142.765	124.646	60.018
15	48.790	44.354	33.468	14.874

the cup-shaped subchondral sclerosis in the patella is replaced by a thin dense ribbon underlying the articular surface, the embodiment of an even distribution of reduced stresses (Fig. 37).

When the patella is laterally subluxated, a medial displacement must be combined with advancement of the tibial tuberosity. This distributes the compressive force R_5 over larger load-transmitting sur-

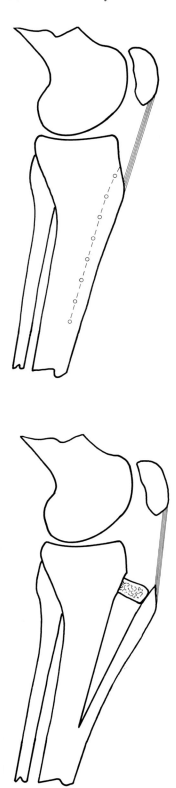

Fig. 35. Anterior displacement of the patella tendon by splitting and moving forward the tibial crest

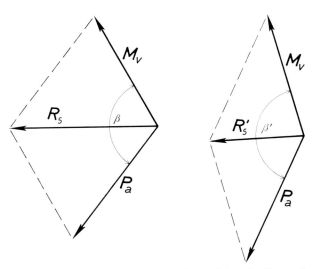

Fig. 36. Opening of the angle β formed by the lines of action of M_v and P_a decreases the magnitude of resultant force R_5

faces and thus further decreases the resultant stresses (Fig. 38). Anterior and medial displacement of the tuberosity is carried out by inserting an iliac graft in which two notches have been cut, one anterior to retain the lateral cortex of the tuberosity, and the other posterior to abut against the lateral cortex of the main fragment (Fig. 39). The clinical and radiological outcome again confirm the diminution of the stresses in the patello-femoral joint (Fig. 40).

This operation can complement an osteotomy of the lower femur when patello-femoral OA is associated with femoro-tibial OA with a valgus deformity.

The anterior displacement of the distal fragment with the tibial tuberosity, obtained by means of the barrel-vault osteotomy, as described above, achieves the same goal of reducing the compressive forces R_5 and R. The post-operative change in the structure of the patella demonstrates that this aim is attained.

Advancement of the tibial tuberosity, if necessary combined with a medial displacement, is indicated both for severe OA of the patello-femoral joint and for persisting chondromalacia patellae. It has been combined with total synovectomy in RA of the knee with some very good results. It is used after a patellectomy to improve the efficiency of the quadriceps muscle by lengthening the lever arm of its tendon (KAUFER, 1971; Fig. 41). It has a mechanical effect opposite to that of a patellectomy.

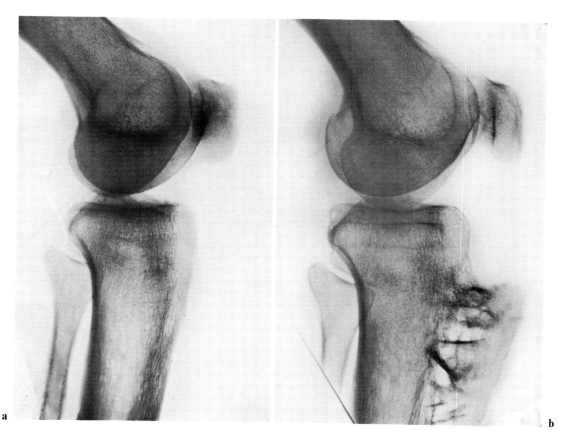

Fig. 37 a and b. 53-year-old female patient before (**a**) and 5 years after (**b**) an anterior displacement of the tibial tuberosity. The cup-shaped density in the patella has regressed

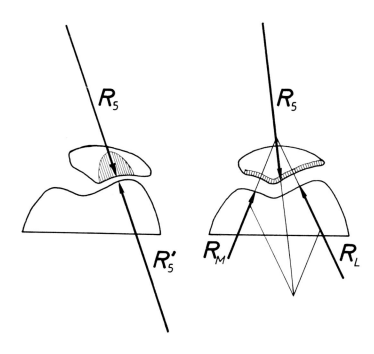

Fig. 38. Brought back into the intercondylar groove, the patella transmits the load to the medial condyle as well as to the lateral

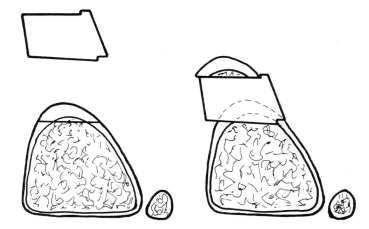

Fig. 39. Anterior and medial displacement of the patella tendon. Horizontal cross-section of the proximal extremity of the lower leg

Post-operative Tissue Changes

The author's experience has been that during the months following a barrel-vault osteotomy of the tibia, a supracondylar osteotomy of the femur, or an anterior displacement of the tibial tuberosity, provided these have redistributed the stresses appropriately in the joint, not only do the subchondral scleroses and the structure of the cancellous bone under the articular surfaces return to normal, but a large joint space reappears between those parts of the bones that were previously in direct contact. It must be remembered that all the AP X-rays upon which this conclusion is based were taken with the patient standing with full weight on the knee. The reappearance of a joint space on the X-rays during standing implies the growth of tissue. It was thus of some interest to determine what kind of tissue regenerates in a joint restored to tolerable pressures, probably of physiological magnitude. To this end, FUJISAWA et al. (1976) carried out a series of arthroscopies of the knee just before surgery and 2 years later. They also biopsied the load-transmitting surfaces of the joint in the area that was pre-operatively overstressed. Before surgery, the eburnated bone was seen on both femoral and tibial articular surfaces (Fig. 42a). In those cases in which overcorrection of the deformity had been sufficient, white smooth tissue similar to cartilage covered the joint surfaces 2 years after surgery (Fig. 42b). Under the microscope, this tissue appeared to be fibro-cartilage with a tendency to remodel into hyaline cartilage in its deep layers (Fig. 43).

This outcome demonstrates the capacity of the tissues of the skeleton for repair. When subjected to appropriate stressing, these tissues regenerate and differentiate into specific varieties such as cartilage. This again confirms the concepts of PAUWELS (1965, 1973a and b).

Clinical and Radiological Results

A follow-up of 201 knees, 100 treated for medial OA (Table 2), 41 for lateral OA (Table 3), and 60 for patello-femoral OA (Table 4) has been published elsewhere (MAQUET, 1976). The classification of the results is oversimplified but still permits practical conclusions.

	Clinical	Radiological
Excellent	Relief of pain, range of movement maintained or improved, stability	Disappearance of the dense areas indicating excessive pressure, reappearance of a joint space
Good	Relief of pain, range of movement slightly diminished, stability	Disappearance of the dense subchondral areas, persistence of a narrow joint space
Fair	Intermittent pain, range of movement diminished, stability	Diminution of the dense subchondral areas, persistence of a narrow joint space
Poor	Deterioration or no amelioration	

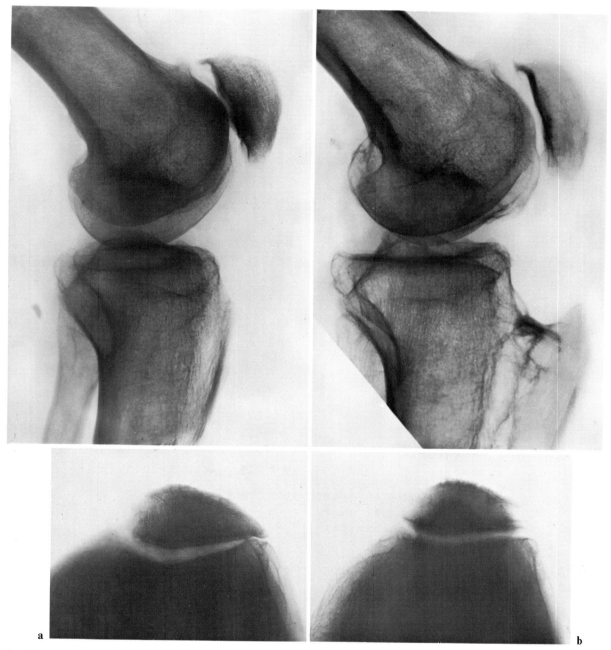

Fig. 40a and b. 43-year-old patient before (**a**) and 5 years after (**b**) an anterior and medial displacement of the tibial tuberosity

The follow-up ranged from 1 to 12 years. Most of the tibial and femoral osteotomies had been carried out according to the procedures described above and some according to other methods previously in use. From this review one conclusion appeared obvious: exact restitution of the anatomical alignment of the knee (i.e., no residual varus or valgus deformity) gives only a small percentage of satisfactory results (6 out of 16 operations). Undercorrection leads to failure as a rule (5 poor and 2 fair results out of 7 operations). When surgery recreates a proper distribution and diminution

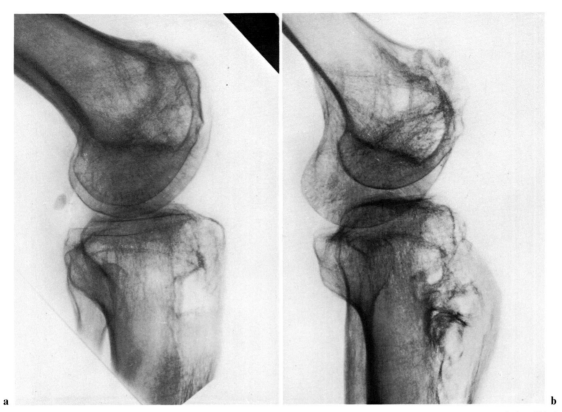

a   b

Fig. 41 a and b. 39-year-old patient after patellectomy (**a**) improved by an anterior displacement of the tibial tuberosity (**b**)

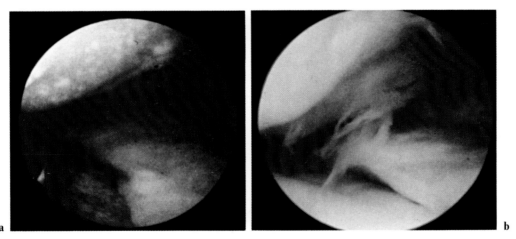

a   b

Fig. 42a and b. Arthroscopy of the overstressed compartment of an osteoarthritic knee with a varus deformity (**a**). Arthroscopy of the same area 2 years and 3 months after an osteotomy of the upper end of the tibia overcorrecting the deformity (**b**): the meniscus appears between the two articular surfaces covered by smooth white tissue [Y. FUJISAWA, K. MASUHARA, N. MATSUMOTO, N. MII, H. FUJIHARA, T. YAMAGUCHI and S. SHIOMI: The effect of High Tibial Osteotomy on Osteoarthritis of the Knee. An Arthroscopic Study. Clinical Orthopaedic Surgery., **11** (576–590) 1976]. Permission to use these pictures has been granted by the authors and by Igaku Schoin Ltd

Table 2. Results of treatment of osteoarthritis with varus deformity (100 knees) (MAQUET, 1976b).

Old techniques: 12 knees

Results:	excellent	good	fair	poor	dead
after restitution of anatomical form	—	1	1	1	—
after overcorrection	—	5	—	1 (complication)	—
after loss of correction	—	—	1	2[a]	—

Present technique: 88 knees

Results:	excellent	good	fair	poor	dead
after restitution of anatomical form	1	—	—	1	—
after overcorrection	68	9	2 (complication)	3	1
after loss of correction	—	—	—	3[b]	—

[a] One case was revised with success by the present technique. The other (85 years old) died after reoperation.
[b] 2 Reoperated on with early success

Table 3. Results of treatment of osteoarthritis with valgus deformity (41 knees) (MAQUET, 1976b).

Proximal tibial osteotomy: 21 knees

Old techniques: 8 knees

Results:	excellent	good	fair	poor	dead
after restitution of anatomical form	1	—	—	2	2
after overcorrection	2	1	—	—	—
after loss of correction	—	—	—	—	—

Present technique: 13 knees

Results:	excellent	good	fair	poor	dead
after restitution of anatomical form	3	—	—	2	—
after overcorrection	3	3	1	—	1
after loss of correction	—	—	—	—	—

Distal femoral osteotomy: 20 knees

Results:	excellent	good	fair	poor	dead
after restitution of anatomical form	2	2	1	—	—
after overcorrection	5	5	—	2	2
after loss of correction	—	—	1	—	—

Table 4. Results of treatment of patello-femoral osteoarthritis, chondromalacia of the patella, and osteoarthritis involving the whole knee. 60 knees (MAQUET, 1976b).

Anterior displacement of the patella tendon:

by elevating the tendon or the tibial crest: 58 knees
cases reviewed: 57

Results:	excellent	good	fair	poor	death
	48	8	—	1	—

by proximal tibial osteotomy: 2 knees

Results:	excellent	good	fair	poor
	1	—	—	1

of the articular compressive stresses, usually by overcorrecting the deformity, the results are excellent or good in the majority of patients (167 out of 184 operations). These results confirm the biomechanical theory proposed, in that they show that the mechanical effect of surgery is the decisive factor, rather than the biological effect obtained merely by dividing the bone.

Anterior displacement of the tibial tuberosity improved OA of the patello-femoral joint in most cases. The results obtained are significantly better than those in other reported series (BANDI, 1972).

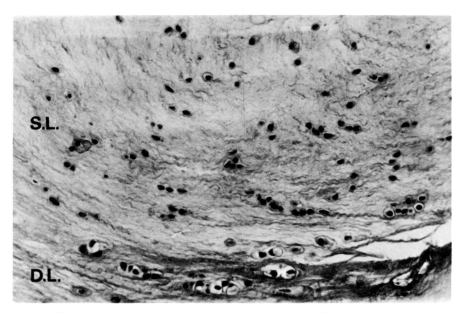

Fig. 43. Histologic appearance of a post-operative biopsy from the tissue covering the articular surfaces of a pre-operatively overstressed compartment [Y. FUJISAWA, K. MASUHARA, N. MATSUMOTO, N. MII, H. FUJIHARA, T. YAMAGUCHI and S. SHIOMI: The effect of High Tibial Osteotomy on Osteoarthritis of the Knee. An Arthroscopic Study. Clinical Orthopaedic Surgery., 11 (576–590) 1976]. Permission to use these pictures has been granted by the authors and by Igaku Schoin Ltd.

The difference probably depends on the magnitude of the anterior displacement. Displacement of 2 cm is the minimum; with any lesser displacement the risk of a poor result increases considerably.

In the author's series, the most common complication after tibial osteotomy has been paralysis of the extensors of the foot, temporary in nine cases and persistent paresis in seven. Two of these patients have been explored. On re-operation yellow degenerative tissue was found in the anterior compartment of the lower leg, the nerves appearing intact. The complication seems to result from compression and subsequent necrosis of the anterior muscles of the lower leg, and particularly of the tibialis anterior, probably by a haematoma induced either by the introduction of the lower Steinmann pin or by the osteotomy itself. To avoid this complication, the distal Steinmann pin is now introduced by hand, avoiding the air-powered drill, and post-operative suction drainage is used in the fibular wound as well as at the tibial osteotomy site. Infection of pin tracks has not been a significant problem. Tilting of the upper tibial fragment occurred in three cases in which the anterior displacement of the lower fragment had been exaggerated. Death from pulmonary embolism was related in three cases to prolonged immobilization required by the use of an earlier technique, and in two cases to the use of a tourniquet. This has now been discarded.

These results compare favourably with those of other series if one keeps in mind that the indications in this series extend to severe deformities and even to subluxated joints, which most authors consider inappropriate for osteotomy. Furthermore, this type of surgery was often carried out on elderly patients, some of them being very poor operative risks.

COVENTRY claims 76 good results (88%) in 86 knees with a follow-up of 1–9 years, although "The changes observed on these roentgenograms[1] showed little or no correlation with the clinical findings postoperatively, in contrast to the roentgenographic changes after subtrochanteric osteotomy for osteoarthritis of the hip." For his planning, COVENTRY relied on X-rays showing part of the femoral and tibial shafts. Therefore his corrections cannot have been accurate. His results are evaluated only from a clinical point of view. They would not be as good if the X-ray changes were

---

[1]   One year or more after operation.

also considered. These changes are actually the only objective signs that forecast the future of the knee.

DEBEYRE and ARTIGOU reviewed 260 knees, 192 varus and 68 valgus, most of which had been treated with an osteotomy below the tibial tuberosity. They found 71.1% of the clinical results were good, with 77.4% showing stabilization or improvement and 22.5% deterioration of the X-ray picture. The follow-up ranged between 18 months and 19 years. It appeared that 55% of the cases had been properly corrected, 30.7% undercorrected, and 14.2% overcorrected. But again the measurement of the deformity was not carried out on X-rays of the whole leg, so that it cannot have been accurate.

Of 51 knees (45 varus, 6 valgus) treated with osteotomy above the tibial tuberosity and followed-up for at least 5 years, INSALL claims complete or nearly complete relief of pain in 30 (59%). Ten were undercorrected. INSALL attributed the failure to the severity of the deformity and recommended the avoidance of osteotomy for malalignment of more than 10°. More than 15° would definitely be a contra-indication. Actually 12 of the 15 knees that INSALL regarded as failures are associated with undercorrection, and only 3 with overcorrection. "All of the bad results were associated with under- or overcorrection and most became obvious in the first year." Since the deformity is measured on X-rays covering only part of the femoral and tibial shaft, the accuracy of this evaluation must once again be doubted. Nevertheless, undercorrection seems to share a greater responsibility for the failures than the degree of initial deformity.

In a series of 70 knees subjected to surgery, JACKSON et al. found 50 pain-free (70%), 17 improved, and 3 unimproved. They carried out the osteotomy below the tibial tuberosity, which may be the cause of the three delayed unions, which required bone grafting. Here again pre-operative planning and the evaluation of the deformity do not seem to have been very accurate.

MACINTOSH and WELSH (1977) also restricted the upper tibial osteotomy to cases "with a reasonably stable ligament structure": "The deformity corrected ranged from zero to 20 degrees of genu varum." The authors operated "in order to transfer the load from the worn to the comparatively normal compartment." They carried out a simultaneous débridement, the usefulness of which the present author doubts in view of his own results

in knees that were not opened. Among 135 knees with a follow-up of at least 1 years, MACINTOSH and WELSH claim 82.2% good or satisfactory results (78 good, 33 satisfactory, 24 poor). They judge these results only from a clinical point of view ("relief from pain, correction of deformity, and improvement in function") and do not mention radiological changes as the criterion of evaluation.

Reviewing 57 knees after BENJAMIN's double osteotomy, TRICKEY (BENJAMIN, 1969), reports 22 knees greatly improved among 36 knees with OA and 14 greatly improved among 21 knees with RA. This is based on the patients' final assessment. But "it was found to be impossible to measure a valgus or varus deformity before operation in the presence of a flexion deformity" and "the operation was not undertaken in cases with severe deformity... Radiographs showed that mild deformities had been corrected." The results are judged according to relief of pain, range of movement, and stability, assessed by the patient. "In only one case did there appear to be any improvement in the radiographic appearance and this was slight." By the present author's rating system, these results would be poor. Such poor results should be expected, however, since the operation fails to alter the mechanical situation significantly. In view of the theory put forward above, and confirmed by consistent clinical and radiological results, double osteotomy no longer seems rational to the present author.

Conclusions

The results of osteotomy, as carried out by the present author and by others, seem to confirm the biomechanical theory proposed in this Chapter. These results therefore suggest the following conclusions:

1) In OA of the knee the aim of surgery must not consist simply in restoring the anatomical alignment of the knee, but rather in reducing the mechanical stresses in the joint sufficiently to make them tolerable for the tissues. This is often achieved at the price of producing a slight deformity in the direction of over-correction.

2) A sufficient reduction of the mechanical stresses generally leads to a regression of the clinical symptoms and of the radiological signs of OA. This is the equivalent of healing.

3) To achieve such results, each case must be carefully analysed, the operation planned with drawings, and the surgical procedure carried out with the utmost accuracy.

Acknowledgement. I would like to thank Mr. R.J. Furlong, FRCS, for his help in phrasing the text of this Chapter.

References

Bandi, W.: Chondromalacia patellae und femoro-patellare Arthrose. Helv. Chir. Acta Suppl. 2 (whole issue) (1972)

Benjamin, A.: Double osteotomy of the painful knee in rheumatoid arthritis and osteoarthritis with an independent assessment of results by E.L. Trickey. J. Bone Joint Surg. (Br.) **51**, 694 (1969)

Blaimont, P.: The curviplane osteotomy in the treatment of the knee arthrosis, p. 443. S.I.C.O.T. XIe Congrès, Mexico 1970

Blaimont, P., Burnotte, J., Baillon, J.M., Duby, P.: Contribution biomécanique à l'étude des conditions d'équilibre dans le genou normal et pathologique. Acta Orthop. Belg. **37**, 573 (1971)

Bouilet, R., Van Gaver, Ph.: L'arthrose du genou. Etude pathogénique et traitement. Acta Orthop. Belg. **27**, 1 (1961)

Coventry, M.B.: Osteotomy of the upper portion of the tibia for degenerative arthritis of the knee: a preliminary report. J. Bone Joint Surg. (Am.) **47**, 984 (1965)

Coventry, M.B.: Osteotomy for genuarthrosis, p. 358. S.I.C.O.T. XIe Congrès, Mexico 1970

Coventry, M.B.: Osteotomy about the knee for degenerative and rheumatoid arthritis. Indications, operative technique and results. J. Bone Joint Surg. (Am.) **55**, 23 (1973)

Debeyre, J., Artigou, J.M.: Les indications et les résultats de l'ostéotomie tibiale. Rev. Chir. Orthop. **59**, 641 (1973)

Fick, R.: Handbuch der Anatomie und Mechanik der Gelenke, Vol. III, p. 535. Jena: Fischer 1910

Fujisawa, Y., Masuhara, K., Matsumoto, N., Mii, N., Fujihara, H., Yamaguchi, T., Shomi, S.: The effect of high tibial osteotomy on osteoarthritis of the knee. An arthroscopic. study of 26 knee joints. Clin. Orthop. Surg. (Japan) **2**, 576 (1976)

Guillamon, J.L., Lord, G., Marotte, J.H., Blanchard, J.P.: Traitement de l'arthrose fémoro-patellaire par la transposition antérieure de la tubérosité tibiale (selon Maquet). Rev. Chir. Orthop. **63**, 545 (1977)

Harding, M.L.: A fresh appraisal of tibial osteotomy for osteoarthritis of the knee. Clin. Orthop. **114**, 223 (1976)

Herbert, J.J.: Les techniques d'ostéotomie. Rev. Chir. Orthop. **53**, 173–187 (1977)

Herbert, J.J., Bouillet, R., Debeyre, J., de Marchin, P., Duparc, J., Ficat, P., Gariépy, J., Judet, J., Maquet, P., Masse, P., Ramadier, O., Simonet, J., Trillat, A.: Symposium sur les gonarthroses d'origine statique. Rev. Chir. Orthop. **53**, 107 (1967)

Husson, A.: The functional anatomy of the knee joint: the closed kinematic chain as a model of a knee joint. The knee joint. Amsterdam: Excerpta Medica 1973a

Husson, A.: La chaîne cinématique fermée. Bull. Assoc. Anat. (Nancy) **57**, 159 (1973b)

Husson, A.: Biomechanische Probleme des Kniegelenks. Orthopäde **3**, 127 (1974)

Insall, J., Shoji, H., Mayer, V.: High tibial osteotomy. J. Bone Joint Surg. (Am.) **56**, 1397 (1974)

Insall, J., Falvo, K.A., Wise, D.W.: Chondromalacia patellae. A prospective study. J. Bone Joint Surg. (Am.) **58**, 1 (1976)

Izadpanah, M., Keönch-Fraknóy, S.: Entlastung des medialen oder lateralen Kniegelenkanteiles ohne Varisierungs- oder Valgisierungsosteotomie. Z. Orthop. **115**, 21 (1977a)

Izadpanah, M., Keönch-Fraknóy, S.: Statische Auswirkung der Varisierungs- bzw. Valgisierungsosteotomie bei Genu valgum and varum. Z. Orthop. **115**, 100 (1977b)

Jackson, J.O., Waugh, W.: Tibial osteotomy for osteoarthritis of the knee. J. Bone Joint Surg. (Br.) **43**, 746 (1961)

Jackson, J.P., Waugh, W., Green, J.P.: High tibial osteotomy for osteoarthritis of the knee. J. Bone Joint Surg. (Br.) **51**, 88–94 (1969)

Jackson, J.P., Waugh, W.: Tibial osteotomy for osteoarthritis of the knee, p. 386. S.I.C.O.T. XIe Congrès, Mexico 1970

Jackson, J.P., Waugh, W.: The technique and complications of upper tibial osteotomy. J. Bone Joint Surg. (Br.) **56**, 236 (1974)

Kaufer, H.: Mechanical function of the patella. J. Bone Joint Surg. (Am.) **53**, 1551 (1971)

Kettelkamp, D.B., Chao, E.Y.: A method for quantitative analysis of medial and lateral compression forces at the knee during standing. Clin. Orthop. **83**, 202 (1972)

Klems, H.: Infrakondyläre Tibiaosteotomie. Stabilizierung mit äußerem Spanner. Indikation, Technik, Komplikationen. Z. Orthop. **114**, 26 (1976)

Kummer, B.: Bauprinzipien des Säugerskeletes. Stuttgart: Georg Thieme 1959

Kummer, B.: Gait and posture under normal conditions with special reference to the lower limbs. Clin. Orthop. **25**, 32 (1962)

Kummer, B.: Die Biomechanik der aufrechten Haltung. Mitteilungen der Naturforschenden Gesellschaft in Bern, N.F. 22, Band 1965. Bern: Haupt 1965

Kummer, B.: Biomechanics of bone: mechanical properties, functional structure, functional adaptation. Biomechanics, its foundations and objectives. FUNG, Y.C., PERRONE, N., ANLIKER, M. (eds.), p. 237. Englewood Cliffs, New Jersey: Prentice Hall 1972

KUMMER, B.: Biomechanischer Grundlagen 'beanspruchungsändernder' Osteotomien im Bereich des Kniegelenks. Z. Orthop. 19, 923 (1977)

LANGE, M.: Orthopädisch-chirurgische Operationslehre, p. 660. München: Bergman 1951

MACINTOSH, D.L.: The surgical treatment of osteoarthritis of the knee, p. 400. S.I.C.O.T. XIe Congrès, Mexico 1970

MACINTOSH, D.L., WELSH, R.P.: Joint debridement. A complement to high tibial osteotomy in the treatment of degenerative arthritis of the knee. J. Bone Joint Surg. (Am.) 59, 1094 (1977)

MAQUET, P.: Considérations biomécaniques sur l'arthrose du genou. Un traitement biomécanique de l'arthrose fémoro-patellaire. L'avancement du tendon rotulien. Rev. Rhum. 30, 779 (1963)

MAQUET, P.: Biomécanique des membres inférieurs. Acta Orthop. Belg. 32, 705 (1966)

MAQUET, P., DE MARCHIN, P.: Guérison, par la chirurgie, des arthroses de la hanche et du genou. Méd. Hyg. (Genève) 25, 1440 (1967)

MAQUET, P., SIMONET, J., DE MARCHIN, P.: Biomécanique du genou et gonarthrose. Rev. Chir. Orthop. 53, 111 (1967a)

MAQUET, P., DE MARCHIN, P., SIMONET, J.: Biomécanique du genou et gonarthrose. Rhumatologie 19, 51 (1967b)

MAQUET, P.: Charge et sollicitation mécanique des os. Le principe du hauban. Rev. Méd. Liège 24, 115 (1969a)

MAQUET, P.: Biomécanique du genou et gonarthrose. Rev. Méd. Liège 24, 170 (1969b)

MAQUET, P.: Biomechanics and osteoarthritis of the knee, p. 317. S.I.C.O.T. XIe Congrès, Mexico 1970

MAQUET, P.: Biomécanique de la gonarthrose. Acta Orthop. Belg. [Suppl.] 38 (1), 33 (1972)

MAQUET, P.: Biomechanische Aspekte der Femur-Patella Beziehungen. Z. Orthop. 112, 620 (1974)

MAQUET, P., VAN DE BERG, A., SIMONET, J.: Femoro-tibial weight bearing areas. J. Bone Joint Surg. (Am.) 57, 766 (1975a)

MAQUET, P., PELZER, G., DE LAMOTTE, F.: La sollicitation mécanique du genou durant la marche. Acta Orthop. Belg. [Suppl.] 41 (1), 119 (1975b)

MAQUET, P.: Advancement of the tibial tuberosity. Clin. Orthop. 115, 225 (1976a)

MAQUET, P.: Biomechanics of the knee. Berlin, Heidelberg, New York: Springer 1976b (French edition: Biomécanique du genou. Springer 1977)

DE MARCHIN, P., MAQUET, P., FONTAINE, J.: Quelques remarques sur la radiographie des genoux arthrosiques, Utilité des clichés 'en charge'. Rev. Méd. Liege 18, 148 (1963a)

DE MARCHIN, P., MAQUET, P., SIMONET, J.: Considérations biomécaniques sur l'arthrose du genou. Quelques remarques sur les radiographies. Rev. Rhum. 30, 775 (1963b)

MASSE, Y.: Résultats de 370 ostéotomies tibiales hautes pour déviation axiale fixées par un matériel angulaire monobloc avec plus de deux ans de recul. Acta Orthop. Belg. 42, 471 (1976)

MENSCHIK, A.: Mechanik des Kniegelenkes. III. Teil. Wien: Sailer 1974

MENSCHIK, A.: Mechanik des Kniegelenkes. I Teil. Z. Orthop. 112, 481 (1974). II Teil. Schlußrotation. Z. Orthop. 113, 388 (1975)

MÜLLER, W.: Biologie der Gelenke. Leipzig: Barth 1929

NITSCH, R., JANSEN, G.: Die Stellung der Suprakondylären Korrekturosteotomie in der Behandlung der Altersgonarthrose. Z. Orthop. 114, 226 (1976)

PAUWELS, F.: Gesammelte Abhandlungen zur funktionellen Anatomie des Bewegungsapparates. Berlin, Heidelberg, New York: Springer 1965

PAUWELS, F.: Atlas zur Biomechanik der gesunden und kranken Hüfte. Prinzipien, Technik und Resultate einer kausalen Therapie. Berlin, Heidelberg, New York: Springer 1973a. English edition: Biomechanics of the Normal and Diseased Hip. Theoretical Foundation, Technique and Results of Treatment. Berlin-Heidelberg-New York: Springer 1976

PAUWELS, F.: Kurzer Überblick über die mechanische Beanspruchung des Knochens und ihre Bedeutung für die funktionelle Anpassung. Z. Orthop. 111, 681 (1973b)

PERRY, J., ANTONELLI, D., FORD, W.: Analysis of knee-joint forces during flexed knee stance. J. Bone Joint Surg. (Am.) 57, 961 (1975)

RADIN, E., PAUL, I.: Does cartilage compliance reduce skeletal impact load? Arthritis Rheum. 13, 139 (1970)

RADIN, E.L., PAUL, I.L., LOWY, M.: A comparison of the dynamic force transmitting properties of subchondral bone and articular cartilage. J. Bone Joint Surg. (Am.) 52, 444 (1970)

RADIN, E.L., PAUL, I.L., ROSE, R.M.: Role of mechanical factors in pathogenesis of primary osteoarthritis. Lancet 1972 1, 519

RAMADIER, J.O.: Prévention et arrêt de l'arthrose du genou avec déviation transversale. Mém. Acad. Chir. 24–25, 815 (1965)

RAMADIER, J.O.: Etude radiologique des déviations dans la gonarthrose. Rev. Chir. Orthop. 53, 139 (1967)

Chapter 9

Tibio-femoral Replacement Using Four Components with Retention of the Cruciate Ligaments (The Polycentric Prosthesis)

R.S. Bryan and L.F.A. Peterson

Mayo Clinic and Mayo Foundation, Rochester, Minnesota 55901 USA

The analysis of normal knee motion and the function of the various ligaments, cartilages, and bony and cartilaginous contours in the control of this motion is a controversial subject. Previous attempts at arthroplasty of the interposition type have had limited success, although the McKeever and MacIntosh metallic tibial plateau replacements achieved fairly widespread use (Potter, 1969). Often, however, the opposing surfaces could not tolerate the stresses placed on them, and pain returned. The goal of pain relief with retention of the ligaments and as much bone as possible, to permit later arthrodesis if necessary, led to attempts to design surface-replacement components as typified by the work of Gunston, Marmor, Buchholz, Savastano, and Charnley.

Historical Development

Polycentric knee arthroplasty was developed by Frank Gunston in John Charnley's laboratory, and was first performed in 1968. Gunston attempted to duplicate the combination of rolling, hinging, gliding, and rotating that comprises normal knee motion (Fig. 1a) by placing semicircular metallic femoral runners in polyethylene tibial tracks with grooves larger than the runners. He incorporated a curve from anterior to posterior in the tracks, but the curve was of considerably larger radius than the femoral components (Fig. 1b). Location of the components far posterior placed the axis of motion near the true instant centres of rotation during knee motion. This represented the earliest attempt to replace the knee joint by a metal–plastic, low-friction, nonhinged interface. Gunston reported his early results to the Canadian Orthopedic Association in June 1969, and subsequently (Gunston, 1971)

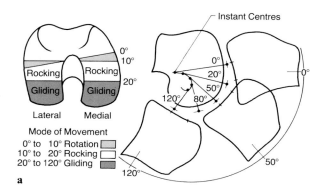

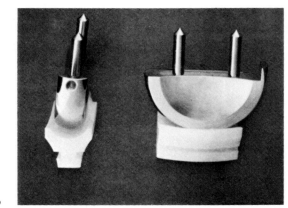

Fig. 1. a Knee motions as depicted by Gunston. Mode of movement: ▨, 0°–10° rotation; □, 10°–20° rocking; ▧, 20°–120° gliding. **b** Original Gunston polycentric knee prostheses. (Gunston, F.H.: Polycentric knee arthroplasty: prosthetic stimulation of normal knee movement. J. Bone Joint Surg. [Br.] **53**, 272–277 (1971). By permission)

reported a series of 22 knees in rheumatoid patients in which the procedure had successfully relieved pain.

After visiting Gunston in December 1969, with his permission we modified the components slightly, making the tibial tracks straight from anterior to posterior and adding fixation grooves

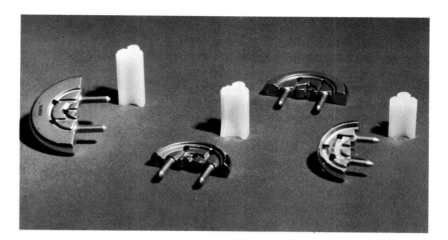

Fig. 2. Mayo variation of polycentric knee prostheses, different sizes

and holes to the femoral prostheses to enhance fixation (Fig. 2). We began clinical use of the modified prosthesis in July 1970 and have operated on 1550 knees since that date. We continue to use this prosthesis in cases of early disease — i.e., in patients without severe bone loss or instability. Initially, the procedure was restricted to rheumatoid patients, but it proved to be even more successful in patients with osteoarthritis (OA). Our early technique embodied several practices, such as creating a posterior wall of cement and drilling holes through the cortex medially and laterally to enhance fixation. These practices subsequently proved to be in error. Despite problems with bone weakening and the application of this method to severe deformities because no other suitable prosthesis was yet available, our success rate has been acceptable.

We have reported our early experiences elsewhere (BRYAN and PETERSON, 1971; BRYAN et al., 1973a and b; PETERSON et al., 1974), including 14 complications in 101 knees. The most worrisome of the complications were anterior subluxation in four knees and deep infection in three. Relief of pain was excellent in 85% of patients.

In 1973, GUNSTON reported on his results in 43 knees operated on during a 5-year interval. Pain was eliminated in 30 knees; there was mild patellofemoral pain in 11, and no relief in 2. Infection in two patients required arthrodesis, and two additional knees were arthrodesed because of technical failure. He reported one patient with component loosening. The range of motion after surgery averaged 91.4° in GUNSTON's series and 97° in ours.

In 1973, we (BRYAN et al., 1973a and b) also reported the early complications in 450 knees: six

deep infections, seven dislocations, six fractures (five stress), three cases of pulmonary embolism, and three cases of clinically diagnosed thrombophlebitis. Four knees developed superficial necrosis, and three had loose tibial prostheses.

In 1976, we reported on 500 polycentric knee arthroplasties in which follow-up was at least 2 years (SKOLNICK et al., 1976). The deep infection rate was 2.8%, with two-thirds of the knees affected requiring arthrodesis. Loosening, usually of a tibial component, was noted in 2.4%, and 10% required re-operation. Relief of pain was achieved in 86%. Early complications involved a rather high rate of abnormal wound healing, which has since been corrected by using a relatively straight incision centered over the medial edge of the patella, extreme gentleness in handling the soft tissues with minimal subcutaneous reflexion of skin, and attention to a careful wound closure over suction drainage. There were eight (1.4%) patients with proved nerve injuries, which were primarily related to the tourniquet or the pressure dressing. Four of the patients recovered completely, and the other four recovered partially.

The clinical incidence of phlebitis was 1.2% and that of pulmonary embolism, 0.5%.

Dislocation occurred in seven knees (1.4%) within 3 months in six patients, and with anterior movement of the tibia in extension in five patients. Most of the dislocations occurred in patients who had severe pre-operative instability and who would not now be considered suitable for this type of arthroplasty.

Seven fatigue fractures (1.4%), usually of the medial tibial plateau, showed us that the bone must be carefully shaped and that the medial components should be as close to the intercondylar notch as possible. Interestingly, in the seven knees with traumatic fracture (five supracondylar and two of the proximal tibia) loosening of the prostheses was rare, and only three required conversion to a different type of knee.

GUNSTON and MACKENZIE (1976) also reported complications in 89 arthroplasties followed for $2–7^1/_2$ years; 77 of the procedures were in rheumatoid patients. There were six infections (7%), with apparent cure in two and arthrodesis in three; all infections were seen early. Loosening occurred in nine knees (10%), posterior subluxation in one, and peroneal palsy (temporary) in three. No late infections had occurred, and the results remained consistent. The authors believed that residual patello-femoral pain was not a major problem in rheumatoid arthritis (RA) and that loosening was related to poor technique or an inappropriate choice of patient.

We reviewed the results of our first 101 arthroplasties, performed in 84 patients between 28 July 1970 and 9 July 1971, after 5 years. These results were reported to the combined meeting of the Orthopedic Associations in London in September 1976 (PETERSON, 1977a and b). Two-thirds of the patients had RA, and information on every patient was obtained by examination, telephone, or letter. Each patient had been examined at 2 years, and 55 patients were examined at 5 years. Seventy-six patients, with 92 arthroplasties, were still alive. Eight patients, with nine arthroplasties, had died of unrelated causes. The results of 80 arthroplasties were satisfactory, without further surgery after 5 years. Twelve patients had been re-operated on, and ten of these had knees that were still functioning well as arthroplasties of some type. Two knees were arthrodesed because of infection. Of the eight patients who died, six had had seven arthroplasties that were excellent, one had fibrous ankylosis, and one had fibrous pseudarthrosis after removal for infection.

The range of motion did not change significantly from 1–5 years after surgery in the patients examined. Relief of pain was complete in 47 patients, and 23 had only mild pain, usually patello-femoral. There were two cases of infection, one superficial and one deep, treated successfully with suction irrigation and antibiotics. Two other infections began after a revision of the total knee and were not related to the primary operation. The last infection occurred $4^1/_2$ years post-operatively due to haematogenous spread from an infected total hip.

Fourteen knees, including those arthrodesed, underwent a total of 23 operations. Most of these were converted to geometric arthroplasties.

Loose components were found in seven re-operations. Pain from the patello-femoral joint or bone impingement also led to re-operation in several patients.

In the year since that report, three additional knees in two of these patients have been re-operated on, two for patello-femoral pain and one for increasing instability due to progression of the RA. One has had polycentric total knee arthroplasty with a patellar replacement of the GUNSTON type, and two have been converted to other types of total knee arthroplasties. None of the tibial tracks in these two patients showed significant wear after 6 years of use, although we were able to define wear in eight knees in the group of 80. We believe that this is most probably due to the methyl methacrylate, because at first we did not understand the necessity for carefully removing any particles that might become loose.

We have now surveyed the second group of 115 arthroplasties (PETERSON et al., unpublished data), performed from July 1971 to January 1972, with the addition of four knee arthroplasties in the same patients performed during spring 1972 (PETERSON et al., 1974). We contacted all the patients. Each patient had been examined at 1 or 2 years (or both) after surgery, and 62 knees were examined at 5 years, while follow-up data on 43 knees were gathered by letter or telephone. Five patients with seven treated knees had died of unrelated causes; three of the knees had been arthrodesed, two because of infection and one because of a Charcot joint. Of the knees in the patients who died, one had been good at 5 years, two good at 3 years, one fair at 3 years, and three good at 2 years.

There were 53 patients with RA, and 24 patients had both knees operated on. An additional 14 of these patients eventually had both knees operated on. Thus, essentially all our rheumatoid patients had progressive disease, and many had three or even four major joint replacements in 5 years. Despite this, 76% of the arthroplasties were considered good by the patient and surgeon after 5 years.

There were 24 patients with 28 affected knees in the OA group. Thus, in only four patients were both knees sufficiently severely involved to warrant replacement, at least in this time span.

As expected, good results were found in 85% of these patients after 5 years, and none of the patients has had further surgery for patellar pain, although this had been predicted by GUNSTON (1973). In contrast, our primary problem with the patella has occurred in our rheumatoid patients as a result of progression of the arthritis in the patello-femoral joint; this is often accompanied by ligamentous laxity and patellar erosion.

All the patients cited above had replacement of both tibio-femoral surfaces, i.e., bicompartmental replacement. Many patients, however, have damage to only half the tibio-femoral articulation, and in 1971 we began to replace only the damaged portion in such patients. These patients were carefully selected and were not suitable for upper tibial osteotomy or other more conservative procedures. Furthermore, they were required to have excellent cartilage on the preserved side of the joint.

The major factors that influenced us to use this method were very advanced patient age, severe unicompartmental laxity (due to bone and cartilage loss), post-traumatic arthritis, and poor vascular status. In addition, we considered valgus deformity to be an indication, because varus osteotomy of the tibia yields less successful results than does a valgus osteotomy for a varus knee.

Recently, we reported on a series involving 214 knees in 179 patients, in which follow-up on unicompartmental replacement ranged from 1–5 years, with a mean of 2.2 years. Previous surgery had been performed in 25% of the knees, and 56% of the patients were men. The ages ranged from 19 to 85 years, with a mean of 65.7. Of 207 knees with follow-up data, 163 (78.7%) were affected by OA, 17 (8.2%) by post-traumatic arthritis, 12 (5.8%) by osteonecrosis, and 8 (3.9%) by RA; miscellaneous diagnoses were recorded in 7 (3.4%). Seven knees were excluded: two of the patients refused follow-up, two died, two were lost to follow-up, and in one case the pre-operative information was inadequate. Unicompartmental polycentric components were used in 91% of the knees and unicompartmental geometric components were used in 9%. Surgical cultures were obtained routinely from 155 knees with primary operations, and isolates were recovered in eight. In addition, positive cultures were obtained from two of the failed knees at revision. None of the 214 knees in this series has at any time shown clinical evidence of infection, but three of the knees with positive cultures eventually failed mechanically and required revision.

Wound healing problems were minor and occurred in only six knees.

Twenty-one (10.1%) of the 207 knees were considered failures, and 16 of these have been revised, at a mean of 26 months after operation. Ten of the failures had a total of 24 prior operations before unicompartmental arthroplasty was done. The reasons for 16 failures requiring revision were loosening in nine, unexplained pain in two, subluxation in two, instability in one, osteochondritis dissecans of the opposite femoral condyle in one, and bony impingement in one. The five knees that were not revised included three with loose tibial components, one that was a technical failure, and one with unexplained pain.

Twenty-five knees (12%) in this series involved wide-track unicompartmental polycentric components. Five of these 25 knees required revision, thus illustrating the unsuitability of this particular design. Of the 16 revisions, 14 involved polycentric components: of the 14 knees, 2 were converted to arthrodesis and 12 involved the use of other components — polycentric bicondylar in 4, geometric in 5, anametric in 1, unicompartmental polycentric in 1, and Crachiola in 1. Two knees with unicompartmental geometric components were converted to geometric total-knee arthroplasties.

Post-operatively, 90% of the patients were relatively free of pain and 96% could walk with no aids or with just a cane. The range of motion averaged 109° but statistically it was not significantly different from the pre-operative range.

Thirteen (62%) of the 21 failures were in varus alignment, and this represented 52% of the knees left in varus after operation. The average post-operative alignment for the failure group was 1.9° varus and for the successful group, 4.5° valgus. Six knees (2.9%) showed radiographical evidence of degenerative changes involving the opposite, unreplaced compartment.

Similar results have been reported by MARMOR (1977) in 87 knees and by SCOTT et al. (1978) in 70 knees with different types of unicompartmental replacements.

This procedure is justified because of the success rate that it has achieved, especially in view of the lessened incidence of complications. The absence of progressive deformity in the remaining anatomical compartment testifies to the careful selection of patients. In this series, the importance of a slightly valgus alignment, which balances one artificial half-joint against the relatively normal half-joint, is convincingly proved. Failures are easily converted into bicompartmental total knee arthroplasties.

Discussion

Justification for the use of unicompartmental arthroplasty was suggested by goniometric tracings of polycentric knee arthroplasties showing comparisons with the normal knee (PETERSON and BRYAN, 1975). The restoration toward normal, with the articular surface velocity being tangential to the point of contact, should theoretically reduce the rate of progression of gonarthrosis in the normal compartment, as implied by FRANKEL et al. (1971). Our experience to date has confirmed this clinically, because progression of arthritis (as evaluated radiographically in the compartment not operated upon) has been found in very few of the 214 knees followed post-operatively for 2–5 years (JONES et al., 1978).

As our experience has increased, we have changed our technique to eliminate problems. The skin incision is now almost straight along the medial edge of the patella, with minimal subcutaneous reflection. The vastus medialis is freed from the quadriceps and the medial border of the patella, and the incision is carried distally on the medial side of the tibial tubercle and extends distal to it for 1–2 in., so that when the patella is reflected and everted laterally the patellar tendon may be partially released in continuity with the periosteum if necessary. The fat pad is partially excised if necessary, and the capsule is reflected medially to give good exposure. The joint is thoroughly debrided of osteophytes, and a synovectomy is done, if indicated. We have found that the osteophytes and the cupping of the tibia and impingement of the tibial spines are the major causes of flexion contractures up to 40°. The femoral prostheses are now placed at an angle of 40°–50° from the horizontal, viewed from the lateral aspect. This does not seem to be critical, but the correction of alignment is, and the various jigs are designed to correct varus and valgus in both femoral and tibial placement.

In practice, the femoral components are fitted so that the knee will only just extend fully with them in place. The anterior edge of the components should be flush with the femur, because this increases the range of flexion and avoids patellar impingement. The medial prosthesis is placed as close to the intercondylar notch as possible. The two femoral components are parallel and are perpendicular to the coronal plane of the knee; they also point to the hip joint rather than along the line of the femur. The tibial tracks are outlined by first marking the contact point of the femoral components on the tibia at 0° and at 90°. With the knee at 15° of flexion, parallel lines or shallow saw cuts along each side of the femoral prosthesis furnish an approximate compromise to allow rotation, and if the two previously marked points of contact are connected by a line, the true desired track will lie between these two sets of marks. The tracks are then cut to the exact depth of the polyethylene component unless further varus or valgus correction is needed, in which case the depth may be adjusted. The posterior $^1/_8$ in. of cortex is left intact, and the longest possible tracks are used, to increase the support. The bottom of the track is notched and a curette hole is made in each track to prevent migration, which did occur in a few patients early in the series. There should be almost no cement exposed in the joint upon completion of the operation, and the alignment should be 0°–5° of valgus in full extension, with contact of the components maintained to beyond 90° of flexion.

Polycentric total knee arthroplasty is a technically demanding procedure, but permits retention of bone and ligaments while correcting alignment, relieving pain, and increasing stability. Conversion to any other type of total knee arthroplasty may be readily accomplished, and arthrodesis after polycentric arthroplasty has been readily attained by the compression method of CHARNLEY. Dislocations in our series all occurred early, and usually in patients whom we would now consider to be unsuitable candidates.

We believe there are six contra-indications to this procedure: (1) absence or weakness of the posterior cruciate or medial collateral ligament; (2) severe bone loss, especially of the opposing femur and tibia; (3) flexion deformity of more than 40°; (4) varus or valgus deformity of more than 15°; (5) uncorrectable hyperextension; and (6) neurogenic arthropathy. In addition, extreme osteoporosis and previous sepsis require caution and may be contra-indications.

We believe that this arthroplasty, by its design, provides lateral stability while permitting normal knee motion. The wide-track polycentric arthroplasty has been discarded because it did not provide this lateral stability (BLOOM and BRYAN, 1977). GUNSTON's tibial design, by its antero-posterior concavity, provided greater antero-posterior stability, but did so at the expense of increased loosening. Wear has not proved to be a major cause of failure at 5 years, but technical error has. Alignment has proved to be the major factor in late failure, with technique of cementing and progression of arthritis next in importance. Knees that were explored for revision have shown a continuing erosion of bone in the rheumatoid patients and often a fibro-cartilaginous resurfacing in areas where bone-to-bone contact has occurred.

We still prefer this type of arthroplasty in the proper patient, because the results at 5 years, as noted, are most acceptable and because failure permits conversion to other nonhinged types without severe loss of bone. In fact, failures other than those due to sepsis may often be attributed to improper selection of the prostheses for the problems involved or inaccurate performance of the procedure. When total knee replacement is considered, one should always keep in mind the potential difficulties should the procedure fail (PETERSON, 1977a). The goals of the surgery should be tempered by this thought, and in certain patients the goal should be reduced to provide more options should failure ensue.

In 1973, MARMOR reported on a series of 32 patients in whom surface replacement with four components had been performed. The metallic femoral components were curved to the shape of the condyles (Fig. 3), while the polyethylene tibial components were flat and were inset into the tibial plateaus, leaving a rim of cortical bone. This type was called "modular" and was very similar to the St. Georg or sledge knee arthroplasty (Fig. 4) that was developed in Germany in 1969 (ENGELBRECHT et al., 1976). Similar types have been designed in several different centres, with minor modifications and different names attached. MARMOR (1976) reported on 105 patients with 126 knee replacements followed for at least 2 years. Sixty-five knees were rheumatoid and 54 were osteoarthritic, but only 16 RA and 5 OA patients had bilateral arthroplasties. There were 5 deep and 32 superficial infections before he began to use suction drainage and antibiotics. In ten patients loosening occurred, which he considered to be related to use of the thin (6 mm) tibial components. He rated the results as excellent in 52% and good in 36% of the knees at 2 years.

LASKIN (1976) reported on 58 OA patients and 31 RA patients in whom modular replacement had been performed. He eliminated from his series any patients with bilateral replacement. He believed that contra-indications were varus–valgus instability of more than 20°, combined varus–valgus instability with flexion contracture of more than 40°,

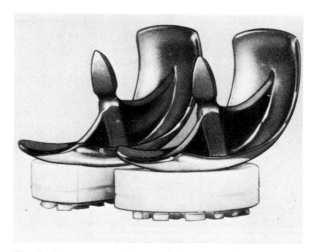

Fig. 3. Marmor modular total knee prostheses. (MARMOR, L.: The modular knee. Clin. Orthop. **94**, 242–248 (1973). By permission of the J.B. Lippincott Company)

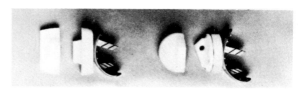

Fig. 4. Sledge, Buchholz, or St. Georg total knee prostheses. (From ENGELBRECHT, E., SIEGEL, A. RÖTTGER, J., BUCHHOLZ, H.W.: Statistics of total knee replacement: partial and total knee replacement, design St. Georg; a review of a 4-year observation. Clin. Orthop. **120**, 54–64 (1976). By permission of the J.B. Lippincott Company)

marked recurvatum, and predominantly patello-femoral symptoms. In about 60% of the patients complete relief of pain was attained, and an additional 35% had only mild pain. Range of motion did not change much, just as in the polycentric knees, but the ability to walk long distances without support was enhanced, also as in the polycentric group.

Both the polycentric and the modular knees are used for unicompartmental replacement successfully and have been equally successful in the range of 90% with a very low infection rate (JONES et al., 1978; MARMOR, 1977). Surface replacement with metal–polyethylene opposing surfaces is an alternative and conservative approach to knee disease, whether RA or OA. Many of the dire predictions made by experts in regard to wear have not proved true, despite point weight-bearing in each of these types. Loosening has been more of a problem with modular than with the polycentric knee arthroplasty, despite its unconstrained surface. MARMOR believes that this is due to the 6-mm tibial component, but it may also be due to increase in tilting forces as the femoro-tibial contact area approaches the periphery of the component, because of its totally unconstrained design. The principal advantages of these types are the utilisation of the normal ligamentous and muscular structures affecting the knee and the preservation of bone.

References

BLOOM, J.D., BRYAN, R.S.: Wide-track polycentric total knee arthroplasty: one year follow-up study. Clin. Orthop. **128**, 210–213 (1977)

BRYAN, R.S., PETERSON, L.F.A.: The quest for the replacement knee. Orthop. Clin. North Am. **2**, 715–728 (1971)

BRYAN, R.S., PETERSON, L.F.A., COMBS, J.J., Jr.: Polycentric knee arthroplasty: a review of 84 patients with more than one year follow-up. Clin. Orthop. **94**, 136–139 (1973a)

BRYAN, R.S., PETERSON, L.F.A., COMBS, J.J., Jr.: Polycentric knee arthroplasty: a preliminary report of postoperative complications in 450 knees. Clin. Orthop. **94**, 148–152 (1973b)

ENGELBRECHT, E., SIEGEL, A., RÖTTGER, J., BUCHHOLZ, H.W.: Statistics of total knee replacement: partial and total knee replacement, design St. Georg; a review of a 4-year observation. Clin. Orthop. **120**, 54–64 (1976)

FRANKEL, V.H., BURSTEIN, A.H., BROOKS, D.B.: Biomechanics of internal derangement of the knee: pathomechanics as determined by analysis of the instant centers of motion. J. Bone Joint Surg. (Am.) **53**, 945–962; 977 (1971)

GUNSTON, F.H.: Polycentric knee arthroplasty: prosthetic simulation of normal knee movement. J. Bone Joint Surg. (Br.) **53**, 272–277 (1971)

GUNSTON, F.H.: Polycentric knee arthroplasty: prosthetic simulation of normal knee movement; interim report. Clin. Orthop. **94**, 128–135 (1973)

GUNSTON, F.H., MACKENZIE, R.I.: Complications of polycentric knee arthroplasty. Clin. Orthop. **120**, 11–17 (1976)

JONES, W., BRYAN, R.S., PETERSON, L.F.A., COVENTRY, M.B., ILSTRUP, D.: Unicondylar knee replacement arthroplasty. Presented at the American Academy of Orthopaedic Surgeons, Dallas, Texas, February 23–28, 1978

LASKIN, R.S.: Modular total knee-replacement arthroplasty: a review of eighty-nine patients. J. Bone Joint Surg. (Am.) **58**, 766–773 (1976)

MARMOR, L.: The modular knee. Clin. Orthop. **94**, 242–248 (1973)

MARMOR, L.: The modular (Marmor) knee: case report with a minimum follow-up of 2 years. Clin. Orthop. **120**, 86–94 (1976)

MARMOR, L.: Single compartment replacement with the Marmor modular knee. Orthop. Rev. **6**, 81 (1977)

PETERSON, L.F.A.: Current status of total knee arthroplasty. Arch. Surg. **112**, 1099–1104 (1977a)

PETERSON, L.F.A.: Gunston polycentric knee arthroplasty revisited: five year follow-up study. Orthop. Trans. **1**, 177 (1977b)

PETERSON, L.F.A., BRYAN, R.S.: Polycentric and geometric total knee arthroplasty: a comparison of indications: In: "Surgical management of degenerative arthritis of the lower limb." CRUESS, R.L., MITCHELL, N.S. (eds.), pp. 186–202. Philadelphia: Lea & Febiger, 1975

PETERSON, L.F.A., BRYAN, R.S., COMBS, J.J., Jr.: Polycentric knee arthroplasty. Instructional Course Lecture American Academy of Orthopaedic Surgery **23**, 6–20 (1974)

PETERSON, L.F.A., BRYAN, R.S., COOMBS, J.J., Jr.: (unpublished data) Polycentric total knee arthroplasty: a 5-year follow-up on 216 knees.

POTTER, T.A.: Arthroplasty of the knee with tibial metallic implants of the McKeever and MacIntosh design. Surg. Clin. North Am. **49**, 903–915 (1969)

SCOTT, R.D., THOMAS, W.H., WELSH, R.F.: Unicompartmental "unicondylar" total knee replacement in osteoarthritis of the knee. Presented to the American Academy of Orthopaedic Surgeons, Dallas, Texas, February 23–28, 1978

SKOLNICK, M.D., BRYAN, R.S., PETERSON, L.F.A., COMBS, J.J., Jr., ILSTRUP, D.M.: Polycentric total knee arthroplasty: a two-year follow-up study. J. Bone Joint Surg. (Am.) **58**, 743–748 (1976)

Chapter 10

Tibio-femoral Replacement Using Two Components with Retention of the Cruciate Ligaments (The Geometric and Anametric Prosthesis)

M.B. Coventry

Department of Orthopedics, Mayo Clinic and Mayo Foundation and Mayo Medical School, Rochester, Minnesota 55901 USA

History

In March 1969, the Food and Drug Administration of the United States approved methyl methacrylate as an investigational new drug for use in total hip arthroplasty. The American orthopaedic surgeon subsequently became familiar with metal-to-polyethylene joint replacement secured by methyl methacrylate. It was only logical that a similar joint replacement for the knee should follow.

The pioneering work of WALLDIUS (1953), with a metal-to-metal hinge prosthesis for the knee, later cemented in with methacrylate as advocated by SHIERS (1965), is well known. At that time, many others were experimenting clinically with similar devices (RILEY, 1976). Endoprostheses and condylar implants were also used. The lower end of the femur was first surfaced with Vitallium by CAMPBELL (1940), and later by the Massachusetts General Hospital group (JONES et al., 1967). Metal coverings or implants of the tibial plateaus were developed by MCKEEVER (1960) and MACINTOSH (1966). These metal endoprostheses of the knee did not achieve the expected goal, however, and their use paralleled the experience in the hip, namely, that in patients with degenerative, rheumatoid, or traumatic arthritis, it was not enough to cover one side of the joint only. The cup arthroplasty, as a metal interpositioning substance (SMITH-PETERSEN, 1939), and the prosthesis to replace the femoral head, as pioneered by JUDET et al. (1954) in France and by MOORE (1957) in this country, did nothing to the opposite side of the joint and often resulted in destruction of any cartilage remaining in the acetabulum and in protrusion into the pelvis or sinking into the femur, or both. Generally, pain was not permanently relieved. Thus, the parallel between the hip and the knee became apparent. If replacing the head of the femur with metal and the acetabulum with polyethylene (or metal, as MCKEE and WATSON-FARRAR [1966] did) would relieve pain, a similar arrangement in the knee might be possible.

In 1970, five orthopaedic surgeons in the United States who had similar ideas on this matter joined to cooperate in a metal-to-polyethylene design for the knee. These orthopaedic surgeons (L.H. RILEY, G.A.M. FINERMAN, J.E. UPSHAW, R.H. TURNER, and M.B. COVENTRY, unpublished data), working with an experienced designer from an instrument manufacturing company, set about the task. There were two ways to go — either imitate the normal anatomy (and thus the function) of the knee joint as closely as possible or depart from the anatomical and use the concept of a mathematical, geometric design. The latter was chosen, partly because of difficulty at the time in manufacturing an anatomical prosthesis with its multiple radii. The goal was to articulate chrome cobalt with ultrahigh-molecular-weight polyethylene (UHMWP). It was elected to make this a two-part design: one to re-surface the femoral condyles and the other to surface the tibial plateau. Because of our previous experience with hinged prostheses, such as YOUNG's (1971), which was modified from WALLDIUS' (1953) and in which there was a high incidence of loosening and delayed infection, nonlinkage of the components was elected, and metal-to-metal contact was considered to be undesirable. By not linking the femoral and tibial components, we could duplicate the normal shift of instant centres as the knee flexed. Building the femoral radius somewhat smaller than the tibial radius would result in enough laxity to allow for at least 15° of rotation of the tibia on the femur. Yet the knee needed to be moderately constrained, because, at this time, we had no clear knowledge of how much constraint would be necessary and we feared the possibility of dislocation.

After many alterations in design, based chiefly on logic and what relatively meagre biomechanical knowledge of the knee was then available, the prostheses were first implanted in cadaver specimens. The geometric knee was then inserted in a patient in March 1971. This original prosthesis has served as a prototype, for good or bad, for future developments, not only in the geometric system but also in many other, somewhat similar designs. Prior to our work, GUNSTON (1971), with CHARNLEY, was pioneering a total-knee arthroplasty based on the same principle of metal-to-polyethylene, and he did the first polycentric knee arthroplasty in February 1968 at Wrightington.

In Europe, the St. Georg unit was reported to be first used in September 1969 (ENGELBRECHT, 1973), and the first Freeman–Swanson unit was implanted in March 1970 (RILEY, 1976).

The Evolution of the Geometric Prosthesis

As replacement of the knee joint with a prosthesis became a reality, bioengineers stepped up their studies and laboratory experiments. In the laboratory, knowledge lagged behind clinical endeavours. At the present time of writing, however, biomechanical knowledge of the knee has caught up and even forged ahead, as it rightfully should. Early workers in the field of total joint replacement were thus handicapped by minimal bench testing. Knee simulators, which were totally inadequate, were of little help; and thus design was based largely on clinical impressions. Rightly or wrongly, the patient became the laboratory, to a large extent. The original (Mark I) geometric prosthesis consisted of a Vitallium femoral condylar unit and a polyethylene tibial plateau unit (Fig. 1). The femoral unit had two hemispherical weight-bearing surfaces with a single radius of 23.8 mm, joined by a cross-bar to make them one, thus obviating the need for separate alignment of each femoral condylar component during insertion. The bony contact surface of the femoral unit allowed adequate fixation to the distal femur by means of two studs and the cut-out undersurfaces. The tibial unit of UHMWP was made concave to nearly match the convex femoral condyles. This was also joined by a polyethylene bar to make it a single unit. Fixa-

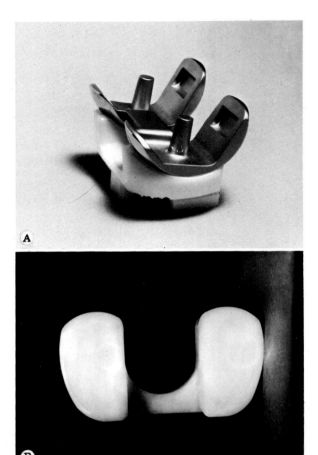

Fig. 1. A Geometric prosthesis. Mark I femoral unit on a Mark II tibial unit. **B** Articulating surface of tibial unit

tion of the tibial component was by parallel runners in an antero-posterior direction and by a cut-out and scored undersurface. Both components were "cemented" with methyl methacrylate. When the units were mated, slight rotation of the tibia on the femur was permitted, because the radius of the femoral component was designed to be less than that of the tibial one. Much thought went into the design of these prostheses, and the fact that the femoral unit has not presented a problem in respect to loosening attests to its basic integrity.

Within a year after the insertion of the first geometric prosthesis, tibial loosening was observed. Flexion of the knee beyond 90° caused a posterior compressive force that resulted in tension on the anterior portion of the tibial prosthesis — an "opening-up" phenomenon. So the first change in design was made, namely, incorporation of a fixation bar on the anterior portion of the

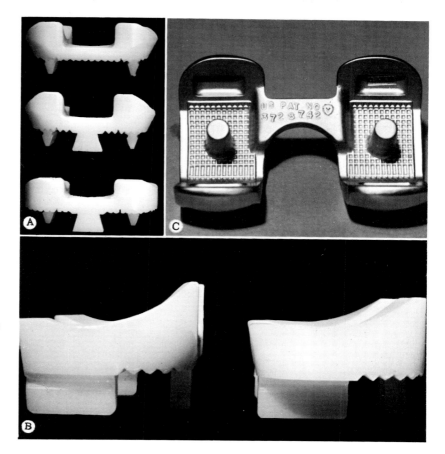

Fig. 2. A Mark I, II, and III geometric tibial units (*top* to *bottom*). Note dovetail added to Mark II, and vertical sides to Mark III, and also shorter anterior lips on Mark III. **B** Lateral profile of Mark II (left) and Mark III (right) tibial units with shortened anterior lips to prevent impaction against femur on hyperextension. Later, posterior portion of runners was bevelled to prevent impingement against posterior cortex of tibia during insertion. **C** Undersurface of geometric femoral unit (Mark III)

tibial unit. This was made in a dovetail shape to provide secure anchorage. The dovetail fits just inside the anterior cortex of the tibia into firm cancellous bone. At the same time as this change was made, the connecting bar of the femoral unit was found to be over-designed and heavier than necessary; impingement of this bar on the anterior cruciate ligament could occur when the knee was in full extension. Thus, its posterior edge was cut out and made concave. This design was termed the Mark II geometric prosthesis.

The Mark III tibial unit evolved from the Mark II. The sides of the tibial unit were originally slanted to conform to the taper of the normal tibial condyles. This was found to be unnecessary, so the sides of the unit were made vertical. Almost a third more surface was thus placed in contact with the underlying tibia, and additionally, the contact surface would bear more directly on stronger, peripheral cortical bone rather than on softer more central medullary bone. In addition, the constraint achieved in the antero-posterior plane was

more than necessary, and so the anterior flare of the prosthesis was lowered. A further reason for this was that re-operation of a few knees revealed that the anterior lips of the tibial unit impinged against the femur if the knee went into hyperextension. This repetitive impact could be a cause of loosening. The evolution of the design of the geometric unit is illustrated in Fig. 2.

Minor alterations also have been made. The metal marking wires were placed differently to prevent migration. The posterior lip of the antero-posterior anchoring runners was bevelled to prevent impingement against the posterior cortex of the tibia during insertion.

Was as much constraint as was originally thought desirable really necessary? Only one of the first 119 knees operated on and followed for a minimum of 2 years dislocated (SKOLNICK et al., 1976). This dislocation occurred in a patient with rheumatoid arthritis (RA) who had no cruciate ligaments at the time of the arthroplasty. The dislocation was in an antero-posterior direction and occurred only when the patient was relaxed, as in sleep. Six years later the patient had no problem with his knee, but he can still luxate the tibia posteriorly on the femur when the knee is in flexion and when he contracts the hamstring muscles. We now believe that we built too much constraint into the prosthesis, and perhaps this contributed to the four loose tibial units that we noted in our combined experience involving 317 knees, although follow-up was brief (COVENTRY et al., 1973). Later, in the Mayo Clinic experience involving 119 knees followed up for a minimum of 2 years, ten tibial units were judged on radiographic examination to be loose (SKOLNICK et al., 1976). This will be discussed later, but the trend was toward less constraint as experience was gained.

The capsule–collateral ligament complex, so often emphasised by FREEMAN et al. (1977), really provided most of the constraint for the knee. This, together with the posterior cruciate ligament (and this is still a controversial point), might provide enough stability with no need for stability to be built into the prostheses themselves. Thus, when the constraint was lessened, stress could be decreased at the bone–cement interface, which would decrease the possibility of loosening. And by making the prostheses more anatomical, this might perhaps lead to a wider range of motion.

The mechanics of the knee were becoming better defined with added experience in this field, both clinically and in the laboratory. So we now took a further step, namely duplication of the anatomical configuration of the normal knee; by so doing, we hoped to increase the range of motion and to decrease the stress at the bone–cement junction. Thus, we moved from a geometric design to an anatomic one.

The six different radii of the femoral condyles were duplicated. The anatomic variation in size and in cant of the femoral condyles was reproduced. The tibial unit was flattened so that there was minimal cupping — just enough to simulate the constraint provided by the menisci in the normal knee. The undersurface of each component was virtually unchanged, and we continued to try to avoid intramedullary projections of much depth, in view of the possibility of later salvage by replacement or arthrodesis. The tibial runners were left to control rotation, as originally designed. The dovetail, which had proved to be so successful, was also left as it was. This prosthesis was the Mark IV design of the geometric system. It was named the "anametric" prosthesis to connote its anatomical rather than its geometric nature. The unit was first inserted in April 1976. The tibial unit was further stabilized by adding an intramedullary stem (the Mark V design) and, soon after, by making the entire unit a metal "T-tray" supporting the articulating polyethylene. To date, this is the final design (Mark VI) (Fig. 3).

L.H. RILEY and J.E. UPSHAW (personal communication) reported no difference in the indications for the anametric as against the geometric design, and believed that it was as intrinsically stable as the geometric. They reported more than 90° of flexion routinely with its use, and no dislocations. R.H. TURNER (personal communication) similarly used the anametric rather than the geometric design, as did FINERMAN, and confirmed the finding of more motion with it. Yet T.A. POTTER (personal communication) did not find an increase in clinical motion. My experience must await a close comparison with a similar group with geometric III prostheses — similar in pre-operative range of motion, diagnosis, age, weight, and so forth. But at this time I can and do use the anametric prosthesis in all instances where I formerly used the geometric. Dislocation, which was formerly considered to be a problem, is definitely not one now. Whether, as expected, there will be less tendency for the tibial unit of the anametric design to loosen, only further observation will tell.

Biomechanics as They Relate to the Geometric Prosthesis

Studies in Mayo Clinic Biomechanical Laboratory

The knee joint is unique and complex in its anatomy and function. It must sustain high dynamic loads and attenuate shock; it must provide a wide range of motion; it must maintain stability during function; and it must produce a propelling strength for body movements. Mechanical knee simulators designed to test these requirements fall far short of the ideal and yet are helpful to verify theoretical findings and to substantiate clinical observations related to component failures.

Gait studies on patients before and after total knee arthroplasty of the geometric and polycentric types have assessed the in vivo function of these implants according to well-defined criteria (DE-

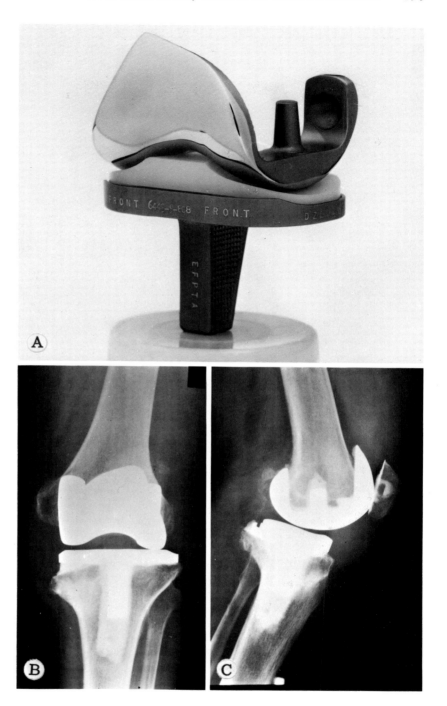

Fig. 3. A Anametric total knee prosthesis, articulated.
B Anametric prosthesis in patient with OA. Antero-posterior view.
C Lateral view

WEERD et al., 1976; GYÖRY et al., 1976; STAUFFER et al., 1977). Although there are variations from normal, the post-operative group has a gait pattern remarkably close to the normal pattern obtained by KETTELKAMP et al. (1970). A comparison of the most significant gait parameters for each type

of knee with normal values is summarised in Table 1. The normal values are well established, based on a group of control subjects matched closely with the patients for both sex and age.

Loosening of the tibial unit has occurred in all types of total knee joint arthroplasty. Experiments

Table 1. Most significant gait parameters for patients with geometric total knee arthroplasty

Parameter	Percentage of normal	
	Pre-op.	Post-op.[a]
Sagittal motion	54	79
Stance flexion	66	103
Standing flexion[b]	208	100
Walking velocity	49	65
Cadence	75	94
Aft shear force (% of body weight)	92	150

[a] These include both the polycentric and the geometric knees. The difference in gait evaluation results between the two types of knees is not statistically significant.

[b] Higher percentage than normal (over 100%) indicates flexion contracture.

Table 2. Mode of failure in 21 cases of geometric total knee arthroplasty

Failure mode	No. of cases	
Components loose		17
Tibial	13	
Femoral	1	
Both	3	
Components not loose		4
Dislocation	2	
Pain and valgus	1	
Pain and varus	1	
		21

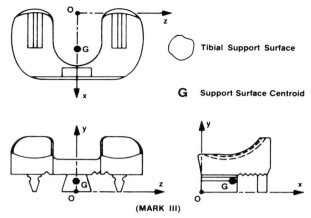

Fig. 4. Tibial supporting surface geometry and location of support surface centroid G. From CHAO, E.Y., MULLEN, J.O.: Theoretical and experimental analyses of the interface strength in geometric total knee replacement. Closed Loop, **6**, 3–16 (1976). By permission of MTS Systems Corporation

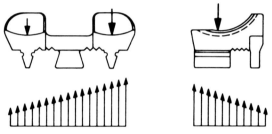

Fig. 5. Tibial contact force imbalance and bone–cement reaction force distribution in geometric total knee prosthesis (Mark II design). From CHAO, E.Y., MULLEN, J.O.: Theoretical and experimental analyses of the interface strength in geometric total knee replacement. Closed Loop **6**, 3–16 (1976). By permission of MTS Systems Corporation)

have been carried out by CHAO and MULLEN (1976) to determine some of the causative factors involved in loosening. Loosening is not related solely to the magnitude of the contact forces acting through the joint, but rather to an imbalance in the distribution of these contact forces on various portions of the components. If these forces can be defined, the design of the prostheses can be modified and changes can be made in the technique of orienting and positioning the prostheses.

We analysed 21 cases of re-operation involving geometric knee arthroplasty. Sixteen re-operations were related to tibial loosening (Table 2) (CHAO and MULLEN, 1976). A theoretical analysis was first attempted, based on the supportive area geometry of the Mark III geometric tibial component (Fig. 4) (CHAO and MULLEN, 1976). Uneven distribution of plateau contact forces, based on altered placement of the prosthesis, causes nonuniform stresses, which may cause loosening (Fig. 5) (CHAO and MULLEN, 1976). Variations through possible ranges of placement were made, and the best orientation that would minimise the loosening potential was found (Fig. 6). The following conclusions can be made on the basis of the results obtained: (1) The minimal loosening moment appears when the tibial component has been placed 0.3 in. medial to the midline of the knee joint; (2) There should be no upward posterior tilting of the tibial prosthesis, and an anterior tilt up to 9° is allowable.

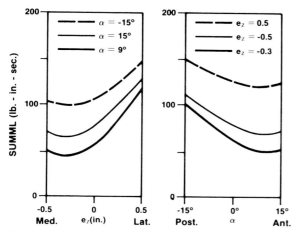

Fig. 6. Variation of loosening moment sum (SUMML) with respect to medio-lateral placement (e_z) and antero-posterior tilting (α) of tibial component. Left: ---, $\alpha = -15°$; —, $\alpha = 15°$; —, $\alpha = 9°$. Right: ---, $e_z = 0.5$; —, $e_z = -0.5$; —, $e_z = -0.3$. (From Chao, E.Y., Mullen, J.O.: Theoretical and experimental analyses of the interface strength in geometric total knee replacement. Closed Loop **6**, 3–16 (1976). By permission of MTS Systems Corporation)

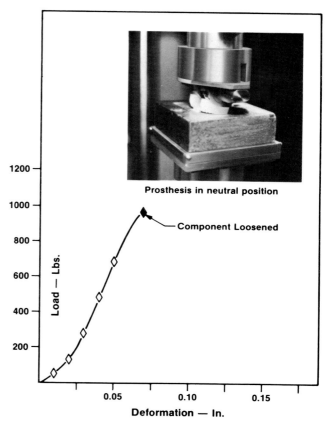

Fig. 7. Load–deformation curve for geometric total knee prosthesis tested under neutral placement. Slope of the straight portion of curve is defined as fixation stiffness of prosthetic interface. Higher stiffness should correspond with lower loosening moment predicted through theoretic analysis. (From Chao, E.Y., Mullen, J.O.: Theoretical and experimental analyses of the interface strength in geometric total knee replacement. Closed Loop **6**, 3–16 (1976). By permission of MTS Systems Corporation)

To verify this theoretical analysis, the tibial unit was loaded after first being implanted in a holding block and then compressed in an axial direction (Figs. 7 and 8). The results were in general agreement with the theoretical analysis. It was additionally verified that any medial or lateral tilt of the tibial unit was detrimental.

Finite element analysis was carried out for the internal and boundary stresses in the tibial component under different loading conditions (Chao et al., 1977). The results revealed that tensile stress can develop at the posterior base of the prosthesis–cement junction and that this stress may lead to loosening. The compressive stress at the loading surface exceeds the yield stress of the polyethylene.

The Cruciate Ligaments

Should the cruciate ligaments, particularly the posterior cruciate ligament, be retained for their stabilising effect? Or should they be removed, as in the total condylar or the initial Freeman–Swanson (ICLH) units? Freeman et al. (1977) summarised their research in this area, testing in situ the knees of 100 consecutive patients with total condylar prostheses (the cruciate ligaments were sacrificed). They found less than 1 cm of antero-poste-rior excursion in 93 of the knees, and only in 7 knees was there over 1 cm of excursion. Even in these seven, though some relative motion was possible between the two components of the prosthesis there were no dislocations, and in only three was instability noted by the patient. Thus, they concluded that removal of the entire upper tibial surface, including the cruciate ligaments, for implant of the prosthesis should not decrease stability.

Designers of total knee units that retain the cruciates (particularly the posterior ligament) believe, however, that the constraint and stability offered by the posterior cruciate ligament cannot be completely tested by anterior and posterior forces placed on the flexed knee. More subtle methods

Effect of tilting angle to load-deformation curve

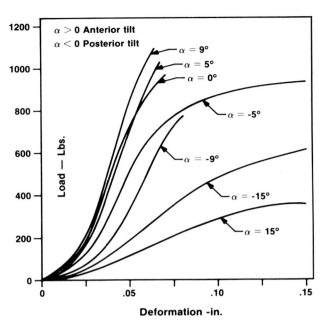

Fig. 8. Load–deformation curves based on varying antero-posterior tilting angle α. α > 0 implies anterior tilt, α < 0, posterior tilt. Slope of straight portion of curve is defined as stiffness and is compared with calculated loosening moment. (From CHAO, E.Y., MULLEN, J.O.: Theoretical and experimental analyses of the interface strength in geometric total knee replacement. Closed Loop **6**, 3–16 (1976). By permission of MTS Systems Corporation)

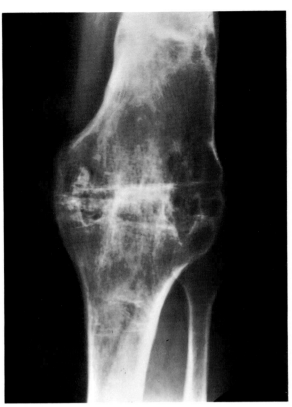

Fig. 9. Antero-posterior radiograph of knee after removal of geometric prosthesis (for infection) and arthrodesis. Mortice and tenon at femur–tibia junction centrally can be clearly seen

must be devised to determine the function, and thus the value, of the posterior cruciate ligament.

There are positive reasons for retaining the cruciate ligaments with some of the intercondylar island of bone containing the ligaments. The geometric (COVENTRY et al., 1972), the anametric (COVENTRY, unpublished data), the University of California, Irvine (UCI) (WAUGH et al., 1973), the Freeman-Swanson bicompartmental with cruciate retention (now withdrawn) (FREEMAN et al., 1973), the Townley (TOWNLEY and HILL, 1974), the Kodama-Yamamoto (KODAMA and YAMAMOTO, 1975), and other similar replacements all allow for retention of the cruciate ligament. Saving all possible stock remains a viable thesis to apply to any joint replacement. Any retained central island of bone, even a small amount posteriorly, makes an excellent tenon to place in the mortice created in the intercondylar area of the femur. The central island markedly increases the bone-to-bone contact

so necessary for fusion (Fig. 9). However, the need for cruciate retention (and retention of the bone between the tibial plateaus) has not yet been fully determined.

Tibial Unit Anchorage

Fixation of the femoral unit has proved to be secure, with virtually no loosening, unless gross technical errors are made or infection has supervened. The anchorage of the tibial unit depends on many factors — only one of them being the design of the component. If less constraint at the femoro-tibial articulation is present, as in the UCI and the anametric prostheses, there will be less shear stress at the bone–cement junction and less tendency to loosen. Rotary stress is controlled by the dovetail anchoring peg placed anteriorly in the geometric and early anametric units, the two vertical runners, and the central island of bone. The addition of a central peg, as in the total condylar prosthesis and the Mark V and VI anametric prostheses, will further restrain the tibial prosthesis. The forces acting on this central peg must be more carefully analysed and their retention abilities determined. If the stem-to-cement and cement-to-bone strength is adequate, the flexion–extension and medial–lateral tilt forces should be lessened with a central stem, although rotary forces may not be (INSALL et al., 1976).

Should the tibial components of polyethylene be supported, in turn, by a metal plate? N. EFTEK-HAR (personal communication) has designed such a unit, and the anametric and total condylar prosthesis is also now available with this alteration in design. Adjustment of load on a metal plate is so critical however, that overload on one part of the plate causes tension effects on the opposite portion, and this tilt effect may be more harmful than be beneficial effects of the supporting metal plate (J.L. LEWIS, personal communication). Yet, many of the problems of loosening are related not so much to design as to indications for the surgery — i.e., the type of person (age, activity, weight, and so forth) who is to receive the prosthesis and the type of bone (osteoporotic, post-operative defects, etc.) into which the prosthesis is to be placed. And even more importantly, the technical aspects of the procedure must be meticulously followed if axial load is to be optimised and secure fixation of the tibial unit is to be obtained.

Indications

Initially, total knee arthroplasty was indicated only for those patients who were strictly limited in activity, required aids for walking or standing, or could not walk at all; who had uncontrolled pain; and whose alternatives would be a bed-to-chair existence or arthrodesis. These indications have gradually broadened as we have developed more confidence in the procedure. However, they have changed in a negative way, as unanticipated problems have emerged. Present indications include those patients afflicted with RA, OA, and traumatic arthritis. Poor candidates are patients who stress their knees because of occupational or avocational demands or because of excessive body weight (perhaps 180 lb is considered an upper limit). In addition to the patient's activities that produce stresses on the knee, the patient's goals (real and imagined) must be defined and, hopefully, met. Obvious contra-indications to the operation are lack of muscular control, e.g., absent quadriceps; infection; a very poor ligament–capsule structure (and here a totally constrained prosthesis or an arthrodesis seem to be the only alternatives); and extensive loss of bone substance, making adequate support for the prosthesis impossible. This would also include the patient with severe osteoporosis, though we have seen very few such patients, because severe osteoporosis usually limits activity and lessens the resulting stress to the bone–prosthesis junction.

The goals of surgery must be carefully defined before operation and must be included on the preoperative knee evaluation forms. In reviewing our first 2 years of experience (SKOLNICK et al., 1976), we found that relief of pain was the primary goal in 84% of the patients, increase in the range of motion in 5%, and correction of a deformity in 11%.

Unicompartmental disease tends to be an indication for upper tibial osteotomy rather than for total knee arthroplasty. First, the diagnosis of chiefly unicompartmental disease must be made, and one means of doing this is the technetium scan (Fig. 10). The advantages of upper tibial osteotomy are now proved, and 19 years of experience in this area convince the author that upper tibial osteotomy, properly indicated and carried out in a correct technical fashion, is a pain-relieving procedure that is conservative, "burns no bridges behind it", and can be converted to a total knee replacement if and when the degenerative arthritic process continues or worsens. Excluded almost entirely from consideration for osteotomy is the rheumatoid patient. In most series of total knee arthroplasty, rheumatoid patients predominate, mostly for this reason. The present controversy is, in part, whether unicompartmental arthritis of the knee should be treated by joint replacement or by osteotomy. If relative contra-indications for osteotomy include a shift of the tibia by more than 1 cm laterally on the femur, rather extensive loss of bone from the tibial plateau, pronounced instability, knee stiffness, and, as is now emerging, a knee with more than 12° or 14° of valgus, then — when these contra-indications exist — a unicompartmental total knee procedure is strongly indicated if the opposite compartment is relatively uninvolved. IN-SALL and WALKER (1976) obtained their best results

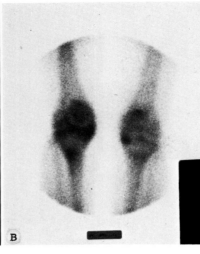

Fig. 10. A Antero-posterior standing radiographs in patient with OA. Lateral compartment of right knee is of good width, but shows cyst in tibial condyle. Technetium scan was performed for confirmation. **B** Scan shows high uptake in both medial and lateral compartments of right knee. Left, however, shows abnormal uptake only medially. Thus, total knee arthroplasty was done on right, and upper tibial osteotomy was done on left

with unicompartmental prostheses in patients with lateral compartment involvement. They believe that when the medial compartment only was involved, osteotomy was probably the treatment of choice. EWALD and SCOTT (unpublished data), reporting on their experience with 70 knees that had unicompartmental total knee replacement, found 61 patients with medial compartment disease and 9 patients with lateral compartment disease–all with OA. By contrast, they found that their results with arthroplasty were equal if not superior to those with upper tibial osteotomy, especially in the elderly patient. They cautioned, however, against using unicompartmental replacement to correct angular deformity of more than 25°.

The entire matter of indications for unicompartmental prostheses, then, is tenuous at this time, but conservatism is strongly recommended. The emergence of all the complications inherent in introducing foreign bodies into a knee joint, and the salvage of such procedures if they should fail because of loosening, foreign-body reaction, infection, and so forth, should determine a careful course in this direction.

Are there specific indications for two-part unhinged components with retention of the cruciate ligaments? Cruciate retention has not yet been totally evaluated, and thus its importance is still not known. One unit for the femur and one for the tibia compared with three- or four-piece units have the distinct advantage of being technically easier to insert, and there is thus less chance of error in placement. If, as in most of these units, a mini-

mal amount of bone is removed from the lower end of the femur and upper tibia and minimal intramedullary invasion is carried out, then bony stock is preserved so that salvage is easier if this is necessary. The amount of constraint necessary in the specific knee to be operated on is a determining factor in selection of the type of prosthesis to be used. If the knee is excessively loose, a constrained prosthesis, or even arthrodesis, is probably necessary. If there is moderate laxity, a minimally constrained unit can be utilised, such as the anametric prosthesis.

An additional determining indication for total knee replacement is the age of the patient. Again one can draw a parallel with the hip. Now, with more than 18 years of experience with total hip arthroplasty, age restrictions for the operation have been lowered. But we must be extremely cautious about total knee replacement in younger people until total knee arthroplasty has been better defined as to its longevity and complications. The younger the patient, the more conservative we must be, conceding, however, the very crippled, juvenile rheumatoid patient who cannot mobilise because of painful, contracted knees. And in these patients, total knee arthroplasty of one type or another is truly a blessing regardless of age, as long as the epiphyses are closed.

Thus, for example, in a male patient of more than 75 years of age with mostly unicompartmental involvement and with pain commensurate with the radiographical findings, a replacement procedure is justified. Recovery after upper tibial osteotomy is slower in the elderly than in the middle-aged, in whom osteotomy is most commonly used. So, in the very elderly, the indications for osteotomy lessen and those for total knee replacement increase.

Results

Experience with total knee arthroplasty is so relatively recent that all results must be evaluated on the basis of this short follow-up period. The many changes in indications, design, and surgical technique make total knee arthroplasty an extremely dynamic subject. It has been said that we are at about the halfway mark in development when compared with total hip arthroplasty. Careful evaluation of the results is imperative to our knowledge — especially so because of the tenuous, changing, rather new character of the procedure. In the simplest terms, if the goals of the operation have been defined, then the orthopaedic surgeon and the patient must decide jointly whether the goals have been achieved. Achieving the goal of pain relief is subjective, whereas range of motion, strength, stability, and other parameters can be tested objectively, as can the radiographic image. Complications are extremely important in the long-term evaluation of results.

As in our experience with hip arthroplasty, we must have a prospective study for any patient in whom we insert total knee components. Our data sheet includes the pre-operative examination and the 8-week, 1-year, 2-year, and subsequent follow-up examinations. From these data, we determine whether our selection of patients for the operation is correct, whether technical aspects of the operation emerge to change or influence the results, and whether the design of the prostheses reveals problem areas. In addition, all complications are carefully noted and evaluated. Many such data recording systems exist. Our data analysis forms have been published (COVENTRY et al., 1973). As in all such studies, for the most part the amassed data can be computerised.

Our study of 119 geometric total knee arthroplasties followed up for 2 years or more (SKOLNICK et al., 1976) included only the Mark I and the Mark II prostheses, and none of the Mark III or anametric types. The ages of the patients ranged from 25 to 84 years, with a mean of 61 years. Of the patients, 38% were men and 62% were women. Rheumatoid involvement was found in

Table 3. Pain after geometric total knee arthroplasty (110 cases)

Pain	Knees			
	Before operation		After operation	
	No.	%	No.	%
None	2 ⎱	4	51 ⎱	92
Mild	2 ⎰		31 ⎰	
Moderate	42 ⎱	96	7 ⎱	8
Severe	64 ⎰		0 ⎰	
	110	100	89	100

From SKOLNICK, M.D., COVENTRY, M.B., ILSTRUP, D.M.: Geometric total knee arthroplasty: a two-year follow-up study. J. Bone Joint Surg. (Am.) **58**, 749–753 (1976). By permission.

53% of the knees, and 41% were osteoarthritic. Forty-eight percent of these patients had had at least one previous surgical intervention. Relief of pain was the primary goal, and 92% of the patients had no pain or had only mild pain after the operation (mild indicated no limitation of activity, no walking aid, but occasional aspirin), while before surgery, 96% had moderate to severe pain (Table 3). There was no difference in relief of pain between the RA and the OA patients. Before surgery 80% of the patients required a cane, crutch, two canes or crutches, or a walker, and 5% could not walk. After surgery, 49% used no aids. Six patients were unable to walk before surgery, and one continued unable to walk after surgery. The post-operative findings were statistically different ($P < 0.001$) from the pre-operative values. Satisfaction with the results of total knee replacement was expressed by 93% of the patients.

In a second study (ILSTRUP et al., 1976), data on 75 knees in 56 patients followed up for at least 2 years were analysed to determine whether there was a significant change in function from the pre-operative state in patients with OA and in those with RA. The mean range of pre-operative motion for the osteoarthritic knee was 86.6°. Post-operatively, it was 87.8°. The rheumatoid motion was 68.3° before operation and 75.8° after it. Thus, the overall range of motion did not significantly change, and the OA patients did not differ significantly from the RA patients. Knees that were stiff before surgery gained motion, and knees that had good motion before surgery lost motion.

Pain on weight-bearing was evaluated to determine whether there was a difference in the osteoarthritic and the rheumatoid knee. All of the OA patients had pain graded as moderate or severe pre-operatively. Post-operatively, 15% had moderate or severe pain, a significant ($P < 0.001$) reduction. Of the knees with RA, 97% had pre-operative pain graded as moderate or severe, while only 8% had moderate or severe pain 2 years after surgery ($P < 0.001$). The groups did not differ significantly from each other in this respect.

The rheumatoid patient required more use of aids after surgery than did the OA patient, although each improved markedly in this respect.

Seventy percent of the OA patients could not walk four blocks before operation. Two years after surgery, only 35% were limited to less than four blocks. Half those who were limited in walking pre-operatively could still not walk four blocks 2 years after surgery. Eighty-nine percent of the rheumatoid patients could not walk four blocks pre-operatively, and 78% could not walk four blocks post-operatively. Of those who were limited pre-operatively, 85% were still limited post-operatively. Thus, the RA patients were significantly more limited as to walking distance than were the OA patients. The use of aids and the distance walked reflect the multiple joint and muscle involvement of the RA patient.

The OA patient had an 85% chance of relief of severe or moderate pain, and the RA patient had a 92% chance of relief of severe or moderate pain after geometric total knee arthroplasty at least 2 years after the surgery.

EVANSKI et al. (1976) analyzed 83 knees (UCI arthroplasties) in 62 patients according to the Modified Larson Knee Analysis Form. There was an average follow-up of 33 months. The average age at surgery was 59 years. OA or post-traumatic arthritis was present in 50 knees, RA in 31, and miscellaneous arthritis in 2. After surgery, 83.3% of the knees were better, 9.6% were not changed, and 12.1% were worse. Knee function as rated by the Larson knee score method (Table 4) showed little change. The average overall pre-operative score with the modified Larson form was 46 (100 being normal), and the average post-operative score was 70.

In a review of those patients treated jointly by the geomedic group (RILEY et al., unpublished data), 361 knees were available for a 2-year follow-up, with an approximately even distribution of rheumatoid and osteoarthritic knees. These results

Table 4. Comparison of knee function after geometric total knee arthroplasty (83 cases)

Method	Normal	Pre-op.	Post-op.
Patient's rating	100%	55%	79%
Modified Larson knee score	100 points	46 points	70 points
Subtotal			
Function	40	18	26
Pain	40	12	27
Anatomy	10	8	9
Motion	10	8	8

From EVANSKI, P.M., WAUGH, T.R., OROFINO, C.F., ANZEL, S.H.: UCI knee replacement. Clin. Orthop. **120**, 33–38 (1976). By permission of J.B. Lippincott Company.

were based on the first 2 years of experience with the geometric prosthesis, and thus the Mark I and Mark II prostheses only were available. Pain relief (rated as poor, fair, good, or excellent) was poor to fair in 17% and good to excellent in 83% at the end of 2 years.

WHITEHURST et al. (1977) analysed 49 geometric total knee arthroplasties, in which the average follow-up was 32 months. Thirty-six of the knees were rheumatoid and 13 were osteoarthritic. Evaluating their results in a similar way, namely by the relief of pain, they found that 6% of this group achieved poor to fair relief and 94% had good to excellent relief. In evaluating motion, they found that 55% of the patients had a gain in motion, 33% had a loss, and 15% had no change.

TIETJENS and CULLEN (1975) reviewed their early experience with 23 geometric total knee arthroplasties over a 2-year period. They stated that all but two patients had significant relief of pain. Only three patients had an increase in range of motion, however, and two patients had less motion than before surgery. The overall function was rated as improved in 21 of the 23 knees.

LOTKE et al. (1976) reviewed the results of 76 geometric total knee replacements, 92% of the patients having been followed up for 1–3 years. The data were amassed from the knee clinic at the University of Pennsylvania and arranged for computerisation. The Mark II tibial component was used. The authors utilised their own knee clinic data form, with 100 points as normal, 90 points or more as excellent, 80–89 points as good, and 70–79 points as satisfactory. They summarised their data by saying that relief of pain has been satisfactory, but not complete, in most of their patients. The post-operative pain was diffusely located over the proximal portion of the medial tibia or about the patella. Twelve knees had scores of over 90 points post-operatively and thus were rated excellent; 24 knees had scores of 80–89 points and were rated good; 12 knees had scores between 70 and 79 points and were considered satisfactory; and 13 knees had scores less than 70 points, but all knees showed some improvement in the knee index. In a subsequent report, LOTKE and ECKER (1977) correlated positioning of the prostheses with the clinical results mentioned and stressed positioning of the components as being the single most important factor in obtaining a satisfactory result.

KODAMA and YAMAMOTO (1975) have reported their experience with their prosthesis, which is a two-part type in which the cruciate ligaments are spared and the components are uncemented. Their later design had a flange for articulation with the patella. The follow-up period ranged from 5 months to 2 years. The scoring system gave 100 for a perfect score: 30 points for evaluating pain, 30 points for evaluating motion, and 40 points for evaluating walking ability. Their patients had significant relief of pain in all knees, with 24% having no pain after surgery and 31% having only occasional pain after prolonged walking. As in all other studies, there was no statistically significant change in the average range of motion before and after surgery.

LACEY (1977) has reported on 100 consecutive patients with UCI total knee replacements and found 90% with no pain or only mild pain.

We have analysed other function modalities as they relate to geometric total knee arthroplasty, namely, motion and the ability to climb stairs and to rise from a chair. The entire group of OA patients and RA patients was compared. None of the OA patients could climb stairs normally before arthroplasty; 43.5% could do so with the aid of a banister; 43.5% could do so by "any method"; and 13% could not climb stairs at all. After total knee arthroplasty, 65.2% could climb stairs normally, 26.1% could climb with the aid of a banister, 0% could climb by any method, and 8.7% could not climb stairs at all. Thus, 87% of the patients functioned better in regard to climbing stairs and 13% were the same; none was worse.

Pre-operatively, none of the RA patients could climb stairs normally, 10.8% could do so with the aid of a banister, 21.6% could do so by any method, and 67.6% could not climb at all. After

total knee arthroplasty, 10.8% could climb stairs normally, 27% could do so with the aid of a banister, 43.2% by any method, and 18.9% could not climb at all. Thus, 59.5% functioned better in regard to climbing stairs, 35.1% were the same, and 5.4% were worse.

The ability to rise from a chair is important to patients. They depend, however, on several factors for this ability — the height of the chair relative to the length of the lower extremities, the strength of the quadriceps, and the amount of knee flexion, in addition to the pain that rising elicits. Before surgery, none of the OA patients could get out of a chair with ease if the chair had no arms, but if there were arms, 17.4% could rise with ease and 82.6% could rise with difficulty. After surgery, 65% could rise with ease from a chair without arms, whereas when a chair with arms was used 78% could rise with ease and 21.7% could rise with difficulty, and no patient was unable to rise. Thus, 78.3% were better, 17.4% the same, and 4.3% worse.

The RA patient fared less well, as would be expected. Before surgery, none could rise from a chair without push-off, and only three patients could rise with ease if they used their arms. Twenty-five percent could rise with difficulty, and 9% were unable to rise. After arthroplasty, 13.5% could rise easily from a chair without arms, 37.8% could rise easily from a chair with arms, 40.5% could rise with difficulty, and 8.1% were unable to rise. Thus, 56.8% were better, 40.5% were the same, and 2.7% were worse.

There was a good statistical correlation between the ability to rise from a chair and the ability to climb stairs.

Patients with mean flexion of 96° after surgery (minimum 75°, maximum 115°) could rise with ease. If mean flexion was 86° (minimum 45°, maximum 110°), the patient needed to use his arms. And patients with 80° of flexion (minimum 20°, maximum 105°) rose with difficulty.

Nearly 86% of the patients with single knee arthroplasty could rise from a chair with ease, with or without arm push, whereas only 48.7% of the patients with bilateral arthroplasties could do this.

Complications

In a 2-year follow-up study at the Mayo Clinic (SKOLNICK et al., 1976), we classified complications as early and late. There were significant numbers of patients who had abnormal wound healing, i.e., failure of perfect primary-intention healing by the 12th post-operative day. EVANSKI et al. (1976) had a 2.9% incidence of abnormal wound healing. By using a relatively straight incision rather than the curved one that was formerly employed, we improved the status of our patients. There was a 3.4% incidence of peroneal nerve palsy, which eventually resolved in all cases. These palsies were traced directly to the use at that early period of a Thomas splint with a Pearson attachment, creating pressure against the peroneal nerve when the patient rotated the extremity externally. Since we changed to the Jones bandage and posterior plaster slab, this problem has been virtually eliminated.

Infection

The late complications are particularly worrisome. The most serious of these is infection, and infection in knee replacement (COVENTRY, 1975b) does not differ widely from infection in other joint replacements. Deep infection developed in two patients (1.8%) in our series. One was a patient with RA who suffered persistent drainage with failure of the wound to heal, although cultures were never positive. Eventually, the patient underwent arthrodesis, and at that time, cultures of her tissue also were negative. Yet we believe that this was a "sterile" infection. The second patient also had RA, and she had a history of three previous operations. She had taken no steroids for 6 months before surgery. The routine cultures from the synovium at the time of surgery were negative, but postoperatively, *Staphylococcus epidermidis* was cultured from her wound. The wound healed, but because of persistent pain, an arthrodesis was performed 1 year later, and *S. aureus* was cultured from the tissues at this time. INSALL et al. (1976) found three late infections in 50 patients with geometric total knee prostheses. WHITEHURST et al. (1977) found six deep infections that required removal of the prostheses.

EVANSKI et al. (1976) noted a deep infection rate of 1.9% in their series. TIETJENS and CULLEN (1975) noted no infections in their 23 patients. Three of 76 patients with geometric total knee replacements reported by LOTKE et al. (1976) had deep infections that required subsequent surgery. FOX (1976) found one deep infection in 74 knees. KODAMA and YAMAMOTO (1975) reported no infections.

GOLDBERG et al. (1977) reported a 2.5% incidence rate for deep infections in 200 total knee operations of various types. LACEY (1977) found three deep infections in 94 knees with UCI prostheses in which the average follow-up was 1.6 years.

PETTY et al. (1975) reviewed 1045 consecutive polycentric and geometric total knee arthroplasties performed at the Mayo Clinic and found an infection rate of 2% at a minimum follow-up of 1-year. Four of the 21 infections were diagnosed (not necessarily appeared) between the first and the second year. Sixty-five percent were in RA patients, who comprised only 48% of the entire series. More than 50% of the knees had been subjected to previous surgery. Continued clinical monitoring of our patients with total knee replacement may show a delayed infection problem much like that seen in the hip (FITZGERALD et al., 1977). The metal-to-metal hinged knee prostheses have shown a special predilection for such delayed infection (DEBURGE, 1976).

Dislocation and Subluxation

In our reported series (SKOLNICK et al. 1976), one of 110 knees dislocated after surgery. But KODAMA and YAMAMOTO (1975) noted no dislocations, nor did LOTKE and ECKER (1977). INSALL et al. (1976) reported one dislocation in 750 geometric total knee prostheses. BRADY et al. (1977) reported two dislocations of geometric prostheses in nine that had failed for various reasons. But six (5.8%) patients in the series reported by EVANSKI et al. (1976) showed such problems and required supportive bracing.

Dislocation seems to be a rather rare phenomenon (except in the report of EVANSKI et al. (1976) on the UCI prostheses), and perhaps the constraint built into the geometric and similar designs is not as necessary as formerly believed. Lax ligamentous structures can be tightened by taking off less bone or by using a thicker tibial unit, both of which will tighten the whole ligament–capsule complex. The patient with dislocation in our series had no posterior cruciate ligament, yet we have operated on other patients with no ligament who have not had dislocation. A highly unstable knee found at the time of surgery should be protected in a cylinder cast for as long as 3 weeks before motion is allowed.

Subsequent to our initial report, there has been an additional dislocation in an osteoarthritic knee that was in rather severe valgus before surgery, and the dislocation of the tibia was lateral on the femur. This was due to the overpull of the vastus lateralis and to a tight ilio-tibial band. Since this was corrected at re-operation, the knee has remained stable and properly positioned.

Loosening

In our report of September 1976, 13 patients (11.8%) had what appeared on the radiograph to be tibial loosening, and in ten patients, loosening was confirmed by re-operation. The other three patients had mild symptoms that were not directly traceable to the apparent loosening. All 13 patients had OA, indicating that the biomechanical demands are more severe in this group than in the RA group. An uncorrected varus alignment of the knee was thought to be the primary cause of loosening in eight knees — again emphasising the absolute need for proper axial alignment. Besides proper axial alignment, inadequate bone medially leads to overstress on the medial tibial plateau, and failure to place the tibial unit in the centre of the knee (i.e., move it laterally enough) puts undue stress on the medial tibial condyle.

Evanski et al. (1976) reported a 5.8% rate for "deformation or loosening" of the tibial components in their series of knees with UCI prostheses, and Lacey (1977) reported 10 cases of loosening in 94 UCI knee replacements. Insall and associates' (1976) report contained four cases of loosening of the tibial component — two associated with infection and two with tibial component loosening and resulting varus deformity — but no symptoms were serious enough for re-operation. Brady et al. (1977) found three loose tibial components of nine failed geometric arthroplasties that they studied.

The whole problem of tibial component loosening is extremely complex and, as will be discussed later under "Operative Technique", is very closely correlated with rigid technical requirements.

What is the significance of lucent lines? Any lucent line is undesirable, although lucent lines are common. If lucent lines increase in width, then they are worrisome, but if their widths remain the same and are less that 2 mm, the lines are probably clinically insignificant. A review of our cases (considering that slight variations in X-ray technique prevent accurate comparison) revealed that about 80% of our patients had lucent lines at some point in the bone–cement interface during their post-operative course.

Patellar Dislocation

The patello-femoral relationship will be discussed later. If the patella impinges against the femoral component, this is a technical error, because the design of these prostheses does not allow patellar impingement. Patellar dislocation in the geometric prostheses is extremely rare. In fact, we had none in our review series.

Failure of Angular Correction

Another complication is emerging, however, namely recurrence of the varus or valgus deformity, whichever existed pre-operatively. This is usually varus (most of the knees were originally in varus) and is due to failure at surgery to restore the axial alignment to at least 5° or 7° of valgus. Thus, the medial condyle continues to be overloaded (Fig. 11). A second complication associated with this failure of axial correction is sinking of the tibial component, with loosening and even fracture of the tibial plateau. Fracture is a combination of failure to align properly and of placing the tibial component too far medially, where the bone is of inferior quality. This is a technical problem again, and the problem is usually due to poor lateral exposure of the knee, which prevents the operator from seeing the entire medial and lateral tibial condyles clearly.

Lotke and Ecker (1977) found that four of the five instances of mechanical failure involving fracture of the medial tibial plateau showed varus angulation, thus confirming our strong feeling that failure to correct axial alignment is the most frequent cause of failure in total knee arthroplasty. Brady et al. (1977) found two patients with medial plateau stress fractures.

Although fracture occurred only once in our original series, a few subsequent knees have shown it.

Chao and Mullen (1976) defined the factors leading to loosening of the tibial unit as follows: The tibial femoral angle should be restored to normal anatomical variation of 5° to 8° of valgus. The tibial unit should be placed in

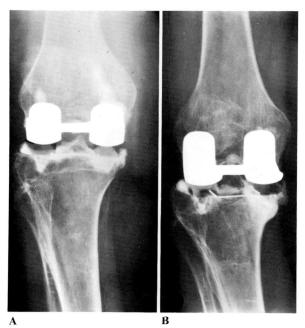

A   **B**

Fig. 11. A Antero-posterior radiograph of Mark I geometric prosthesis inserted for post-traumatic medial compartment OA. One year after insertion. Note medial placement of tibial unit and failure to correct varus axial deviation. **B** Same patient 3 years later. Marked reactive sclerosis developing at medial tibial condyle due to overload. Patient asymptomatic, but it is expected that loosening will ultimately occur

the centre of the tibia or just slightly medial of centre. Rotational alignment should be proper and normal for that patient. (The normal can often be found by examining the opposite extremity.) The antero-posterior placement of the tibial unit should be at right angles to the tibia or up to 7° of anterior tilt. We have found posterior tilt to be detrimental, in contrast to the findings of others (WILDE et al., 1975). Technical aspects of cementing include inserting the tibial unit first and supporting it with firm finger pressure only. The cement should be allowed to set before the femoral unit is put in. If, while the tibial unit is being cemented, the femoral unit is allowed to impact against the tibial unit, very high stress concentrations may occur on one portion of the tibial unit, with tension forces on another.

Wear

Implant wear has not been detected clinically or radiographically in any geometric prosthesis to date. Prostheses that have been removed, however, show some deformation of the plastic ("cold-flow"), and loosened prostheses have shown indentation, scoring, and pitting of the polyethylene due to loose methacrylate particles in the joint.

Re-operation

Analysis of re-operation data (SKOLNICK et al., 1976) revealed 17 of 110 knees (15.5%) required re-operation. EVANSKI et al. (1976) found a re-operation rate of 17.4%.

Comparing the re-operation data of the rheumatoid and osteoarthritic knees (ILSTRUP et al., 1976), we found that 19% of the knees with OA and 5% of the knees with RA required re-operation. Loosening was responsible for re-operation in five of the six osteoarthritic knees. A migrating marker wire in one knee was of no real significance, but a persistent flexion deformity in a rheumatoid knee was. This was corrected by removing more bone from the femur and re-inserting the femoral unit. Three years later, the patient has a serviceable and well-functioning, painless knee and the flexion contracture has changed from 30° to 5°.

GOLDBERG et al. (1977) had to revise 7% of their total knee arthroplasties, but they included seven different types of components. BRADY et al. (1977) analysed nine geometric failures needing revision, and HUNGERFORD and RILEY (1976) performed re-operations on 3.5% of 58 rheumatoid patients with geometric total knee arthroplasties.

Whether future evaluation of our patients will show a higher or a lower rate of re-operation is unknown. Clearer indications regarding patient selection, advances in technique with increased knowledge and better instrumentation, and improvements in design will all lessen the early errors and complications. This improvement is now becoming evident as we study our more recent patients. Placement of the prostheses, particularly, is more accurate. And to date, after more than a year's experience with the anametric knee prosthesis, no loosenings have become evident and no re-operations have been necessary.

Yet it is also obvious that, with further time, knees that have been operated on will exhibit problems such as wear, delayed infection, and perhaps evidence of delayed loosening. And thus, the two factors that produce the need for re-operation may cancel out.

The Future

Now, after 8 years of experience at our institution and a vast accumulation of clinical experience throughout the world, there is no question at all that knee arthroplasty, with metal-to-polyethylene, will be with us for a very long time. There is also no question that improvements in design and technique will naturally evolve. Along with clinical experience will go a comparable, and hopefully even greater, laboratory experience. The biomechanical engineer and physiologist will be able to guide the further development of total knee arthroplasty. Methyl methacrylate has been a most fortunate discovery and is an extremely useful adjunct to the operation.

Without it, the operation could not have been carried out, at least as originally conceived for the nonhinged prostheses. Whereas the Kodama–Yamamoto prosthesis uses no methacrylate, long-term results with its use are not available. No doubt different methods of securing the prostheses to bone will evolve, as they have in the hip and elsewhere in the body, and sintered and porous metals will perhaps eventually prove to be useful. Certainly, in the foreseeable future there will be no marked changes in the composition of the metallic portion of the prostheses, which will be stainless steel, chrome cobalt, or other alloys containing titanium. Ultrahigh-molecular-weight polyethylene seems almost ideal. Change from its use will occur only if, with further time, the polyethylene particles are found to be carcinogenic or otherwise harmful to the body.

Total knee replacement began with the hinged, metal-to-metal units. It then evolved to four-compartment polycentric resurfacing, as developed by GUNSTON (1971). Next came the two-component prostheses (geometric and anatomical) that retained at least the posterior cruciate ligament, and the two-component, more anatomical units in which the cruciates were sacrificed. The linked, but not truly hinged, prostheses gained prominence when constraint was needed. Design has been altered considerably in each of the separately developed total knee arthroplasties, and new designs are constantly emerging.

Prostheses are referred to as biomechanically nonconstrained, semi-constrained, or constrained; the trend is moving away from the semi-constrained prosthesis to either a minimally or nonconstrained prosthesis or a totally constrained prosthesis. There now seems little need for the semi-constrained units.

All prostheses, the ones in this chapter included, are at the centre of continuing efforts to improve design, based on laboratory and clinical testing; to develop more secure methods of anchorage without sacrificing too much bone either at the joint surface or in the intramedullary region; to lessen the incidence of infection common to all implants; and to gain a better range of motion — something that all the present implants are, in some measure, lacking.

Operative Technique

As the evolution of the total knee arthroplasty continues, better means of applying an accurate surgical technique during insertion becomes a major concern. The very involved function of the knee, based on its anatomy and on the needs of the body, demands much of any implant. As failures have been analysed by ourselves and others (COVENTRY, 1975a; EVANSKI et al., 1976; HUNGERFORD and RILEY, 1976; INSALL et al., 1976; SKOLNICK et al., 1976; BRADY et al., 1977; GOLDBERG et al., 1977; LACEY, 1977), the complications of loosening, uncorrected deformity both in flexion–extension and axial alignment, dislocation, stress fractures under the components, and other such problems seem to be related specifically to technical errors. As WAUGH (1975) has stated, "The technical errors were largely related to incorrect placement of the prosthesis...."

What is the correct placement of the prosthesis? Emerging from all these experiences, in some instances verified by laboratory experimentation, the prostheses discussed in this chapter should all be placed with careful regard for axial alignment, that is, restoration of the normal anatomic valgus. This is the one primary key to long-term success. The tibial component in turn must be placed at a right angle to the tibia, i.e., parallel to the ground in the frontal plane. The femoral component must be placed so that the resulting femoral–tibial angle is approximately normal (5°–7° of anatomical valgus) (KETTELKAMP and NASCA, 1973). In the lateral plane, the tibial prosthesis should be placed either in a neutral (right angle) position to the axis of the tibia or with a slight anterior tilt, up to 7°.

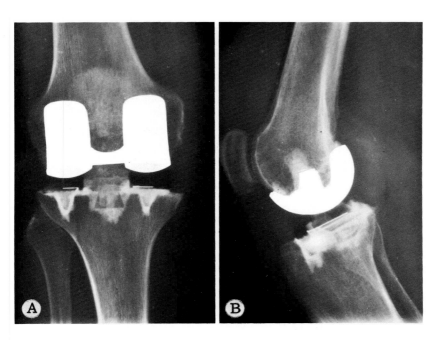

Fig. 12 A and B. Geometric Mark III prosthesis properly positioned, with axial alignment of 7° of valgus. Note that tibial unit is centered on tibial condyles; no lucent lines are present. There is no excess methacrylate. **A** Antero-posterior view; **B** lateral view

A common source of late complication is failure to place the tibial unit away from the high-stress concentration. In other words, if the knee is in varus, the tibial unit should be placed at least in the midline of the knee rather than allowing it to be more medial, where the previous varus has produced bone reaction to stress with sclerosis and even cystic formation (see Fig. 11). Later collapse and even fracture of this portion of the medial tibial plateau can occur. This error occurs because of the relative difficulty in getting good lateral exposure. And the truism, as in all surgery, is that adequate exposure is the key to a successful operation. Excessive or uneven stresses on the tibial component while it is being cemented may be extremely harmful. The tibial unit should be held in firmly with finger pressure during its cementing and should never be cemented in after the femoral component has been placed and with the knee extended. There is no way to create even compression on the tibial component if it is not held in with finger pressure. Figure 12 is an illustration of the geometric Mark III prosthesis properly placed, and Fig. 13 of an anametric total knee prosthesis.

How tight should the knee be when the components are cemented in place? This will depend largely on how tight it was before the operation and how much axial angulation existed. A difficult and not fully resolved problem is the varus knee with a relatively relaxed and stretched lateral collateral ligament. Once this knee has been converted to the desired valgus of between 4° and 7°, there will be relative snugness of the medial collateral ligament. The knee will tend to be unstable as the patient bears weight and a varus strain occurs. Release with cephalad "sliding" of the medial collateral ligament from the tibia is practiced by us as advised by some (J. INSALL, personal communication). Others may tighten the relatively lax lateral collateral ligament. It has been our experience that tightening the ligaments by advancing, reefing, or other measures works poorly with total knee arthroplasty because the need to rest the knee long enough after operation for ligament healing may result in stiffness.

The entire problem of the ligaments in total knee arthroplasty is not yet resolved and needs further study. We have already referred to the posterior cruciate ligament in this regard. The success of the operation itself depends on sufficient knowledge by the operator to master its technical aspects and to know the technical pitfalls (COVENTRY and BRYAN, 1975). Adequate exposure and meticulous attention to detail are absolutely essential. And of extreme importance and often neglected, because there is inadequate instrumentation for this, is the rotary alignment of the tibia on the femur.

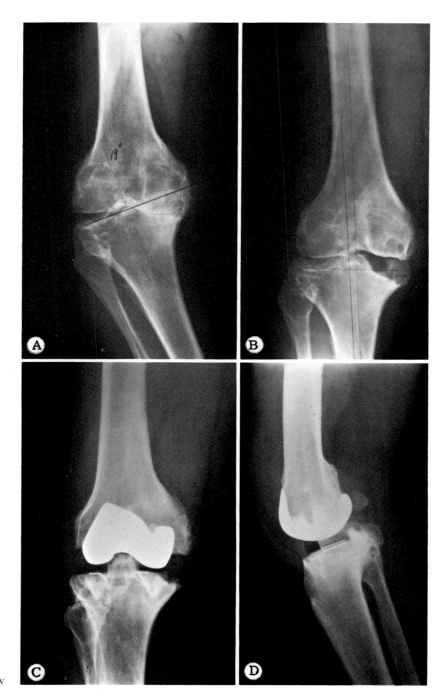

Fig. 13. A–D Anametric total knee arthroplasty for OA. **A** 19° varus angulation pre-operatively; **B** assessment of bone loss from medial tibial plateau by stressing the knee in valgus; **C** antero-posterior radiograph with anametric prosthesis in place; **D** lateral view

We prefer to consider the other side as being normal — if it actually is. If it is not, one should try for approximately 5° of external rotation of the tibia on the femur. Excessive rotary variation will transmit rotatory stresses to the components and create loosening, deformation, and wear.

These problems are intensified when there are extremes of varus or valgus or with flexion contractures. Various limits of deformity for total knee arthroplasty have been suggested. But there are too many problems involved with each patient to state accurately that a specific degree of deformity can or cannot be corrected with any one procedure.

Certainly we have had problems in achieving full correction of more than 30° of flexion contracture. However, because as much as 10° or 12° of flexion is still compatible with reasonably good function, full extension is not essential. Knees with varus of as much as 25° have posed no great problem in correction. Valgus knees are more difficult because of the very tight lateral structures. Mandatory procedures in these patients are release of the ilio-tibial band; very occasionally, lengthening of the vastus lateralis; and certainly always, release of the lateral retinaculum.

Finally, closure of the knee after insertion of the prosthesis requires due regard for the quadriceps mechanism. The quadriceps–patellar tendon angle must be restored. The patella must track properly in the intercondylar notch or on the metal flange of the femoral component, if such exists. Particular care should be taken in resuturing the portion of the patellar tendon that may be partially removed from its attachment during the operation. Release of any restricting structures laterally must be carried out. The oblique fibres of the vastus medialis should always be carefully restored or, in some instances, advanced distally and medially. If these procedures are carefully observed and if the axial alignment has been properly restored, patellar subluxation or dislocation should not occur.

Patello-femoral Replacement

Our continuing experience with upper tibial osteotomy for degenerative arthritis of the knee has so far revealed a relative paucity of patello-femoral problems (BOWMAN and COVENTRY, unpublished data). Now, 19 years after first doing this operation, I have done only two subsequent patellectomies, because few patients present with incapacitating symptoms of patello-femoral arthritis. The reason postulated for this infrequency of patello-femoral joint symptoms after osteotomy is that the patient generally does not make severe demands on the knee. Yet these patients do climb stairs and engage in most normal activities, and some ski and play tennis.

After upper tibial osteotomy, in which axial deviation is corrected, there is a change in the quadriceps–patellar tendon angle and a retracking of the patella not only in a medial–lateral position but also in an inferior–superior one. The patellar

tendon is relatively lengthened by approximately 0.5 cm, depending on the size of the wedge. There may be more subtle changes in the dynamics of the knee relating to the antero-posterior position of the patellar tendon attachment on the tibial tubercle (MAQUET, 1972). The early development of total knee arthroplasty omitted resurfacing of the patella. But axial alignment changes were accomplished just as they are in osteotomy, and perhaps for this reason, relatively few patients presented with patello-femoral symptoms after a geometric type of total knee arthroplasty, although most of them, just as after upper tibial osteotomy, had the radiographic changes of patello-femoral arthritis.

In our first 2 years of experience with geometric total knee arthroplasty, no patient had specific patello-femoral pain. As our experience increased, however, the diagnosis was occasionally made (and as the duration of the replacement in the patient increased, the knee continued to "age" and any degenerative arthritis probably increased). Because of the possibility of patello-femoral symptoms, J. UPSHAW (personal communication) altered the femoral component of the geometric prosthesis and put on an anterior flare for patello-femoral articulation. This allowed patellar surfacing with a button of polyethylene. In designing the anametric total knee system, the femoral unit has a flange for patellar articulation, and the patella can be resurfaced if the surgeon wishes.

Just how great is the problem of patello-femoral pain after total knee arthroplasty? The incidence may relate to the importance that the examiner places on the patient's symptoms. If the history is suggestive of pain occurring in front of the knee on quadriceps contraction and patello-femoral motion, such as in climbing stairs, and if one accepts patellar compression against the femur as a diagnostic sign to determine symptomatic patello-femoral arthritis, the problem may be more prevalent than we have found and certainly may increase as time continues. INSALL et al. (1976) found that, when they compared the duocondylar, unicondylar, Guépar, and geometric prostheses in the 50 knees with geometric prostheses, 29 had pain on patello-femoral compression and 5 showed evidence of patellar "erosion." No mention is made of the radiographic findings in the 29 knees with pain or of whether they were compared on radiographs with knees that were without pain. They found that with the Guépar prostheses, in which there is a femoral flange for the patellar but the patellar is not specifically resurfaced, the clinical findings of pain and erosion were similar. These observations probably led to the development of the total condylar arthroplasty, which allows the patella to be resurfaced. GOLDBERG et al. (1977) diagnosed patello-femoral pain in 25% of their patients with total knee arthroplasties without patellar surfacing, and LACEY (1977) found that 25 of 94 patients with UCI prostheses had patellar erosion. In their follow-up study, WHITEHURST et al. (1977) found that patello-femoral pain was less frequent with the geometric than with the modular prostheses, although the geometric group included more rheumatoid patients (who thus possibly placed less stress on the knee than was the case with the modular prosthesis).

Any future total knee arthroplasty should really be total and should include not only the tibio-femoral joint but also the patello-femoral joint — at least there should be an option for the surgeon to resurface the patella with polyethylene, and the femoral component should have a corresponding gliding surface of metal for its articulation with the patella. Whether all patellae should be resurfaced, regardless of their appearance at surgery, the age of the patient, and the demands on the knee, is still a moot question and must be left to the discretion of the orthopaedic surgeon.

Apart from whether the patella is resurfaced or not, there is the problem of patellar luxation or dislocation. As described under "Operative Technique," very careful attention must be paid to restoring a normal quadriceps–patellar tendon alignment. This is particularly necessary in the valgus knee, because in this type of knee the patella may continue to ride laterally. Luxation of the patella is not an infrequent problem, as emphasised initially be the GUÉPAR group (DEBURGE, 1976). These workers emphasised the distinction between pain at the patello-femoral articulation and patellar malalignment. These two situations are related, but they are also different. Sixty-two of their 103 patients complained of patellar pain pre-operatively, and 43 of these patients had residual pain post-operatively. Eight knees were painless pre-operatively and became painful after surgery. In these cases, however, one must be very careful to interpret the cause of the anterior knee pain and not assign it simply to patello-femoral disease. They found that patellar malalignment, including complete dislocation, existed in 20 patients before surgery. Correction was accomplished in only nine. In most, when only lateral patellar retinaculum

resection was performed, malalignment persisted or recurred. The authors transferred the tibial tubercle in some patients to maintain correction of severe malalignment. They also emphasised the difficulty in assessing malalignment problems by the use of radiographic evidence alone unless a true antero-posterior projection was made both before and after operation. INSALL et al. (1976) frequently observed patellar subluxation in the Guépar prosthesis, in spite of wide lateral release of the patellar retinaculum. They believed that it was an incidental finding and was not symptomatic, because the subluxation did not necessarily correlate with complaints of post-operative pain. Nonetheless, subluxation, which is almost always a lateral riding of the patella, cannot be deemed a "good" thing, and as time goes on, it may produce increasing symptoms. Will patellectomy relieve such symptoms? Again, INSALL et al. (1976) found that this did not lessen the symptoms in the anterior aspect of the knee.

If, however, the patella impinges against the femoral component of the geometric prosthesis, patellectomy will relieve the symptoms. Thus, the operative technique should be accurate and allow for no impingement of the patella on the femoral unit. What often appears to be X-ray evidence of impingement on the lateral view is usually overlap of the femoral unit condyles and the patella, which occupies the intercondylar space. Only the operating surgeon can tell at surgery just how the patella tracks. It will not impinge in any of the geometric, UCI, or other prostheses of this nature if the technique is correct.

Is there a place for revision, therefore, if the surgeon believes that patello-femoral arthritis is the cause of considerable pain after a total knee arthroplasty? Patellectomy does not seem to be the complete answer, as mentioned. Realignment more medially may help if definite malalignment can be demonstrated. The patella should not be surfaced without a comparable surfacing of the juxtaposing femur; but a separate metal component for the femur is available and can be used in certain patients. A patelloplasty, using the infrapatellar fat pad, can be carried out and may be successful in certain patients (CAVE and ROWE, 1950). Another alternative is to anteriorise the patellar tendon insertion at the tibial tubercle to decrease the compressive forces on the patello-femoral joint (MAQUET, 1972).

EVANSKI et al. (1976) reviewed their results with 83 arthroplasties. Two patients had patellar impingement and subsequent patellectomy, and two patients had dislocation of the patella post-operatively. In a separate study of re-operation after total knee arthroplasties, including both the polycentric and the geometric types (PETTY et al., unpublished data) and with a follow-up ranging from $1-3^1/_2$ years, 109 re-operations were performed in 68 knees. None of the patients had patellar problems of malalignment, subluxation, dislocation, or patello-femoral pain. The patients have not been subsequently studied by us to determine whether patello-femoral arthritis has since become a problem.

Thus, subluxation and dislocation of the patella after knee arthroplasty are caused chiefly by technical error, as is impingement of the patella on any part of the femoral component. Patellofemoral arthritis, however, is basically a separate problem and in the future may be obviated by resurfacing the patella. The particular complications that may emerge from resurfacing the patella are problematic. Loosening of the polyethylene patellar button is one. There may be an increase in the incidence of patellar luxation. Wear particles will increase as more polyethylene is exposed to wear in the knee joint, and their ultimate fate in the body and harmful effects cannot now be assessed.

References

BOWMAN, P., COVENTRY, M.B.: Unpublished data

BRADY, T.A., RANAWAT, C., KETTELKAMP, D.B., RAPP, G.F.: Salvage of the failed total knee arthroplasty (abstract). Orthop. Trans. 1, 101–102 (1977)

CAMPBELL, W.C.: Interposition of vitallium plates in arthroplasties of the knee: preliminary report. Am. J. Surg. 47, 639–641 (1940)

CAVE, E.F., ROWE, C.R.: The patella: its importance in derangement of the knee. J. Bone Joint Surg. (Am.) 32, 542–553 (1950)

CHAO, E.Y., MULLEN, J.O.: Theoretical and experimental analyses of the interface strength in geometric total knee replacement. Closed Loop 6, 3–16 (1976)

CHAO, E.Y., WONG, H.W., FRAIN, W.E., COVENTRY, M.B.: Stress analysis of the geometric knee under static loading. New York: American Society of Mechanical Engineers 1977

COVENTRY, M.B.: Geometric knee arthroplasty. Curr. Pract. Orthop. Surg. 6, 10–21 (1975a)

COVENTRY, M.B.: Treatment of infections occurring in total hip surgery. Orthop. Clin. North Am. 6, 991–1003 (1975b)

COVENTRY, M.B., BRYAN, R.S.: Technical pitfalls in the polycentric and geometric total knee arthroplasties. In: Total knee replacement, pp. 163–168. London: Mechanical Engineering Publications for The Institution of Mechanical Engineers 1975

COVENTRY, M.B., FINERMAN, G.A.M., RILEY, L.H., TURNER, R.H., UPSHAW, J.E.: A new geometric knee for total knee arthroplasty. Clin. Orthop. 83, 157–162 (1972)

COVENTRY, M.B., UPSHAW, J.E., RILEY, L.H., FINERMAN, G.A.M., TURNER, R.H.: Geometric total knee arthroplasty. II. Patient data and complications. Clin. Orthop. 94, 177–184 (1973)

DEBURGE, A.: GUEPAR hinge prosthesis: complications and results with 2 years follow-up. Clin. Orthop. 120, 47–53 (1976)

DEWEERD, J.H., Jr., STAUFFER, R.N., CHAO, E.Y., AXMEAR, F.E.: Functional evaluation of pre and postoperative total knee arthroplasty patients (abstract). Transactions of the 22nd annual meeting of the Orthopaedic Research Society 1, 77 (1976)

ENGELBRECHT, E.: The intra-articular total endoprosthesis of the knee joint (design "St. Georg") (abstract). Excerpta Medica International Congress Series No. 298, 33–34 (1973)

EVANSKI, P.M., WAUGH, T.R., OROFINO, C.F., ANZEL, S.H.: UCI knee replacement. Clin. Orthop. 120, 33–38 (1976)

EWALD, F., SCOTT, R.: Unpublished data

FITZGERALD, R.H., Jr., NOLAN, D.R., ILSTRUP, D.M., VAN SCOY, R.E., WASHINGTON, J.H., II, COVENTRY, M.B.: Deep wound sepsis following total hip arthroplasty. J. Bone Joint Surg. (Am.) 59, 847–855 (1977)

FOX, K.W.: Geometric total knee arthroplasty: local complications. Tex. Med. 72, 92–97 (1976)

FREEMAN, M.A.R., SWANSON, S.A.V., TODD, R.C.: Total replacement of the knee using the Freeman-Swanson knee prosthesis. Clin. Orthop. 94, 153–170 (1973)

FREEMAN, M.A.R., INSALL, J.N., BESSER, W., WALKER, P.S., HALLEL, T.: Excision of the cruciate ligaments in total knee replacement. Clin. Orthop. 126, 209–212 (1977)

GOLDBERG, V.M., RASHBAUM, R., FRANKEL, V.: Complications of total knee arthroplasty (abstract). Orthop. Trans. 1, 102 (1977)

GUNSTON, F.H.: Polycentric knee arthroplasty: prosthetic simulation of normal knee movement. J. Bone Joint Surg. (Br.) 53, 272–277 (1971)

GYÖRY, A.N., CHAO, E.Y.S., STAUFFER, R.N.: Functional evaluation of normal and pathologic knees during gait. Arch. Phys. Med. Rehabil. 57, 571–577 (1976)

HUNGERFORD, D.S., RILEY, L.H., Jr.: Total knee replacement in rheumatoid arthritis (abstract). J. Bone Joint Surg. (Am.) 58, 731 (1976)

ILSTRUP, D.M., COVENTRY, M.B., SKOLNICK, M.D.: A

statistical evaluation of geometric total knee arthroplasties. Clin. Orthop. **120**, 27–32 (1976)

INSALL, J., WALKER, P.: Unicondylar knee replacement. Clin Orthop. **120**, 83–85 (1976)

INSALL, J.N., RANAWAT, C.S., AGLIETTI, P., SHINE, J.: A comparison of four models of total knee-replacement prostheses. J. Bone Joint Surg. (Am.) **58**, 754–765 (1976)

JONES, W.N., AUFRANC, O.E., KERMOND, W.L.: Mold arthroplasty of the knee (abstract). J. Bone Joint Surg. (Am.) **49**, 1022 (1967)

JUDET, J., JUDET, R., LAGRANGE, J., DUNOYER, J.: Resection-reconstruction of the hip: Arthroplasty with an acrylic prosthesis. NISSEN, K.I., (ed.), Edinburgh: Livingston 1954

KETTELKAMP, D.B., NASCA, R.: Biomechanics and knee replacement arthroplasty. Clin. Orthop. **94**, 8–14 (1973)

KETTELKAMP, D.B., JOHNSON, R.J., SMIDT, G.L., CHAO, E.Y.S., WALKER, M.: An electrogoniometric study of knee motion in normal gait. J. Bone Joint Surg. (Am.) **52**, 775–790 (1970)

KODAMA, T., YAMAMOTO, S.: Internal publication. Okayama, Japan: Okayama University, Medical School 1975

LACEY, J.A.: A statistical review of one hundred consecutive "U.C.I." low friction knee arthroplasties with analysis of results (abstract). Orthop. Trans. **1**, 102–103 (1977)

LEWIS, J.L.: Personal communication

LOTKE, P.A., ECKER, M.L.: Influence of positioning of prosthesis in total knee replacement. J. Bone Joint Surg. (Am.) **59**, 77–79 (1977)

LOTKE, P.A., ECKER, M.L., MCCLOSKEY, J., STEINBERG, M.E.: Early experience with total knee arthroplasty. J. Am. Med. Assoc. **236**, 2403–2406 (1976)

MACINTOSH, D.L.: Arthroplasty of the knee in rheumatoid arthritis (abstract). J. Bone Joint Surg. (Br.) **48**, 179 (1966)

MAQUET, P.: Biomécanique de la gonarthrose. Acta Orthop. Belg. [Suppl.] **38**, (1), 33–54 (1972)

MCKEE, G.K., WATSON-FARRAR, J.: Replacement of arthritic hips by the McKee-Farrar prosthesis. J. Bone Joint Surg. (Br.) **48**, 245–259 (1966)

MCKEEVER, D.C.: Tibial plateau prosthesis. Clin. Orthop. **18**, 86–94 (1960)

MOORE, A.T.: The self-locking metal hip prosthesis. J. Bone Joint Surg. (Am.) **39**, 811–827 (1957)

PETTY, W., BRYAN, R.S., COVENTRY, M.B., PETERSON, L.F.A.: Infection after total knee arthroplasty. Orthop. Clin. North Am. **6**, 1005–1014 (1975)

PETTY, W., BRYAN, R.S., PETERSON, L.F.A., COVENTRY, M.B.: Unpublished data

RILEY, L.H.: Evolution of total knee arthroplasty. Clin. Orthop. **120**, 7–10 (1976)

SHIERS, L.G.P.: Hinge arthroplasty of the knee (abstract). J. Bone Joint Surg. (Br.) **47**, 586 (1965)

SKOLNICK, M.D., COVENTRY, M.B., ILSTRUP, D.M.: Geometric total knee arthroplasty: a two-year follow-up study. J. Bone Joint Surg. (Am.) **58**, 749–753 (1976)

SMITH-PETERSEN, M.N.: Arthroplasty of the hip: a new method. J. Bone Joint Surg. **21**, 269–288 (1939)

STAUFFER, R.N., CHAO, E.Y.S., GYÖRY, A.N.: Biomechanical gait analysis of the diseased knee joint. Clin. Orthop. **126**, 246–255 (1977)

TIETJENS, B.R., CULLEN, J.C.: Early experience with total knee replacement. N. Z. Med. J. **82**, 42–45 (1975)

TOWNLEY, C., HILL, L.: Total knee replacement. Am. J. Nurs. **74**, 1612–1617 (1974)

WALLDIUS, B.: Arthroplasty of the knee joint employing an acrylic prosthesis. Acta Orthop. Scand. **23**, 121–131 (1953)

WAUGH, T.R.: Knee arthroplasty using the UCI tibiofemoral prosthesis. Curr. Pract. Orthop. Surg. **6**, 21–28 (1975)

WAUGH, T.R., SMITH, R.C., OROFINO, C.F., ANZEL, S.M.: Total knee replacement: operative technic and preliminary results. Clin. Orthop. **94**, 196–201 (1973)

WHITEHURST, L., MCCOLLUM, D.E., GOLDNER, J.L.: Which total knee? Comparative results of the modular and geometric replacements (abstract). Orthop. Trans. **1**, 91 (1977)

WILDE, A.H., COLLINS, H.R., EVARTS, C.M., GREENWALD, A.S., DEHAVEN, K.E., BERGFELD, J.A.: Report on the geometric knee prosthesis. Contemp. Surg. **6**, 37–41 (1975)

YOUNG, H.H.: Use of a hinged Vitallium prosthesis (Young type) for arthroplasty of the knee (abstract). J. Bone Joint Surg. (Am.) **53**, 1658–1659 (1971)

Chapter 11

Tibio-femoral Replacement Using a Totally Constrained Prosthesis and Cruciate Resection (The Guépar Prosthesis)

J.H. AUBRIOT

Centre Hospitalier Universitaire de Caen, Service de Chirurgie Orthopédique,
Avenue George-Clemenceau, Caen, France

Historical Account and Introduction

The reduction of the physiology of the knee to its essentials — a simple movement of flexion–extension around a hinged axis — was in use well before the advent of surgeons and engineers, as is illustrated by Fig. 1, a terra-cotta sculpture from Ancient Greece. The first attempt at an endoprosthesis of the knee was a hinged prosthesis made by GLUCK. In Berlin 1890, three cases were published of tumor albus of the knee, which were operated upon to fit hinged ivory prostheses (Fig. 2) fixed in the femoral and tibial diaphyses by means of Cellophane, pumice stone, and plaster of Paris (cited in BUCHHOLZ and ENGELBRECHT, 1973). It appears that this attempt was abandoned, if not forgotten, and the history of hinged prostheses of the knee does not resume until 1947, when the Judet brothers made a model in acrylic resin. Anyone seeking precise information and references on the history of the development of these hinged prostheses should refer to the important review compiled by WAGNER and MASSE (1973) for the Belgian Congress of Orthopaedics in 1972, and to the abbreviated but very full analysis by RILEY (1976).

Without returning to these articles and without relating the vicissitudes of this type of surgery, we should like to stress that this historical account enables us to understand why this procedure took some time to become widespread and popular. It is to the credit of surgeons such as WALLDIUS (1960), from 1951, and SHIERS (1954), from 1953, that they continued with their work despite the many initial complications, and that they contributed — like other surgeons who invented prostheses, such as YOUNG (1963) and McKEE (1974) — to making treatment with total endoprostheses

acceptable and credible. These pioneers had several problems to solve:

1) *The choice of material:* The use of acrylic resin, at first, and then stainless steel did not result in prostheses that were sufficiently resistant to the stresses imposed by the principle of the hinge. The risk of fatigue fracture was minimised by the adoption of chrome–cobalt alloys and a better understanding of the shape of the prosthesis.

2) *The considerable rate of infection*, related especially to the problems of wound healing: at first it was not exceptional for amputation to be reported. The superficial situation of the knee and the dramatic consequences of infection explain why many surgeons were unwilling for a long time to use total prostheses of the knee, even though they already had wide experience of total prostheses of the hip.

3) *The results as regards mobility* were often poor, more especially when there were complications and re-operation. Interest was then lost in total prostheses in favour of arthrodesis, with its safety and relative simplicity.

4) *Fixation of the prosthetic components to the bone* was inadequate. The use of methyl methacrylate cement, as advocated by CHARNLEY, provided one solution to this problem, and after its adoption the number of prostheses inserted increased rapidly. It must be emphasised, however, that even such an experienced surgeon as WALLDIUS now rarely makes use of cement for fixation.

The pioneers of this kind of surgery, and the first surgeons who adopted their prostheses, published analyses of their results that were sometimes reviewed after a considerable time — even up to

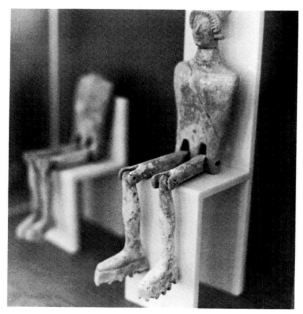

Fig. 1. Greek sculpture in terra-cotta (325 B.C.)

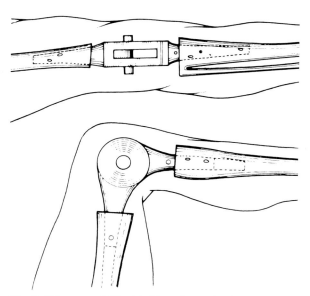

Fig. 2. Diagram of Gluck's hinged prosthesis (1890)

the past 5 years. In this respect it is significant to compare the publications in two issues of *Clinical Orthopaedics and Related Research* that were devoted to prostheses of the knee and appeared 3 years apart:

1973. 11 papers: Results with six models of hinged prosthesis

10 papers: Results with six models of non-hinged prosthesis

1976. 3 papers: Results with three hinged models

9 papers: Results with eight nonhinged models

The aim of this Chapter is not to contrast these different types of prosthesis, but to take stock of the problems posed by the hinged prostheses, especially the frequency of complications and their treatment, and the quality of the functional results. Considerable space will be allotted to findings from the literature, but particular attention will be paid to the experience acquired with the Guépar prosthesis by the GUÉPAR group (*Groupe d'Utilisation et d'Etude des Prothèses Articulaires*), which was founded in 1969. The Section on the possible indications for the hinged prosthesis will more particularly reflect my own present position.

Mechanical Findings on Total Hinged Prostheses

The use of a fixed-axis hinged prosthesis at the knee modifies the physiology of the joint by suppressing the movements of rotation and varus–valgus displacement in the frontal plane. This brings about modifications of the working conditions of the knee, and it might be feared that these would favour loosening of the components of the prosthesis, especially in view of the considerable rotation forces on the flexed knee so much emphasised by BLUNDELL JONES.

The theoretical calculations of the forces, the measurement of stresses upon the bone, and the measurement of friction and wear of the components carried out in the laboratory setting on simulators (FREEMAN et al., 1973) are certainly far removed from the conditions under which prostheses function in vivo, but nevertheless these studies have facilitated an approach to the problem and they give some idea of the quantitative dimensions involved, which is useful in deciding the size

10 or 15 years. This gives us a good idea of the complications and results of hinged prostheses at present and enables us to assess the improvements contributed by the other types of prosthesis that have been suggested SCALES and LETTIN (1973), AUBRIOT (1974), BUCHOLZ and ENGELBRECHT (1973). From 1968, however, total prostheses without hinges began to be invented, and their number has increased very rapidly, especially in

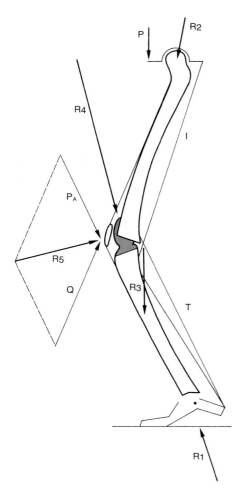

Fig. 3. Vectorial breakdown of forces acting upon a lower limb fitted with a total hinged prosthesis of the knee. (After J. WAGNER)

and shape of implants. We shall report here the principal conclusions from the work of WAGNER and co-workers (1973a, b).

The diagram in Fig. 3 shows the breakdown of forces acting upon a lower limb provided with a hinged knee prosthesis. Force R4 is the one that acts upon the hinge axis: for a load P of 100 kg on a knee flexed to 45°, force R4 is increased over that in a normal knee without a prosthesis (438 kg), but very variably, depending on the type of prosthesis: 523 kg (+19%) for the Guépar prosthesis, 600 kg (+36%) for the Shiers' prosthesis, 703 kg (+60%) for Walldius' prosthesis. At 90° of flexion the percentages of increase are identical; for example, force R4, which is thus

supported by the hinge, is 1043 kg in Walldius' prosthesis. This has two consequences. Firstly the axis of the hinge must be sufficiently stiff to give minimum deformation; secondly the friction of this axis increases with the load that it supports, and the amount of wear debris will be greater in the case of prostheses entirely made of chrome–cobalt alloy (FREEMAN et al., 1973).

In his study, WAGNER also indicated the value of force R5, involving patello-femoral pressure (WAGNER et al., 1973a and b). These clinical results are well known and will be dealt with in the section on complications and results. The extent of the force R5, involving patello-femoral pressure, varies with the type of prosthesis, essentially because of the placing of the axis of the hinge in relation to the prosthesis and to the knee: for example, at 90° of flexion, as compared with the normal knee, in which this force is estimated at 603 kg for a load of 100 kg, R5 is 864 kg with the Guépar prosthesis (an increase of 43%) and 1282 kg with the Walldius' prosthesis (an increase of 112%).

The cortical deformation of the femur and tibia of a cadaver's knee equipped with a cemented Walldius' prosthesis was measured by means of strain gauge rings. Figure 4, also taken from the work by WAGNER, summarises the deformation recorded at different levels of the cortical bone, against the standard deformation of the knee of the cadaver before insertion of the prosthesis. The differences are marked, particularly in the areas near the ends of the intramedullary stems of the prosthesis. WAGNER repeated these measurements, varying the properties of the prosthesis, and concluded that the deformations were less pronounced and more regular when a valgus deviation was set up in the assembly and when the shafts of the intramedullary stems were made longer.

This approach is interesting, since it clearly demonstrates the nonphysiological character of a hinged prosthesis that can carry considerable stresses: these stresses were responsible for the fatigue breakages observed with the earliest models in acrylic resin or stainless steel, which put a strain upon the neighbouring bone and possibly encouraged fractures or loosening.

These studies also show that there are important differences between prostheses. We shall now describe a few models that are still in use and we will try to see, by considering the complications and results, whether these are influenced by the type of prosthesis, the type of patient, or even the surgeon himself.

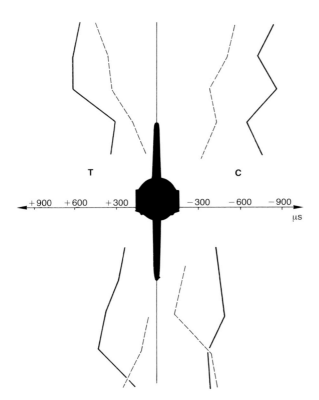

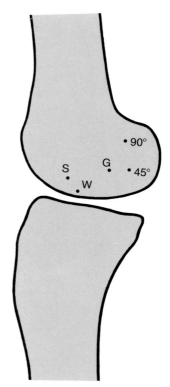

Fig. 4. Maximum bone deformation around a knee that has had a Walldius prosthesis placed in valgus deviation (*continuous line*), compared with that of an intact lower limb (*dotted line*). T, tensile strain; C, compressive strain. (After J. Wagner)

Fig. 5. Position of axis of rotation of hinged prostheses of Shiers (S), Walldius (W), and Guépar (G). (After J. Wagner)

Types of Hinged Prosthesis

Operative Technique

Several factors have to be considered if an attempt is to be made to classify the models of hinged prostheses that have been published or made commercially available. We have chosen as an arbitrary criterion the situation of the axis of the hinge in relation to the spongy bone of the femur.

In the majority of prostheses, this axis and its supporting system are placed outside the bone and the prosthesis is put in place after resection of the femur and tibia. The minimum height of resection is variable, depending on the type of prosthesis (Fig. 5) (Shiers, 35 mm; Stanmore, 35 mm; Walldius, 28 mm; Guépar 18 mm).

These variations are important, since should the prosthesis fail, the difficulty of performing a cor-rective arthrodesis is inversely related to the amount of spongy bone that remains.

Apart from Shiers' prosthesis, the models in this group usually comprise an anterior femoral shield, which stabilises the femoral piece in rotation and offers a sliding surface to the patella. There is also an anti-rotation stabilisation system on the tibial component provided by a fin situated either behind the diaphyseal shaft (Walldius, Guépar No. 1) or else at the level of the shaft (Stanmore, Guépar No. 2).

In this group of prostheses the axis of the hinge is placed at variable sites, as indicated in Fig. 5. To come closer to the physiological axis, limit the effect of anterior gaping of the joint, and discourage a posterior buffer in flexion, this axis has been placed above and behind in the Guépar prosthesis, with complete flexion made possible by the design of the prosthesis. It might be mentioned that there is a Silastic buffer on the tibial component in this prosthesis, to limit the movement of extension of the knee (see the experimental study in the article by WAGNER et al. (1973a and b)).

In another group, the axis of the hinge and its housing are placed within the spongy mass at the lower end of the femur, with the theoretical advantages that, first, only a minimum of epiphyseal bone need be resected and second, the dead space will be reduced, which may have some effect on the occurrence of haematomas.

Link arthroplasty, as conceived by DEVAS (1973), is one of the smallest hinge prostheses. It is also peculiar in not having a fixed axis, this movement being obtained by reciprocal jointing without a bolt. The GSB hinge, which also has a mobile axis, is described in Chap. 14.

The St. Georg prosthesis (BUCHHOLZ and EN-GELBRECHT, 1973) has a more definitely intracondyloid situation, in spite of which this group did succeed with an arthrodesis after one of these prostheses had been removed for infection. The St. Georg prosthesis has two variants: one is made completely of chrome–cobalt alloy except for the contact surfaces between the axis of the hinge and the femoral component, which are made of polyethylene to avoid wear debris; while the other has a femoral component that is itself made entirely of polyethylene to diminish the stresses at the end of the diaphyseal shaft. It seems that the latter prosthesis has been a failure, since the authors did not observe any fewer diaphyseal fractures with it; on the contrary, numerous metaphyseal fatigue fractures appeared (40 cases out of 106 prostheses).

In this second group of prostheses, which also includes the Lagrange–Letournel prosthesis (LA-GRANGE and LETOURNEL, 1973), no piece of the prosthesis replaces the patellar surface of the femur. The patello-femoral surfaces are not altered by the prosthesis, unless of course by the play of increased stresses recorded at this level, as already mentioned in the section on mechanics.

Each of these prostheses can be inserted by particular methods related to their design and conception. The operative technique has in general been widely described in the papers given as references in the publicity leaflets; we shall merely list the different operative phases of the Guépar prosthesis that we use.

1) *Place the patient in the dorsal decubitus position,* with the iliac crest clear.

2) *Apply a sterile Esmarch's bandage* at the root of the thigh.

3) *Make a medial patellar incision* to expose the knee joint after section of the plicae alaris. This is necessary to slacken the patella and diminish the risk of subsequent patellar subluxation.

4) *Use a guiding rasp and cutting gauge.* The average depth of section is 15 mm over the femur, 5 mm over the tibia. If there is substantial fixed flexion, it is advisable to increase the bone resection up to 25–30 mm to avoid paralysing the external popliteal nerve.

5) *The only technically difficult point* is the arrangement of the prosthetic components in rotation. The trochlear resection surface over the femur should be parallel to the anterior surface of the inferior metaphysis of the femur. Care should be taken not to make a mistake if the ipsilateral hip has reduced mobility with a fixed rotation deformity.

Over the tibia, the guide marks for rotation are the anterior tibial tuberosity (but this is sometimes in an abnormally lateral position) and the flexion–extension axis of the ankle, which should be slightly in external rotation in relation to the chosen axis of flexion of the knee.

6) *Usually the Esmarch's bandage is slackened* before cement fixation, which is done separately for each of the components; it is easier to begin with the femoral component.

7) *The two components should be joined* and placed in position without force. An easily handled metal clip will prevent the axis from leaving its housing. It can easily be removed in the event of re-operation necessitating dismantling of the prosthesis.

8) At present we tend more and more to *complete the operation by applying a triangular polyethylene insert,* which can easily be cemented into the patella (Fig. 6).

9) *The wound is closed with an aspirating drain in it.* It is important to insert the sutures with the knee flexed at a right angle so that the sutures will not yield during post-operative mobilisation of the knee.

10) *The post-operative course* is usually characterised by extreme simplicity:

a) Surgeons vary in their attitude to antibiotics and as to when anticoagulants should be given. The present author recommends post-operative continuation of the heparin anticoagulants that were started pre-operatively, and in the case of a knee that has not previously been operated upon, gives no antibiotics;

b) Rehabilitation with active extension can begin the day after the operation. The patient gets up

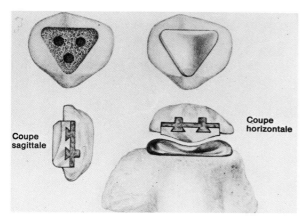

Fig. 6. Patellar insert in RCH 1000 adapted to Guépar prosthesis. Left, sagittal section; right, horizontal section

and can walk from the second or third day. Flexion starts to be recovered from the third or fourth day, the range depending on the progress of wound healing. If mobility does not exceed 70°–80° about the 12th to 15th day, it is advisable to manipulate the knee under a brief general anaesthetic.

Complications

It is important to expand the discussion on complications, which are not always discussed in detail by the pioneers of this type of surgery. However, since this type of surgery has become widespread, quite a number of publications have been devoted to complications, though their presentation has varied a great deal from one paper to another, sometimes even in papers by the same author. The origin of these complications is variable and very intricate, since three factors are involved.

1) *The patient.* The risks involved in surgery of the rheumatoid knee certainly differ considerably from those of an operation for gonarthrosis, for reasons that have often been specified — frailty of the patient, osteoporosis, the condition of the skin, polyarthritis, aggressiveness of general medical therapy.
2) *The type of prosthesis.* Peculiarities of its application, its sturdiness, its effect upon the stresses in the knee, and consequences for the patello-femoral joint all contribute to any complications.

3) *The surgeon.* In this type of surgery, which initially had very limited indications, personal experience is a very important factor, since a particular paper may refer to the problems encountered by an experienced surgeon or may bring together the complications observed by a miscellaneous group of surgeons, each of whom is starting his apprenticeship in this type of surgery.

Nevertheless, it is important to present the principal complications, since every surgeon who states that a total hinge prosthesis is indicated should know the risks that the patient will have to run and should be capable of treating the complications that may occur while trying to attain, at worst, an arthrodesed, stable, and painless knee.

We will deal in turn with the general complications, the intra-operative local and early complications, infections, complications of the extensor apparatus, and the mechanical complications of fractures and loosening.

General

The general complications are related to the clinical situation of these patients, i.e., severe rheumatoid arthritis (RA) and gonarthrosis in elderly subjects. They take the form of pulmonary and urinary infection, cardiorespiratory failure, cerebral conditions, thromboembolic complications, and their incidences are similar for hinged and for non-hinged prostheses. On the other hand there seems to be a problem specific to the hinged prostheses in the extent to which methyl methacrylate cement is utilised to fix the shafts in the diaphyses. Little information on this problem was given by the first users of cemented hinged joints (SHIERS, YOUNG, MACKEE), but within the past few years attention has been attracted to it, especially in France, in papers written by LAGRANGE and LETOURNEL (1973) and by DUPARC et al. (1975). The cases described in these papers were characterised by early operative collapse or early secondary death in coma. These accidents were found much more often (Table 1) than in total prosthetic surgery of the hip, and gave rise to a number of experimental trials (ELLIS and MULVEIN, 1974; KALLOS et al., 1974) that sought to provide an explanation for them. The most important clinical statistics were published in the survey carried out in France by KENESI (1976): there were 36 complications, 21 of them ending fatally, in 758 operations to insert

Table 1. Operative collapse and fat embolism on insertion of cemented hinged prostheses

Author	Prosthesis	Number applied	Operative collapse	Fat embolism	Deaths	
					Total	Percentage
ARDEN, 1973	Shiers	192	2	3	1	0.5
DEBURGE, 1976	Guépar	292	14	1	4	1.4
DUPARC et al., 1974	Shiers	61		3	2	3.3
FREEMAN, 1973	Walldius	74		2	0	0
KENESI (review), 1976	Shiers, Guépar, Trillat	758	36		16	2.1
LAGRANGE and LETOURNEL, 1973	L.L.	62		2	0	0

different types of prosthesis with an intramedullary stem (Shiers, Guépar, Trillat). However, it is curious to discover that BUCHHOLZ' team never observed these complications in 240 hinged prostheses.

Clinically, two types of complication have been described:

1) *Operative collapse within minutes after slackening of the tourniquet,* or when the tourniquet was slackened after cementing. Collapse of this kind often gave rise to cardiac arrest and was often very poorly tolerated by elderly subjects, resulting in death.

2) *Deferred accidents:* after a problem-free operation and a faint hint of coming round, the patient falls into an often irreversible coma after a few hours or days.

When the patient can be observed for a longer time, as in the case reported by BISLA et al. (1976), clinical observation, pulmonary radiography, and biological examinations will often reveal signs of fat embolism, which have sometimes been found on autopsy. But this fat embolism is often a secondary aspect and not the cause of the disorders. Experimental studies have often given contradictory results as to the role of an increased intradiaphyseal pressure in the genesis of this fat embolism, and stress is more often placed upon the cementing and the liberation of the monomer, which passes into the general circulation when the prosthesis is cemented even if a tourniquet is applied. The cardiovascular and pulmonary toxic effects of this monomer are well known experimentally (ELLIS and MULVEIN, 1974); to these may be added

the vasodilator effect of the methyl radicles, which potentiate the circulatory deficit. The frequency of these accidents after a total prosthesis of the knee has been inserted with the use of a tourniquet could be explained by the fact that haemodynamic disorders are much more considerable at the knee than in a hip operated upon for insertion of a total prosthesis.

Uncertainty as to the origin of these complications prevents us from stating that the recommendations advised for their avoidance are certain to prevent the accidents. These recommendations are: check that haemodynamic equilibrium has been attended to at the time of cementing, and whether the tourniquet has been slackened (some patients may have a well-filled, well-oxygenated circulation); cement the tibial and femoral components separately in dried cavities, evacuating the air through a large drain (it seems somewhat aggressive to make a hole in the diaphysis beyond the level of the cement, and not necessarily effective, according to the cases reported); introduce the cement when it is no longer liquid and no longer sticks to the gloves (this is the first recommendation made by SHIERS).

Intra-operative and Early Local

The intra-operative complications are allied either to errors in operative technique or to weakness of the bone in patients affected by RA, and more especially in bed-ridden patients and in those who have been taking cortisone for a long time. These complications include: malplacement of the stem in the diaphysis, metaphyseal fracture, avulsion of the patellar tendon, and skin tears.

The external popliteal nerve is affected almost solely in cases of very deformed knees (flexed and in valgus) where bone resection has not been sufficient. The cases reported practically all recovered without sequelae.

Skin complications (delayed healing and necrosis) may be serious if the planes of closure have been altered so that the tissues do not oppose the spread of superficial infection. Such complications are particularly likely in skin that has deteriorated after prolonged corticoid treatment. It is difficult to obtain from the publications any exact idea of the influence of the type of incision upon healing; we usually prefer the medial para-patellar incision. The incisions that were used when we first started to practise with the GUÉPAR group (median vertical and horizontal transverse) gave rise to complications, and it is surprising to learn that WALLDIUS (1973), continues to use a transverse incision, though this is situated distally, at the level of the tibial tuberosity and that he systematically applies plaster for 2–3 weeks, which we think does not favour the recovery of mobility.

DUPARC et al. (1974) have called attention to the increased fragility produced in the covering tissues by patellectomy performed at the same operation as insertion of the prosthesis. He noted five cases with severe cutaneous necrosis among 61 patients who received Shiers' prostheses and were simultaneously subjected to patellectomy.

In addition to early necrosis, ARDEN (1973) has reported a cutaneous necrosis that occurred 4 years after a Shiers' prosthesis had been inserted. Late skin lesions were observed with Walldius' prosthesis. With haematoma there is a risk that rehabilitation will be retarded, but most of all it is a factor that predisposes to infection.

Deep Infection

Deep infections are the most worrying complication of this type of surgery. Table 2 shows their frequency in the different bodies of statistics available and (where given) their distribution between early and late infections. We do not propose to study all the causes of these infections here, since they are multifactorial and the various writers have given contradictory opinions. For example, as regards the trial made in 1976 in the GUÉPAR group

(DEBURGE, 1977), we do not agree with the currently accepted idea that deep infections are more frequent in RA: 292 prostheses were inserted by this group, and 7.2% of osteoarthritic knees had deep infections, while the corresponding figure was 4.4% in cases of RA.

A previous operation, such as osteotomy, meniscectomy, or patellectomy, is said to involve the greatest risk of infection. But patients with a history of this kind did not have a higher frequency of deep infection in our sample.

On the other hand, re-operation after insertion of Guépar prostheses due to a complication affecting the extensor apparatus was followed on four occasions by suppuration. This approaches the risk of early infection after skin lesions (delayed healing and necrosis) and after a severe haematoma.

The recent review of 179 knees a minimum of 5 years after insertion of Guépar prostheses did not reveal any increase in the incidence of deep infection in the years following the operation: only one case was diagnosed after 2 years (AUBRIOT et al., 1979).

Like other writers, we have observed late deep infection that was undoubtedly related to contamination via the blood or lymphatic system: deep infections following infected corns on the toes of patients affected by RA or, following septicaemia of urinary, bone, or gastrointestinal origin.

As Table 2 shows, the way to treat a deep infection varies according to the different writers. To avoid overcrowding of the table, the treatment is not indicated on it according to whether the infection is early or late. Some writers appear to have a clear-cut policy, i.e., remove the prosthesis and the cement (if present). WALLDIUS then performs an arthrodesis, but his total cases have included two amputations. SHIERS does not attempt to obtain fusion, perhaps because in his case, after removal of the prosthesis and cement there is little effective spongy bone left, especially in patients with RA. His policy is to try antibiotic therapy for 6 months, with irrigation and hyperbaric oxygen. If the infection persists, he removes the material through a small incision, so as not to destroy the fibrous adhesions; and he immobilises the patient in plaster. Rehabilitation is prolonged, so as to enable the quadriceps to bring about fibrous ankylosis. He does not state the quality of the results obtained in the three patients treated in this way. But the other surgeons (ARDEN, 1973) who have adopted this attitude with Shiers' prosthesis mention only results in which the patients'

Table 2. Deep infection and its progress with total hinged prostheses

Author	Prosthesis	Number applied	Deep infection		Early infection	Late inf.	Prostheses retained	Fused arthrodesis	Fibrous ankylosis	Amputation	Miscellaneous and insufficient follow-up
			Total	Percentage							
ARDEN, 1973	Shiers	192	13	6.7	10	3	6		4	2	1 deceased
BAIN, 1973	Walldius Cemented	100	10	10	3	7	3	3	4		
DEBURGE, 1976	Guépar	285	19	6.6	9	10	5	3	7		4
ENGELBRECHT et al., 1976	St. Georg	240	4	1.7			3	1			
FREEMAN, 1973	Walldius Cemented / Not cemented	74 / 6	2} 2}	5				1	3		
JONES B.J., 1973	Walldius Not cemented	120	12	10	9	3		9	2	1	
PHILLIPS and TAYLOR 1975	Walldius Not cemented	67	4	4.8	2	2	3	1			
SHIERS, 1973	Shiers	140	3	2.1					3		
SLEDGE, 1976	Walldius Cemented / Guépar / Shiers	111 / 31 / 2 }144	10	7	3	7	5	2	2	1	
WALLDIUS, 1974	Walldius Not cemented	156	12	7.7				10		2	

knees were so unstable that they required a leather or plastic artificial limb to walk with.

We think that this policy is not a good solution, especially since not all the infected tissue can be excised with certainty on re-operation with a minimal exposure. In addition, if fusion is not obtained this will certainly encourage persistence of the infection. It is noteworthy that among six patients who had an infected Shiers' prosthesis removed ARDEN had to perform two amputations, one because of a persistent sinus and the other due to septicaemia.

When it has definitely been decided to remove the prosthesis, an attempt must therefore be made to obtain an arthrodesis. Quite apart from Shiers' prosthesis, there are many reasons why this is not easy to do. In the review of the cases of the GUÉPAR group (DEBURGE, 1976), of ten attempts in which the result could be assessed, fusion was obtained in only three. In the seven cases of fibrous ankylosis, the patients had to walk with an orthosis. In a more recent trial (DEBURGE et al., 1977) published by the GUÉPAR group, arthrodesis succeeded in 8 of 18 attempts. Of the ten cases of fibrous pseudarthrosis, a sinus persisted in five, showing that the most important elements in combatting infection are good excision and successful immobilisation.

It seems to us that intensification of the technical precautions should make it possible to improve the figures: all suspect tissue should be rigorously excised, the arthrodesis should be firmly fixed by a double external fixation frame, spongy bone should be added either secondarily, when healing has been obtained, or initially by Papineau's open method, as in two cases that were reported by the GUÉPAR group (DEBURGE et al., 1977).

Table 2 shows that another therapeutic policy is possible in deep infections of hinged prostheses, namely preservation of the prosthesis even in cases of late infections with manifest loosening. This conservative treatment is carried out in various ways:

1) *Systemic antibiotic treatment,* with nothing applied locally or merely lavage and irrigation. This has given some success in early deep infections, as proved by three of BAIN's cases (1973) and one of those reported by PHILLIPS and TAYLOR (1975), but the functional result was poor, with a stiffened knee in all cases. In late deep infections this treatment resulted in failure in six of BAIN's cases, the prosthesis finally having to be removed; while in two of the cases of PHILLIPS and TAYLOR (1975) the infection appears to have been cured but the functional result was poor, due to the persistence of considerable pain.

2) *Surgical excision of all the infected tissue,* followed by irrigation or drainage and then general antibiotic therapy, appears to us to be the solution of choice, since the possibility of preserving the prosthesis and keeping the knee mobile can then be envisaged. For a full surgical excision of the infected tissues the approach must be wide, allowing excision of the sinus and dismantling of the prosthesis. Another prosthesis can be inserted if the first has loosened; it can be cemented with antibiotic cement as recommended by BUCHHOLZ' team (ENGELBRECHT et al., 1976), who were able to keep three prostheses out of three in which this was attempted.

In the recent review carried out by the GUÉPAR group (DEBURGE et al., 1977) (not reported in Table 2), 14 revision operations were performed. Six were failures, but attempts at arthrodesis were then rapidly resorted to; in eight cases the infection resolved with a follow-up of at least 1 year, and often between 2 and 4 years. In five of these cases mobility reached or exceeded 90°. Our cases of failure seemed especially to be due to an insufficiently prompt re-operation in the early infections, or else to insufficient excision without changing of the prosthesis.

We therefore think that this serious problem of deep infections in hinged prostheses can be effectively treated without permanent loss of the prosthesis even in delayed cases with loosening

and marked radiographic signs, provided the revision operation is rigorous and bold enough.

Affecting the Extensor Apparatus

Rupture of the Extensor Apparatus

There are two possible forms of rupture of the extensor apparatus, namely early avulsion of the tibial tuberosity in cases of osteoporotic RA, and secondary rupture of the patellar tendon, especially, it seems, with Shiers' prosthesis, due to attrition of the tendon against the prosthesis (5 of 192 of ARDEN's cases). The poor quality of the ruptured tendon often makes it necessary to resort to plastic methods of repair, using neighbouring tendons, plastic surgery with autologous tendons, or synthetic material. The effect on movement is variable.

Dislocation and subluxation of the extensor apparatus can easily be demonstrated by axial radiography of the patella. Their frequency has been very variously reported in the different series. In the GUÉPAR series 20 patellae that were dislocated or markedly subluxed were found.

There are three possible causes of this complication: poor positioning in rotation of the tibial component, with a leg placed in external rotation in relation to the prosthesis; a tibial tuberosity in an initially lateral position, not corrected at the end of the operation by transposition; or considerable mobility in flexion of a knee fitted with a prosthesis. The Guépar prosthesis has no limit to flexion, as have the Walldius, Young, and MacKee prostheses; we have observed that dislocations occurred in knees whose mobility exceeded 100°. Because of the absence of internal rotation in flexion, and because physiological valgus is allowed for in the prosthesis, the patella tends to sublux laterally beyond a certain degree of flexion, to shorten its course and perhaps also its stresses. We have observed cases in which the patella was well centered during the first few weeks, and then subluxed when flexion of the knee increased.

The patient's tolerance of these lateral displacements is variable and sometimes surprising. However, in the Guépar sample, 8 knees of 20 with considerable lateral displacements had to undergo re-operation for transposition of the tibial tuberosity. No secondary patellectomy was performed. At present, when re-operating to transpose the tuberosity, this group also replaces the articular sur-

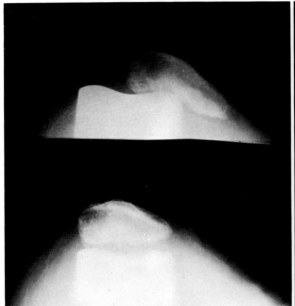

Fig. 7. a *Above:* lateral subluxation of patella 2 years after fitting of a Guépar prosthesis for OA of the knee in a woman aged 66; *below:* result of re-alignment by transposition of tibial tuberosity. Skyline radiograph at 60°. **b** Same patient, antero-posterior and lateral radiographs of the knee 3 years after fitting of the prosthesis, 3 months after transposition. Mobility of knee 0°–100°, painless

face of the patella, using a small patellar inset (Fig. 7). These re-operations have made it possible to re-route the patella, without losing movement.

Mechanical

Aseptic loosening, secondary bone fractures, breaking of the material, and wear on the axis may be considered as mechanical complications of hinged prostheses.

Aseptic Loosening

Table 3 shows the frequency of aseptic loosening in the main published series; but these reports are not all comparable, some of them mentioning only loosening that was followed by re-operation

(SHIERS, 1973; WALLDIUS, 1974; ARDEN, 1973; BAIN, 1973).

The percentages found are not very high, although some authors (SHIERS, 1973; WALLDIUS, 1974; ARDEN, 1973; BAIN, 1973) have reviewed their cases after at least 5 years and very often after 10 years. This somewhat contradicts the biomechanical findings, from which it might be feared that this complication would occur much more frequently. From the clinical point of view it is absolutely essential to distinguish two types of cases: those in which the prosthesis has been cemented, and those in which it has not.

The examples of noncemented prostheses have essentially been provided by writers who have used the Walldius prosthesis — WALLDIUS himself in most cases, and also BLUNDELL JONES (1973), PHILLIPS (1975), and WILSON and VENTERS (1976), (Ta-

Table 3. Painful aseptic loosening and its progress in hinged prostheses

Author	Prosthesis	Number followed-up	Painful aseptic loosening		Not operated on	Re-op. for prosthesis	Arthrod-esis
			Total	%			
ARDEN, 1973	Shiers	192	14	7.3	4	9	1
BAIN, 1973	Walldius cemented	100	5	5		5	
BLUNDELL JONES, 1973	Walldius Not cemented	34	7	20.6	7		
DEBURGE and GUÉPAR, 1976	Guépar	285	6	2.1		6	
DUPARC et al., 1974	Shiers	46	4	8.7		4	
ENGELBRECHT et al., 1976	St. Georg	240	5	2.1	4	1	
FREEMAN, 1973	Walldius cemented	74	4	5.4		4	
PHILLIPS and TAYLOR, 1975	Walldius Not cemented	83	3	3.6	1	1	1
SLEDGE, 1976	Walldius cemented	106	5	4.7	1	4	
WALLDIUS, 1974	Walldius Not cemented	156	7	4.5		7	
WILSON and VENTERS 1976	Walldius Not cemented	42	4	9.5	1	2	1

ble 3). All these writers agree that there is some free movement of the prosthesis within the bone; the prosthesis becomes embedded in the spongy bone and there is evident mobility of its stem. BLUNDELL JONES (1973) found this picture in all 34 knees that he checked when reviewing cases after at least 5 years; WILSON noted these radiographic signs in 34 cases of 42 reviewed after 2–14 years. But it is striking to see that this movement of the prosthesis is usually well tolerated. WILSON noted four cases in which it was poorly tolerated in a total of 34, all with varus deviation. In PHILLIPS' series of 83 prostheses followed up for 1–7 years only three knees were painful, two of which were re-operated upon. In 34 knees, all of which showed radiographic signs at review at least 5 years after surgery, BLUNDELL JONES found five cases with slight pain but with good alignment, and two cases with deformation in the frontal plane, though apparently re-operation was not performed in any of these knees.

WALLDIUS himself (1973) who has had the widest experience as regards the number of patients oper-ated upon with one follow-up, refers to only seven cases out of 156 chrome–cobalt prostheses in which re-operation for fitting of a new prosthesis was required.

Surgeons who cement hinged prostheses with methyl methacrylate rarely specify in precisely which cases they observed a radiolucent line. It is known that this is not manifest clinically but that it may later develop into complete loosening. INSALL et al. (1976) compared four different types of total prosthesis of the knee, and noted that this line occurred in 45% of cases with the Guépar prosthesis, and in a much higher proportion in nonhinged prostheses (80% with the geometric prosthesis).

The published cases and our own experience do not make it possible to state the cause of aseptic loosening, except in the special case of patients affected by Charcot's disease (neuropathic arthropathy). ENGELBRECHT et al. (1976) have stressed that all cases of aseptic loosening with the St. Georg prosthesis have occurred in patients who weighed more than 90 kg.

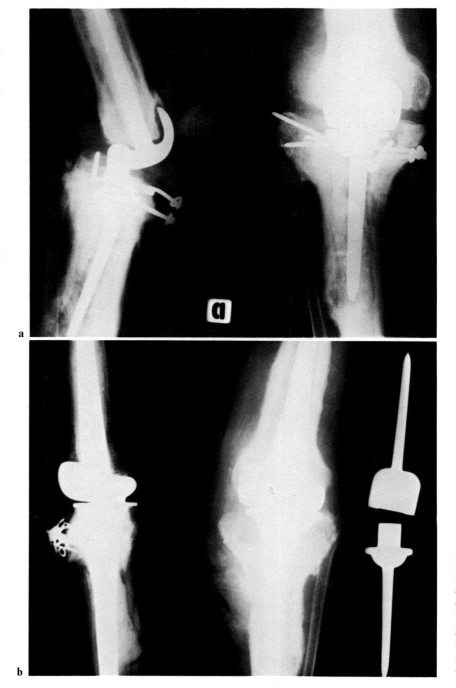

Fig. 8. a Loosening 1 year after fitting of a Guépar prosthesis in a man aged 63 affected by Charcot's disease. **b** Replacement by larger Guépar prosthesis. An antero-posterior radiograph of a standard prosthesis has been taken at the same time in order to show the difference in size

In nearly all the published cases in which loosening of cemented hinged prostheses has made re-operation necessary (Table 3), a new prosthesis has been inserted. The present tendency in the GUÉPAR group is to insert a new hinge, whose intramedullary stems are thickened and extended so that they can be anchored well within the diaphysis (Fig. 8). Some of these prostheses are not cemented, since their shape alone ensures sufficient stability. In some cases they have a madreporic surface, as it is hoped that a fresh growth of bone will infiltrate and improve stabilisation. We are not at present able to give results for this procedure from a sufficiently homogeneous series with an adequate follow-up.

In the review conducted by AUBRIOT et al. (1979) of 179 Guépar hinged prostheses after a minimum of 5 years, ten revision operations had been performed because of painful aseptic loosening (5.6%), and there were two cases of breakage of the femoral stem. At the 2-year follow-up (DEBURGE, 1976) only 2.5% of patients had needed revision operations.

Bone Fractures

Even if bone fractures occur after true trauma, they reflect the changes in distribution of the stresses brought about by the presence of the prosthesis (already studied in the section on mechanics). All those reported at the level of the femoral or tibial diaphyses have proceeded to consolidate, whether the treatment was conservative or by internal fixation with a plate. The fact that this complication did not occur in the 292 cases of the first prostheses of the GUÉPAR group leads us to suggest that the invention of this prosthesis has minimised this complication of hinged prostheses.

The BUCHHOLZ team (ENGELBRECHT et al., 1976) is practically the only one to have described supracondylar fractures of the femur, but only in cases in which the femoral component was made of polyethylene. We have already mentioned the frequency of this complication (in 40 of 106 cases) with this prosthesis.

Fracture of the Prosthesis

Fracture of the prosthesis indicates the magnitude of the stresses sustained by the prosthesis, which led the pioneers of this kind of surgery to modify their models. Because of these modifications, not a single breakage of a Walldius' prosthesis seems to have been reported since 1958. SHIERS says that the only breakages he has observed took place with the stainless steel model. But DUPARC et al. (1974), reviewing 46 Shiers' prostheses, reported fracture of the shaft in three, in addition to four cases of painful loosening. In the sample reported by DEBURGE in 1976, no fractures were observed in 292 Guépar prostheses; but since then two cases have occurred more than 5 years after insertion of the prosthesis, at the lower part of the femoral stem (Fig. 9). Re-operation showed that the prosthesis was well cemented, and that the fracture

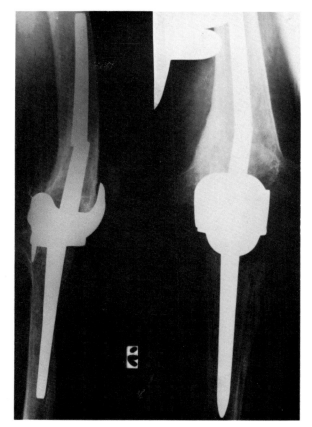

Fig. 9. Guépar prosthesis fitted in a woman aged 73 years for OA of the knee. Fatigue failure at level of femoral stem occurred 5 years later

was not due to a fault in the alloy but to fatigue, a phenomenon well known to metallurgists.

Wear on the Axis of the Hinge

The work of SWANSON et al. (1973), already mentioned in the mechanics section, enabled wear of the axis in hinged prostheses to be dealt with in the laboratory. Clinical publications refer only exceptionally to this problem. The work of GIRZADAS et al. (1968) should be mentioned; he was able, on autopsy, to obtain a Young's prosthesis from a man who had a good functional result 3½ years after the prosthesis had been inserted; there were obvious signs of wear over the axis, and metallic deposits in the joint. We have observed such findings with our Guépar prostheses, but the reason for re-operation was never this slight wear of the axis, or a synovial reaction to the metal debris brought about by wear. YOUNG (1971), who observed this metal debris in the joint, wondered whether it was not a factor that might encourage late infection.

Functional Results

We have not drawn up any summary tables of the functional results published in the literature, since it seems to us that it would be difficult to compare the different statistics published, for the following reasons (among others):

The criteria used vary widely among the different writers

The categories of results do not correspond in any way, since every intermediate is found between PHILLIPS' simplification (results classified only by success or failure) and such scoring systems as that used by WILSON

The initial pre-operative state is often imprecisely stated, especially in RA, where it is difficult to take into account the improvement contributed by the knee operation to these patients, who are handicapped by several concomitant or subsequent conditions of the joints

The role of the complications and their treatment in the functional results is often poorly defined.

To give an idea of these functional results, we shall study the criteria of pain and the arc of movement separately, before attempting to evaluate the influence of certain factors upon the results as a whole.

Pain Alleviation

The majority of publications emphasise the spectacular effect of the operation upon pain: the figures for painless or very slightly painful knees range between 75% and 90%.

Figure 10 shows the results obtained with 103 Guépar prostheses followed up for 2–5 years (DEBURGE, 1976). Different hatching is used for each pre-operative category, so that the precise future of these patients can be followed. It was found that 93% of them showed improvement.

Loosening is certainly the principal cause of persistent pain. Pain of patellar origin is the second most frequent type. The pain varies a little in frequency, depending on the type of prosthesis: for example, the design of Young's prosthesis appears to favour it. This is why HANSLIK (1973), in 46 cases in which 52 Young's prostheses were used, also made use of a patellar prosthesis made of polyethylene, similar to the McKeever one.

In the St. Georg prosthesis neither of the two patello-femoral surfaces is replaced, whilst the use of a hinged prosthesis will increase the stresses at this level. ENGELBRECHT et al. (1976) reported patellar pain in 18% of these patients (240 St. Georg prostheses).

This pain is usually of low intensity and re-operation is rarely necessary. In the same sample of St. Georg prostheses, only five knees had to be re-operated upon for patellectomy. The GUÉPAR group is very reluctant to perform a secondary patellectomy; the present policy is to re-operate, inserting a polyethylene patellar implant and at the same time transposing the tibial tuberosity to re-align the extensor apparatus, which is usually dislocated or subluxed in these painful patellae (Fig. 7).

Restoration of Movement

The aim of arthroplasty, in contrast to arthrodesis, is the restoration of movement. It is all the more important to recover or preserve movement when both knees are affected, as is very often the case with RA; we think a functional result cannot be considered good, even if the knee gives no pain, when flexion does not reach 90°. (In our all-round criteria we insist on 110° of flexion before speaking of an excellent result.) With some prostheses, such as the Walldius or the McKee, flexion was limited to 90° with the earlier models. In the Shiers' prosthesis, flexion is not limited by the prosthesis. However the design of the prosthesis and the position of the axis encourage lifting of the tibial component beyond about 100° of flexion. Post-operatively the patient must, more or less deliberately, restrict flexion to this limit. This is perhaps why, in ARDEN's sample (1973) of Shiers' prostheses, only 20% of the knees had a range of 100°.

Figure 11 shows the results for range of movement (flexion less the extension defect) published by DEBURGE (1976) with 103 Guépar prostheses. The arrangement of Fig. 11 allows consideration of the outcome in each group subjected to surgery. Overall a substantial range was retained: 84% had more than 90° and 26% reached or ex-

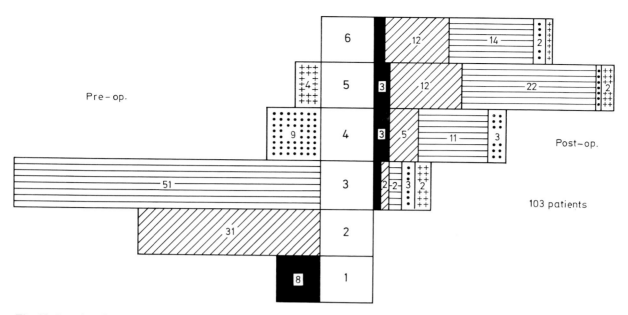

Fig. 10. Results of surgery with respect to pain in 103 patients followed up 2–5 years (standard, 8) after insertion of Guépar prostheses. 1, permanent and acute; 2, acute with total disability; 3, severe with restricted ability; 4, moderate after long walk; 5, slight or occasional; 6, none

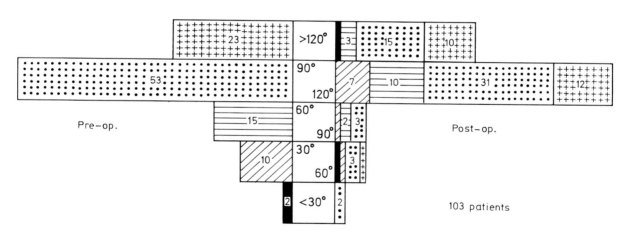

Fig. 11. Results of surgery with respect to range of movement in 103 patients followed up 2–5 years (standard, 8) after insertion of Guépar prostheses

ceeded 120° (Fig. 12). However, knees that were very stiff initially did not always improve. ENGELBRECHT reports that five ankylosed knees were treated by insertion of a St. Georg prosthesis; four of them did not recover flexion of more than 40° and only one reached 60°. It seems to us that a knee prosthesis is not indicated in such cases.

The recovery of extension is usually easy after implantation of a hinged prosthesis, which enables gross pre-operative fixed flexion deformities to be corrected. The difference between active and passive extension is minimal and often disappears after 1 year. In the GUÉPAR group, we have not yet counted the cases in which the Silastic buffer was still working properly after more than a year of walking. We have the impression that in about half these cases the buffer deteriorates and is not effective.

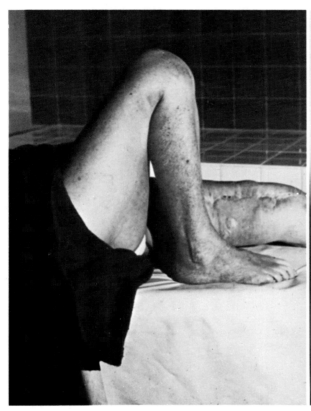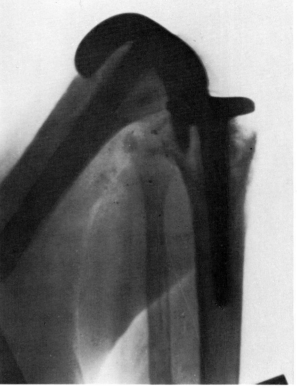

Fig. 12. Example of very good flexion of knee in a woman aged 70 operated upon for OA of the knee. Fiften months before these pictures were taken she had had a new pros-

thesis fitted due to septic loosening; this was still well tolerated 5 years later

Global Function

All-round functional results are dependent essentially upon two criteria: pain and movement. In the long run the overall results are identical with those with regard to pain; the mobility factor affects function on going upstairs or getting up from a chair. Statistically the good and very good functional results are assessed in general at between 80% and 90% (89% in WALLDIUS' statistics for 156 knees operated upon between 1958 and 1972). We have already expressed the reservations we hold regarding these results; in particular we think that truly excellent results are rare (between 5% and 10%), since we insist on complete absence of pain, movement reaching at least 110°, and ability to descend stairs without limping. An operation involving a hinged prosthesis of the knee only rarely restores a level of function that is practically identical with that of a normal knee. Our experience gives us the impression that the percentage

of these excellent results is no greater than with nonhinged prostheses, and that we are far from obtaining the functional quality of a hip replacement. Studies of the gait of subjects with hinged prostheses of the knee by means of objective recordings clearly show that walking is impaired (study on a walk track, HARRINGTON, 1974; electrogoniometric study, VAN HUSSEN, 1973).

Although truly excellent results seem unusual to us, on the other hand our experience confirms the majority of publications that give the percentage of good results at around 75%–80%. Two publications must be cited, however, whose authors do not share this view:

YOUNG (1971) found no good results in RA or in post-traumatic lesions with his prosthesis on review at 10 years, although he obtained good results in 72% of cases of gonarthrosis.

WATSON et al. (1976) used Shiers' prostheses in 38 rheumatoid knees (review after 2–7 years), and obtained only three good or excellent results (al-

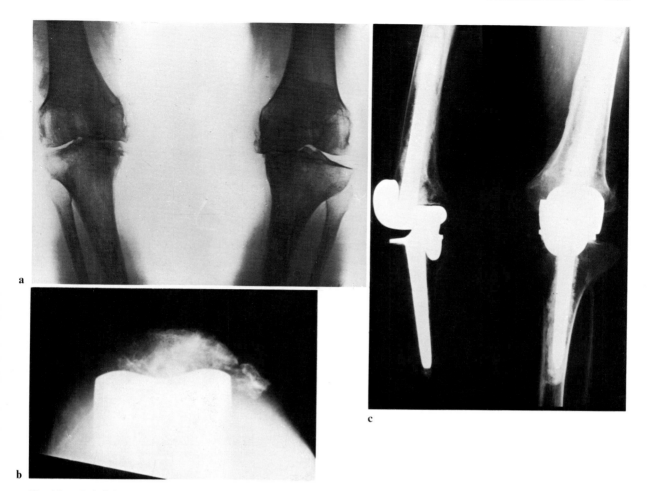

Fig. 13. a Painful and unstable bilateral OA of the knee in a woman aged 63. **b** Radiograph of left side 5½ years after fitting of a Guépar prosthesis. Knee painless; mobility 0°–115°. Patient walks without a stick, can go downstairs normally. **c** Skyline radiograph at 30° in the same patient at 5½ years

though the requirement for this category was only 50° of flexion) and nine fair results. Twenty-six results were poor, and most cases deteriorated at the end of the second year due to aseptic loosening with loss of mobility in flexion. Writers who review their cases after more than 5 years — ARDEN (1973), BLUNDELL JONES (1973), SHIERS (1973), WILSON and VENTERS (1976), WALLDIUS (1974) — in contrast, mention the stability of their results. This is also the impression that we have with the Guépar prosthesis when we review cases after 5 years (Fig. 13).

The following results were recorded in the recent review (AUBRIOT et al., 1979) of patients who had been walking for a minimum of 5 years with one normal knee and one Guépar hinge prosthesis:

Very good	8%
Good	46%
Fair	26%
Poor	11%
No appreciable improvement	8%

These results are very strictly classified: for a result to be classed as fair, mobility is 60°–90°; the patient walks with an uneven gait and limps when going downstairs; and patellar pain is present but tolerable.

Related to Aetiology

The opinion of different writers varies with regard to the results in rheumatoid as against arthrosic knees.

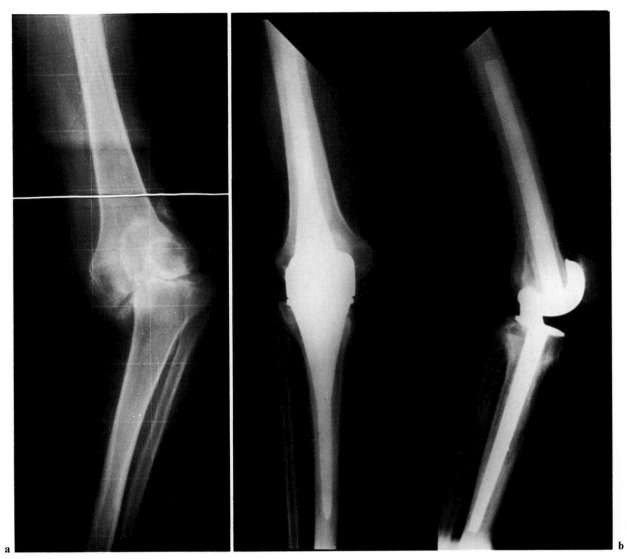

a   b

Fig. 14. a Charcot's disease in a woman aged 65. **b** Radiograph of special, large-size Guépar prosthesis. No pain had recurred after $2\frac{1}{2}$ years; mobility 5°–115°, knee very stable on walking

Some, such as ENGELBRECHT et al. (1976), note no difference. YOUNG had much more satisfactory results in gonarthrosis. In contrast to other series, in the GUÉPAR group (DEBURGE, 1976) we have operated upon many more cases of gonarthrosis (192) than of RA (91). Our impression is that there are fewer complications with the rheumatoid knees, but possibly this is because these patients' walking activity is reduced. SHIERS (1973) has also operated on more cases of gonarthrosis than of RA. He had better results with the latter, which is the reverse of WATSON's experience; he reported 95% good results, 5% moderate, and no failures among 42 cases; while in the 89 cases of gonarthrosis there were 23% good results, 17% moderate, and 10% failures.

Two aetiologies should be mentioned individually:

Charcot's disease. Everyone who has had patients with Charcot's disease has observed aseptic loosening in a considerable number of them; we have found the same. We think that these patients should be provided with a prosthesis with extended shaft, reinforced to achieve bone fixation well up into the diaphysis (Fig. 14).

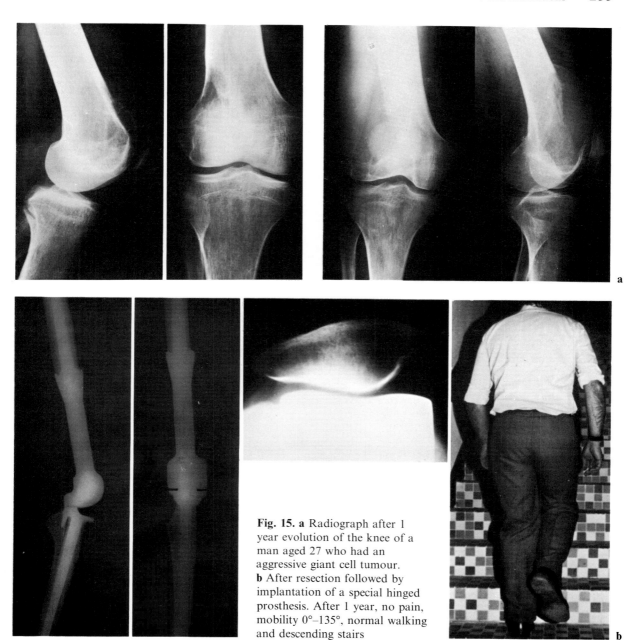

Fig. 15. a Radiograph after 1 year evolution of the knee of a man aged 27 who had an aggressive giant cell tumour. **b** After resection followed by implantation of a special hinged prosthesis. After 1 year, no pain, mobility 0°–135°, normal walking and descending stairs

Tumours of the lower end of the femur. Since 1952 the STANMORE group have used hinged prostheses to replace the lower end of the femur when this is affected by a tumour necessitating extensive bone resection. SCALES and LETTIN (1973) have reported results with nine prostheses. Since 1972, the GUÉPAR group have performed similar operations, adapting the Guépar prosthesis to these resections, especially in cases of giant cell tumour (Fig. 15). Our follow-up and the number of cases are limited, but we have not yet observed fracture of the material or loosening, and in the case shown in Fig. 16 we were surprised to see the quality of the result, which was objectively excellent.

Conclusions and Indications

The findings in the literature and the experience of the GUÉPAR group relative to the complications

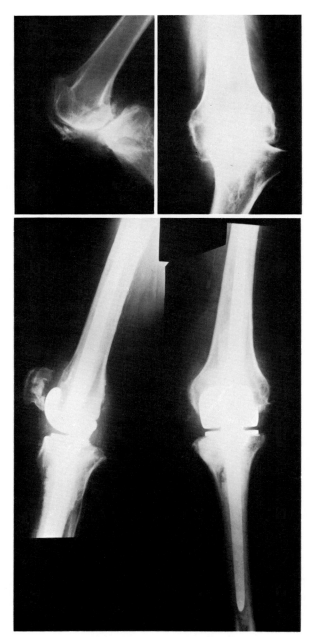

Fig. 16. a Severe OA of the knee causing pain, an unstable genu varum and complete crippling, in a man weighing 75 kg. b After insertion of a Guépar II prosthesis with patellar insert

and to the results of total hinged prostheses of the knee have been analysed in the knowledge that it is not always easy to determine what is attributable to the prosthesis itself and what to the disease. We find an apparent paradox in the fact that the hinged prostheses that are not physiological (as

mentioned in the section on mechanics) are rarely complicated by loosening, even in cases reviewed after more than 10 years. The behaviour of the Walldius prosthesis without cement is particularly surprising, since despite the almost constant presence of radiographic signs of movement between the prosthesis and the bone, the functional results are usually statisfactory. Whether the prosthesis is cemented or not, it is in any case quite easy to re-operate if a Walldius prosthesis becomes aseptically loosened. The fact that, in our opinion, the functional result of the hinged prostheses is often good but rarely excellent is probably due partly to the principle of the hinge itself, but also to the frequency of RA as an aetiological factor. So far, comparison with the functional results obtained with nonhinged prostheses is not unfavourable to the hinged prostheses. The analysis published by INSALL and his co-workers in 1976 is interesting in this respect, since they used the same criteria to compare the Guépar prosthesis and three models of prostheses without hinges, the unicondylar, the bicondylar, and the geometric. We have reproduced their conclusions while stressing that after referring to their misgivings concerning the difficulty of treating an infected hinge, they do say: "In this study, the Guépar prosthesis emerged as superior from many standpoints. This prosthesis was used in the knees with the most severe involvement and yet equalled any of the other prostheses in the quality of results both in rheumatoid arthritis and in osteoarthritis. The Guépar also had the lowest proportion of failures. It was the only model to improve the range of movement significantly, and also gave the greatest percentage improvement rating."

We feel it would be useful to sum up our views on the advantages and disadvantages of the Guépar, which is the hinged prosthesis we prefer; and in conclusion we shall state the indications currently in use.

The Guépar has the following *advantages* as a hinged prosthesis:

1) It is simple to insert, with a minimal risk of malplacement. The only difficult problem is the assessment of rotation
2) Considerable deformation and instability can be corrected
3) The prosthesis can be securely implanted even when the spongy bone is very porotic. With rheumatoid knees we have sometimes abandoned the idea of using a nonhinged prosthesis during the

operation, because of the severity of the osteoporosis, and have inserted a Guépar prosthesis instead

4) The post-operative management is simple, since the patient quickly feels stable because of the hinge and because of the secure anchorage to the tibial and femoral shafts. Rehabilitation is simple and there is no difficulty in recovering complete extension.

In the section on mechanics we have explained the differences in behaviour between the different hinges. Clinically, the Guépar prosthesis seems to resemble models such as the Walldius or the Shiers, and in this respect its *advantages* are:

1) Very good recovery of flexion which probably results in better function, especially in RA

2) An apparently lower frequency of the mechanical complications of loosening, bone fracture, and fracture of the prosthesis itself

3) The ease with which a patellar prosthesis can be added. We find it difficult to discover any obvious difference between the Guépar and an intracondylar prosthesis such as the St. Georg as regards mobility, function, and mechanical complications. But the problem of patello-femoral pain seems to be more easily resolved by an associated implant than by patellectomy, the solution adopted by the Buchholz team.

The *disadvantages* of hinged prostheses are not peculiar to the Guépar prosthesis. The main problems derive from the presence of methyl methacrylate cement in the diaphysis:

1) The general pre-operative and early postoperative complications, with coma, have been described at length without providing any definite explanation as to their occurrence. Various writers have given greatly differing frequencies for these complications

2) The most worrying problem is that of infection. Whatever the type of hinged prosthesis, arthrodesis is difficult to perform successfully; yet Walldius usually does not cement his prosthesis, removes it, and easily obtains bone fusion in case of infection. The policy now most often adopted in the Guépar group and by the Buchholz team is to re-operate, excising all infected tissue, replacing the prosthesis if it is loosened and refixing it with antibiotic cement. In this way it seems we can hope to preserve satisfactory function in a considerable number of cases.

Our knowledge of these complications and of the possibility of treating them has led us to prefer to fix hinged prostheses with methyl methacrylate at present. We have already said that the increased stresses caused by the hinge–cement–bone system is not reflected clinically in a much increased level of mechanical complications.

The present author finds the clinical assessment of hinged prostheses, and especially the Guépar, very satisfactory. If I consider the complications seen in my own patients, I no longer have doubts about using this prosthesis. Since 1972, in private practice, and since the end of 1974, at the Hospital Universitaire at Caen, 14 rheumatoid knees and 43 cases of gonarthrosis (27 genu varum, 15 genu valgum, 1 arthrosis in normal alignment) have been operated upon for implantation of the Guépar prosthesis, with the following principal complications: one case of early post-operative coma, followed by death; one of aseptic loosening, re-operated upon successfully (reviewed after $2\frac{1}{2}$ years), no infection, no fracture. I consider the prosthesis to have broader indications than merely those of salvage. However, it is certain that the *indications* listed below will be modified as time passes and other types of prosthesis appear that can resolve the problems solved by hinged prostheses without involving risks.

Whatever the aetiology of the deterioration in the knee to be operated upon, it seems preferable not to apply a hinged prosthesis in two circumstances:

1) When there is a history of joint infection
2) When the patient is very young.

Another possible contra-indication — stiffness in a more or less fused knee — is less clear, but this condition involves some risk of failure and should be carefully considered.

Having made these general reservations, it seems not unreasonable to envisage the use of a Guépar prosthesis in the following cases:

1) *When semi-constrained prostheses* have failed.
2) *In gonarthrosis* in which it is too late to consider osteotomy; very great instability, tibio-femoral subluxation especially frontally, with destruction of the tibial spines, considerable fixed flexion or on the contrary genu recurvatum, and some forms of chrondrocalcinosis involving considerable destruction of bone. All these anatomical anomalies make a hinged prosthesis more favourable,

especially if the subject is over 70. In fact, if it has been well inserted the hinged prosthesis should allow satisfactory functional activity for at least 10 years. In the elderly, a hinged prosthesis simplifies the problems of functional recovery. In the overweight, it seems preferable to use the recent model (Guépar no. 2), whose diaphyseal shafts are longer and reinforced.

3) *In RA*, with considerable incorrectable deformity, in particular in valgus, or in the presence of marked instability. The use of a hinged prosthesis is particularly appropriate if there is considerable osteoporosis, with poor quadriceps function, in a patient who is no longer young and whose life expectancy is limited.

4) *In Charcot's disease* the hinged prosthesis may be a good solution, provided a model that permits extended diaphyseal anchorage, e.g., Guépar no. 2, is used.

The use of a special hinged prosthesis after the resection of tumours at the lower end of the femur should be considered in relation to the tumour, balanced against amputation, and from the orthopaedic point of view in relation to resection arthrodesis, since these lesions are nearly always unilateral and very often occur in young subjects. The extent of the resection to be undertaken, and the difficulties that can be foreseen if reconstruction by arthrodesis is performed, may lead to a preference for a special hinged prosthesis.

References

ARDEN, G.P.: Total knee replacement. Clin. Orthop. **94**, 92 (1973)

AUBRIOT, J.H.: Les arthroplasties du genou par endoprothèse totale. Conference d'enseignement Sofcot. Expansion Sci. Fr. **2**, 65 (1974)

AUBRIOT, J.H., BADELON, B.: Chirurgie prothétique du genou et medecine de rééducation. In: Genou et médecine du rééducation, p. 194. Paris: Masson 1978

AUBRIOT, J.H., DEBURGE, A., KENESI, C., SCHRAMM, P.: La prothèse Guépar. Acta Orth. Belg. **39**, 257 (1973)

AUBRIOT, J.H., DEBURGE, A., GENET, J.P., et al.: Total hinge prosthesis Guépar: experience with 5-year follow-up. Paper presented at the First International Congress on the Knee, Lyons, 1979

BAIN, A.M.: Replacement of the knee joint with the Walldius prothesis using cement fixation. Clin. Orthop. **94**, 65 (1973)

BISLA, R.S., INGLIS, A.E., LEWIS, R.J.: Fat embolism following bilateral total knee replacement with the Guépar prothesis: A case report. Clin. Orthop. **115** 195 (1976)

BLUNDELL JONES, G.: Arthroplasty of the knee. Modern trends in orthopaedics, p. 210. London: Graham Apley 1972

BLUNDELL JONES, G.: Total knee replacement: The Walldius hinge. Clin. Orthop. **94**, 50 (1973)

BUCHHOLZ, H.W., ENGELBRECHT, E.: Die intrakondyläre total Kniegelenksendo prothese "Modell St-Georg". Chirurg **44**, 373 (1973)

DEBURGE, A.: Guépar hinge prosthesis. Complications and results with two year follow-up. Clin. Orthop. **120**, 47 (1976)

DEBURGE, A., AUBRIOT, J.H., MASSE, Y.: Infections profondes dans les arthroplasties Guépar. Rev. Chir. Orthop. **63** (2) 79 (1977)

DEVAS, M: Link arthroplasty of the knee. The knee joint, p. 248. Proceedings of the international congress. Rotterdam: Excerpta Medica 1973

DUPARC, J., BOUCHER, X.Y., DESMONT, J.M.: Prothèse de Shiers et ses complications. Communications aux journées du genou. Hôpital Bichat Paris 1974

DUPARC, J., DESMONT, J.M., OLIVIER, H., HAGE, J.F., BOCQUET, L.: Accidents généraux et prothèses scéllées du genou. Nouv. Presse Med. **5**, 253 (1975)

ELLIS, R.H., MULVEIN, J.: The cardiovascular effects of methylmetacrylate. J. Bone Joint Surg. (Br.) **56**, 59 (1974)

ENGELBRECHT, E., SIEGEL, A., ROTTGER, J., BUCHHOLZ, H.W.: Statistics of total knee replacement. Partial and total knee replacement design. St. Georg. A review of a 4 year observation. Clin. Orthop. **120**, 54 (1976)

FREEMAN, P.A.: Walldius arthroplasty. A review of 80 cases. Clin. Orthop. **94**, 85 (1973)

GIRZADAS, D.V., GEENS, S., CLAYTON, M.L., LEIDHOLT, J.D.: Performance of a hinged metal knee prosthesis case report with a follow-up three and one-half years and histological and metallurgical data. J. Bone Joint Surg. (Am.) **50**, 355 (1968)

HANSLIK, K.: First experience on knee joint replacement using the young hinged prothesis combined with a modification on the Mac-Keever Patella Prosthesis. Clin. Orthop. **94**, 115 (1973)

HARRINGTON, I.J.: The effect of congenital and pathological conditions on the load action transmitted at the knee joint. Conference on total knee replacement, p. 1. London: Institution of Mechanical Engineers 1974

INSALL, J.N., RANAWAT, E.S., AGLIETTI, P., SHINE, J.: A comparison of four models of total knee replacement prosthesis. J. Bone Joint Surg. (Am.) **58**, 754 (1976)

JONES, B.G.: Arthroplasty of the knee. In: Modern trends in orthopedics, Vol. 8, pp. 210–249. London: Graham Apley 1972

JONES, B.G.: Total knee replacement. The Walldius hinge. Clin. Orthop. **94**, 50–57 (1973)

KALLOS, T., ENIS, J.E., GOLLAN, F., DAVIS, J.H.: Intramedullary pressure and pulmonary embolism of femoral medullary contents in dogs during insertion of bone cement and a prosthesis. J. Bone Joint Surg. (Am.) **56**, 1363 (1974)

KENESI, C.: Complications générales précoces dans les prothèses totales du genou à charnières cimentées. Rev. Chir. Orthop. **62**, 413 (1976)

LAGRANGE, J., LETOURNEL, E.: Principes et réalisations de la prothese totale du genou. Acta Orthop. Belg. **39**, 280 (1973)

MCKEE, G.K.: Total knee replacement since 1957. Conference on total knee replacement, p. 40. London: Institution of Mechanical Engineers 1974

PHILLIPS, H., TAYLOR, J.G.: The Walldius hinge arthroplasty. J. Bone Joint Surg. (Br.) **57**, 59 (1975)

RILEY, L.H.: The evolution of total knee arthroplasty. Clin. Orthop. **120**, 7 (1976)

SCALES, J.T., LETTIN, A.W.F.: The evolution of the Stanmore hinged total knee replacement. The knee joint, p. 284. Proceedings of the international congress. Rotterdam: Excerpta Medica 1973

SHIERS, L.G.P.: Exempta medica. Arthroplasty of the knee. Preliminary report of a new method. J. Bone Joint Surg. (Br.) **36**, 553 (1954)

SHIERS, L.G.P.: Total replacement of the knee joint. Acta Orthop. **39**, 252 (1973)

SLEDGE, C.B.: Constrained total knee prosthesis. Personal communication 1976

SWANSON, S.A.V., FREEMAN, M.A.R., HEATH, J.C.: Laboratory tests on total joint replacement prostheses. J. Bone Joint Surg. (Br.) **55**, 759 (1973)

VAN HUSSEN, F.A.J.: Movement of the knee during locomotion in patients with a Walldius prosthesis. The knee joint, p. 54. Proceedings of the international congress. Rotterdam: Excerpta Medica 1973

WAGNER, J., MASSE, Y.: Historique de l'arthroplastie du genou par implants partiels et totaux. Acta Orthop. Belg. **39**, 11 (1973)

WAGNER, J., BOURGOIS, R., BAILLON, J.M., HALLEUX, J.P.: Etude bioméchanique des prothèses totales à charnière du genou. Acta Orthop. Belg. **39**, 217 (1973a)

WAGNER, J., BOURGOIS, R., HALLEUX, J.P., BAILLON, J.M.: A mechanical study of total knee arthoplasty: Preliminary report. The Knee joint, p. 58. Proceedings of the international congress. Rotterdam: Excerpta Medica 1973b

WALLDIUS, B.: Arthoplasty of the knee using an endoprosthesis. 8 years experience. Acta Orthop. Scand. **30**, 137 (1960)

WALLDIUS, B.: Arthroplasty of the knee using a hinged Vitallium prosthesis. Acta Orthop. Belg. **39**, 245 (1973)

WALLDIUS, B.: A comparative analysis of different methods for arthroplasty of the knee, p. 34. Conference on total knee replacement. London: Institution of Mechanical Engineers 1974

WATSON, J.R., WOOD, H., HILL, R.C.J.: The Shiers arthroplasty of the knee. J. Bone Joint Surg. (Br.) **58**, 300 (1976)

WILSON, F.C., VENTERS, G.C.: Results of knee replacement with the Walldius prosthesis. Clin. Orthop. **120**, 39 (1976)

YOUNG, H.H.: Use of a hinged Vitallium prosthesis for arthroplasty of the knee. J. Bone Joint Surg. (Am.) **45**, 1627 (1963)

YOUNG, H.H.: Use of a hinged Vitallium prosthesis for arthroplasty of the knee. J. Bone Joint Surg. (Am.) **53**, 1658 (1971)

Chapter 12

Tibio-femoral Replacement Using a Semi-stabilised Prosthesis and Cruciate Resection (The Sheehan, GSB, Attenborough and Spherocentric Prostheses)

J.M. Sheehan

St. Vincents Hospital, Elm Park, Donnybrook, Dublin 4, Ireland

The knee joint is characterised by a high degree of stability and a wide range of movement while bearing body weight. Arthrodesis of the knee is a safe, simple operative procedure, which results in a stable pain-free outcome. This is achieved at the expense of movement and occasionally of social acceptability. In proposing arthroplasty one must be confident that the advantages of arthrodesis will be retained, with the added bonus of a functional arc of movement.

The knee joint has long been recognised as a ginglymus or hinge-type joint, and the earliest attempts at prosthetic replacement were based on this simple principle. However, the incidence of biological and mechanical problems following hinge arthroplasties was high, and in a number of instances the risks and complications of surgery proved prohibitive.

It took some years for clinicians to appreciate that the human knee was a much more sophisticated apparatus and that the design of a knee mechanism should ideally simulate the joint it replaces as closely as possible. This does not necessarily imply that the exact anatomical configuration of the intact joint should be copied (as has been done for example by the Leeds group: Seedhom et al., 1974), and in fact this approach can have its own specific disadvantages, e.g., the implantation of an excessive bulk of foreign material in a superficial location. Instead adequate movement and stability can be restored by a mechanical device having a different form but achieving the same function as in the normal knee.

In recent years the knee replacement field has become more complex, because surgeons and designers have advocated different appliances for varying degrees of collapse, deformity, or instability of the joint. Ideally any knee replcement should be applicable to all degrees and varieties of pathological disorders involving the joint. No knee should be considered too destroyed, too

unstable, or too angulated for reconstruction. In addition, reconstruction should be an easy, safe, and reliable procedure.

Because of the difficulties encountered in salvage procedures for large hinge replacements, the pendulum has swung in the opposite direction, so that the current trend in prosthetic knee joint replacement is towards safety should failure occur. This has resulted in a very large number of prostheses appearing on the market that involve minimal bone resection, so that in the event of failure a salvage procedure, i.e., arthrodesis, is technically possible without gross shortening. Such surface-mounted prostheses without intramedullary fixation achieve their stability from the compressive forces acting across the joint. No form of inherent stability can exist in such joints, as their design does not permit tensile forces to be applied without a major risk of dislocation.

The phenomenal success of hip arthroplasty in the latter part of the 1960s emphasised all the more the lack of adequate knee prostheses. In particular, patients with polyarticular disease who had hip arthroplasties performed still remained grossly disabled by their knee arthropathy, and patients with knee arthropathy alone remained unoperated upon as very few surgeons were willing to subject their patients to the fairly major risks entailed in the insertion of a massive hinge prosthesis.

The results of hinge arthroplasty even in the most competent hands were at best only moderately satisfactory. Improved design and better operative technique had certainly increased the success rate, but the comments of Young (1963), an enthusiast in this field, were of special interest. "It should be emphasised that on the basis of available evidence the hinged prosthesis method for arthroplasty of the knee should neither be used promiscuously nor be abandoned because of the failures observed. It is well established that the tissues can tolerate a large mass of inert inorganic material. It behoves us to work out the proper mechanics and design of the prosthesis."

In the same year, AUFRANC recognised the complexity of the normal knee mechanism. "The knee joint is such a functionally complicated mechanism that to substitute a joint with only a hinge factor of motion seems a little less than desirable. In the motion of flexion, the knee has a rotatory element; in the motion of complete extension, it has a locking element through the two arcs of motion that are normally allowed by the femoral condyles. The femoral condyles are rounded in the anteroposterior and lateral planes. I think these shapes need to be incorporated into any prosthesis if we are to get a greater and freer range of motion."

The first departure from the traditional hinge type mechanism was in 1968, when GUNSTON introduced his hingeless polycentric arthroplasty. This was the first real effort to simulate the normal knee mechanism, and heralded a new era in knee reconstruction. The early success in such patients aroused great enthusiasm, but the disadvantages were soon apparent — the technical difficulties encountered in inserting four separate components, the inability to correct varus, valgus, or flexion deformities of any great magnitude, and the difficulties with fixation of the components if bone destruction had occurred — and these and other problems stimulated two other, distinct lines of thought:

1) The development of surface-mounted prostheses without inherent stability

2) The development of intramedullary prostheses with some inherent stability, i.e., semi-stabilised prostheses.

The latter group of prostheses were designed to provide a means of reconstructing not only the moderately involved knee but also the knee with gross destruction where there is a shortage of bone on the articular surfaces and no reliance can be placed on the integrity of the ligamentous structures.

This Chapter will only be concerned with such semi-stabilised prostheses, i.e., with prostheses that have some inherent stability but are of a nonhinged design. Four such prostheses exist: the Sheehan, the Gschwend or GSB, the Attenborough, and the Spherocentric. These prostheses were first implanted in November 1971, June 1972, January 1973, and October 1973, respectively.

Design Features

In the present author's view, a prosthesis for the replacement of the knee should ideally have the following characteristics:

1) Adequate fixation even in soft, osteoporotic, destroyed joints

2) Low-frictional bearing surfaces

3) Preservation of the collateral ligaments and of the lateral and medial margins of the femur and tibia for a two-fold purpose: (a) To allow normal collateral ligament function and thus to preserve the contribution of these ligaments to knee stability; (b) To permit subsequent arthrodesis without shortening if sepsis supervenes and necessitates removal of the implant

4) Anchorage by cement or another, alternative method to permit early mobilisation, with suitable tapered stems on the implant

5) Requirement of minimal skill for insertion

6) Interchangeable plastic component in case of long-term wear

7) Implant largely buried in bone

8) Preservation of patello-femoral mechanism as an essential component of the extensor apparatus.

Individual Prostheses

The four semi-stabilised prostheses considered in this Chapter have the following design features.

Sheehan (Fig. 1)

The range of motion of the Sheehan prosthesis simulates normal knee movement, i.e., $-5°$ to $+130°$ flexion. No rotation is permitted in the extended position but rotation gradually increases to 20° when the knee is flexed to approximately 60°. A varus–valgus movement of about 2° is allowed in the fully extended position, increasing to about 6°–7° when the knee is semi-flexed. The flexion–extension axis of the prosthesis is movable, as the shape of the condylar component is the same as that of the normal knee. No side-to-side movement is permitted, and only minimal backward and forward movement is permitted, to simulate the normal action of the cruciate ligaments.

These complex movements are possible because of the geometry of the high-density polythene tibial stud and reciprocally shaped locating tracks on

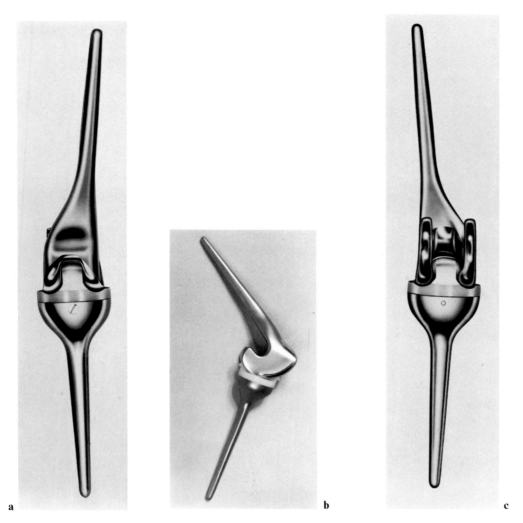

Fig. 1a–c. The Sheehan prosthesis

the inner aspect of the femoral bearing surfaces. The tibial plastic component is firmly anchored in the metal cup, which provides the intramedullary stem for fixation.

When viewed from the inferior aspect, the gap between the femoral surfaces diverges posteriorly, thus allowing increasing degrees of rotation with flexion. The outer surfaces of the femoral bearings are parallel at all times.

When a knee replaced with a rigid hinge is flexed beyond 90°, the compressive force transmitted to the stem is changed to a tensile or distraction force, thus tending to loosen the prosthesis. A similar effect may be obtained by contact between the tibial and posterior femoral surfaces. To obviate distraction forces on one or other component of

the Sheehan prosthesis, there is no firm linkage between the components when the knee is flexed beyond 100°. Thus if apposition of soft tissues occurs on the posterior aspect of the knee, the tibial stud is free to sublux anteriorly from the femoral component.

There is no patellar surface as such on the prosthesis, but the patella approaches the femoral bearing surfaces at approximately 50° of flexion and remains in contact with them for the remainder of the range. By a combination of design and accurate placement of the prosthesis, the transition point where the patella passes from the lower femur on to the prosthesis is very smooth, and beyond 50° of flexion a hemi-arthroplasty of the patello-femoral joint has in fact been achieved.

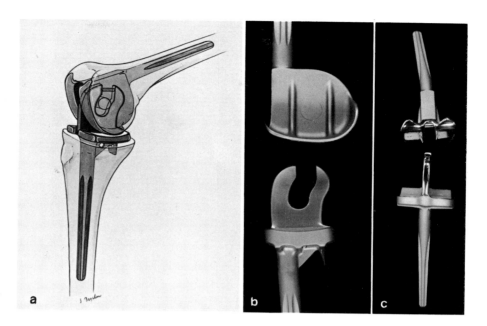

Fig. 2a–c. The Gschwend (GSB) prosthesis

Gschwend; GSB (Gschwend, Scheier, and Bahler) (Fig. 2).

The GSB prosthesis is also polycentric. The connection between the femoral and the tibial component is effected by a central bridge, in which there is a slightly curved slot running from below (anterior) to above (posterior). The slot serves as a guide for the non-load-bearing axis of the femoral component. Rotation proper is absent but there is some clearance between the components, allowing slight antero-posterior movement. In addition, the femoral component can — in analogy to a normal knee joint — be lifted off the tibial component in maximum flexion without disturbing the functional relationship the between the two components. The amount of bone resected is small and the bearing surface of the prosthesis on the bone is very wide.

Attenborough (Fig. 3)

The femoral component of the Attenborough prosthesis consists of a shell for the two femoral condyles attached to a tapered intramedullary stem. A stabilising link exists between the two components. Because of the possibility that stress is transmitted to the other component by this linkage, tapered intramedullary stems are provided. ATTENBOROUGH feels that it is best to have inter-

changeable prostheses fitting either knee, and for this reason the stem length is restricted.

At the base of the stem is a hollow into which is fitted a ball on the end of a rounded stem. This ball is free to rotate and its stem runs in a gap between the posterior parts of the femoral condyles. This gap is only just greater than the stem's diameter at the front, but widens at the back. There is a radius of 40 mm on the normal weight-bearing surface of the prosthesis and a smaller radius of 25 mm posteriorly and anteriorly. These last two curves are long enough at the back to allow for flexion of the knee through about 120° and at the front they are long enough to allow the patella to articulate with the femoral prosthesis and not with the femoral condyles. The tibial component has a tapered, hollowed intramedullary stem into which the rounded linking stem of the femoral component fits. It has a tibial plateau shaped with the same radius as the larger radius of the femoral condyle (40 mm).

Thus in extension the two components fit exactly, but as soon as 20° of flexion is reached the smaller curve of the posterior parts of the femoral condyles comes into apposition with the tibial plateau and some backward and forward movement of each femoral condyle is possible, allowing rotation. At the same time, in this position the linking stem of the femoral component is in a wider gap between the condyles of the femur and

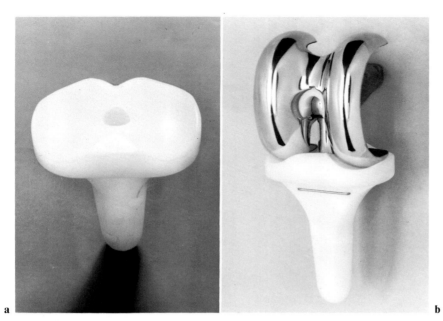

a   b

Fig. 3a and b. The Attenborough prosthesis

is thus able to move sideways, allowing some lateral mobility, which increases with flexion and decreases to nothing in full extension.

The movement of this joint is polycentric because of the different curves of the femoral condyles, and the length of the linking stem projecting below the level of the femoral condyles must therefore vary according to the position of the joint, as the centre of the ball cannot lie at the axis of both radii. Thus there is a longer projection in extension than in flexion. This makes the stem move up and down within the tibial component. There is a hole drilled from just above the weight-bearing surface of each side of the tibial plateau to the bottom of the central hole containing the rounded stem. The stem has one flattened surface. Synovial fluid can run into the bottom of the central hole when the knee is flexed more than a few degrees and on extension the stem acts as a piston, driving the fluid up again and out through the two small lateral holes close to the main weight bearing area.

Recently this design has been altered so that the metal sphere now articulates in a high-density polyethylene (HDP) socket. This simplifies the technique of insertion and also removes the metal-to-metal articulation that previously existed. A patellar surface has also been added. No clinical results with this recently modified prosthesis are yet available.

Spherocentric (Fig. 4)

The spherocentric prosthesis is an intrinsically stable, nonhinged device with three metal-on-ultra-high-molecular-weight polyethylene (UHMWP) bearing surfaces, a ball-and-socket joint located within the femoral component, and two runner-and-track joints between the femoral and tibial condyles. The ball-and-socket joint is composed of a central sphere on top of a column rising from the tibial component. In the articulated prosthesis this sphere is contained within a polyethylene socket. This in turn is fixed within the femoral component by its flat outer posterior surface, which abuts against a reciprocal flat surface within the cavity of the femoral component and by flanges on the femoral component which prevent distal displacement.

The ball-and-socket joint formed by this socket and sphere permits triaxial rotation, but translation (dislocation) is not possible in any direction. The centre of the sphere lies above the joint surfaces and well posterior to the long axis of the femur, thus approximating the location of the average flexion axis of the normal knee. The location, dimensions, and contour of the metal femoral runners and their mated tibial polyethylene tracks serve to guide and control flexion, varus–valgus movement, and torsion, and to increase the total bearing surface of the joint. The contours of the

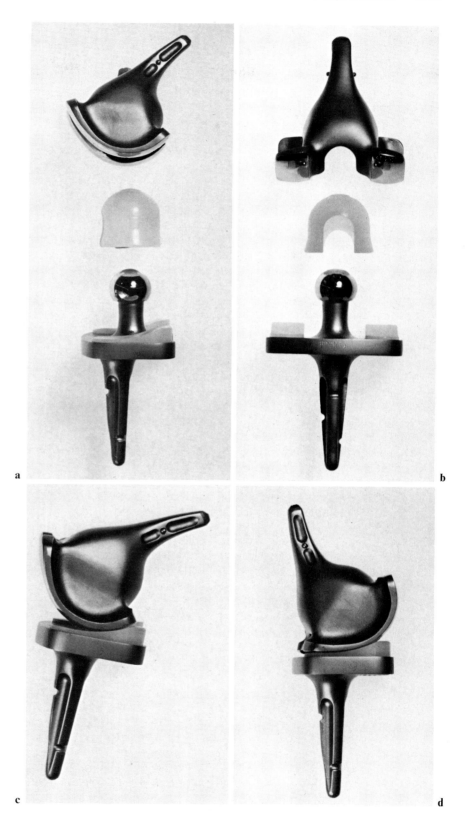

Fig. 4a–d. The spherocentric prosthesis

femoral condylar surfaces of the prosthesis in the sagittal plane include an anterior part with a larger radius of curvature, which is not concentric with the surface of the sphere, and a posterior part with a smaller radius of curvature, which is concentric with the surface of the sphere. As the knee approaches full extension, the anterior surfaces of the femoral condylar runners with their larger radius of curvature bear increasingly on the plastic tibial tracks, thereby unloading the top of the sphere and forcing the underside of the sphere against the surrounding plastic socket. The central pillar is thus placed in tension. Hyperextension is arrested by gradual deceleration due to the cam effect with no rigid extension stop. Impact loading at the end of extension should therefore be minimised and at full extension the prosthesis is fixed and completely stable in all directions except flexion.

As the prosthesis flexes from its fully extended position, the femoral condylar surfaces slowly lift off of the plastic tibial tracks, gradually transferring all the load to the dome of the sphere, thereby permitting triaxial rotation of increasing amplitude as the condylar runners lift further and further off the tibial tracks. At maximum flexion (120°) the prosthesis permits up to 30° of tibial rotation and up to 5° of varus–valgus motion.

All articulating surfaces are metal on plastic. There is no metal-to-metal contact in any position. All plastic (and thus potentially deformable) components (including the press-fit tibial tracks) are supported by metal and are readily replaceable should this be desirable because of wear.

This prosthesis, although consisting of arcs of two different radii, is not truly polycentric, as most of the load is transmitted from the central sphere to its plastic socket. It is only towards full extension that the load is transmitted to the outer condylar surfaces. Thus in normal function, movement is largely uni-axial in a coronal plane.

Intramedullary Fixation

All four of these devices use intramedullary fixation. It is totally impractical to consider a semi-stabilised prosthesis depending on surface fixation: if there is any stability in the prosthesis itself — other than the stability produced by compressive loading — then intramedullary stems become mandatory to achieve adequate fixation.

In soft, osteoporotic bone such as is frequently encountered in RA, the ideal method for both fixation and alignment in the author's view, is the use of intramedullary stems. In patients with normal bone density, intramedullary fixation still has the advantage that it greatly facilitates insertion and accurate alignment. In addition, the degree of destruction or collapse of the condyles does not influence the final stability of the joint.

On the other hand, fatigue failure of femoral hip stems is now becoming a major problem, so that an appreciation of the importance of adequate stem design has been growing for some years. Thus sharp angles form points of stress concentration, which predispose to failure of the stem through fatigue and also cause failure of the acrylic cement with crack propagation starting at these sharp points. The latter phenomenon, if it occurs, causes loosening of the stem in its cement bed. This imposes high loads on certain areas of the stem, and this in turn predisposes to stem failure due to fatigue.

Stem Taper

To achieve ideal stress transmission from the prosthesis to the bone via the cement, an evenly tapered stem is desirable. If the stem taper is less than 5°, the taper is described as a locking taper and such a component requires moderate force to dislodge it from its cement bed.

When stress is transmitted through a straight taper to a surrounding cylindrical structure, so-called hoop stresses are developed in the bone and cement. If excessive, these may cause longitudinal cracks in the cement. To obviate this danger a simple taper can be modified by the provision of a platform, an external collar, or an internal collar (as in the tibial component of the Sheehan prosthesis, in which the upper expanded portion of the prosthesis acts as an internal collar and transmits the stress directly to the upper tibial cortex).

Stem Length

The ideal stem length is still unknown. The stem should be long enough to give adequate cement fixation and alignment. On the other hand, it should be short enough to allow cement to be introduced at its tip and to permit removal of the implant and of its accompanying cement if infection ensues. An additional consideration in decisions concerning femoral stem length is that patients requiring knee arthroplasty frequently also require hip arthroplasty, and both stems must be accommodated in the same bone.

In view of the width of the lower femoral canal a stem length of 25–30 cm is required to give accurate alignment. On many counts this length is impractical, so that a compromise situation results. Experimentally a tibial stem of 11 cm overall in length does not give accurate alignment in all cases, as the stem tip still lies in cancellous bone but if the overall length is extended to 13.5 cm very good alignment can be achieved routinely.

The advantages of short (as against long) intramedullary stems are, firstly, that a zone of cancellous bone can be preserved between the implant and cortical bone: this facilitates fixation with cement, and by retaining the energy-absorbing properties of cancellous bone it should help to prevent failure at the bone–implant interface. Secondly, short stems have the advantage that a single femoral device can be used for either the right or the left side, provided the stem is not off-set. The disadvantage, however, of a straight femoral stem is that load is transmitted eccentrically from the prosthesis to the bone. Thus a bending moment is produced, which will theoretically increase the likelihood of loosening.

The effect of stem length upon the stresses in the femur itself is controversial. In the present author's view short thick stems should be avoided, since such a stem can be expected to increase the risk of supracondylar fractures due to the sudden change in elastic modulus between the bone and the implant. The junction of the lower expanded condylar part of the femur with the thin cortical region is already a weak area, as evidenced by the occurrence of supracondylar fractures in this region in the normal femur. If a stem is to be used, it should therefore pass well into the cortical region of the bone to obviate stress concentration in an area which is already weak.

In contrast to this view, two of the designs described in this Chapter do in fact have short, thick stems, and both designers differ from the view set out above, believing that the likelihood of fracture is greater with longer stems passing into the cortical region.

The alternating transmission of force between the medial condyle during the stance phase and the lateral condyle during the swing phase of gait (MORRISON, 1969) gives rise to obvious design difficulties if one attempts to anchor surface-mounted prostheses to the bone. The see-saw effect transmitted to the cement–bone junction loads the cement with an alternating tension–compression cycle. This predisposes to loosening of one or both components, as acrylic cement is particularly unsuited to cyclically alternating stresses. Short straight stems are also exposed to this mode of failure. From a salvage point of view the stem length is not of great significance, since if the cement has to be removed from the lower femur and upper tibia an extra few centimetres on either side will not appreciably increase the technical problems involved.

In the long term it will be of interest to see whether the short stems of the Attenborough and Spherocentric prostheses will be elongated by their designers or whether the long stems of the GSB and Sheehan prostheses will be shortened.

Systemic Collapse

One obvious disadvantage of intramedullary fixation is the reported incidence of systemic collapse during anaesthesia, associated either with the insertion of the cement or with the release of the tourniquet. The exact cause of this has not been established. It may be associated with monomer passing into the circulation, the release of fat or hypovolaemia following release of the tourniquet, or to a number of these factors acting in combination. A combination of factors appears to be the usual explanation in patients who collapse during hip arthroplasty, and in the author's view is the most likely explanation for collapse after knee arthroplasty.

DOWLING (1976) recently studied the level of monomer passing into the circulation during simulated knee arthroplasty. A series of experiments was carried out to consider the effects of exsanguination on the migration of MMA monomer during total knee replacement (Fig. 5). An experimental model was established, which incorporated the canine tibio-femoral joint and a simulated total knee replacement with intramedullary stems. MMA monomer was tagged with ^{14}C and was readily measured in the inferior vena cava. When implant experiments were performed without an exsanguinating tourniquet MMA monomer migration similar to that found by HOMSY et al. (1969, 1972) and MCLOUGHLIN et al. (1973) for simulated total hip replacement in dogs was seen. However, in the simulated total knee replacement without tourniquet (Series II) a monomer level of up to 7.5 mg% was detected. This indicated a high vol-

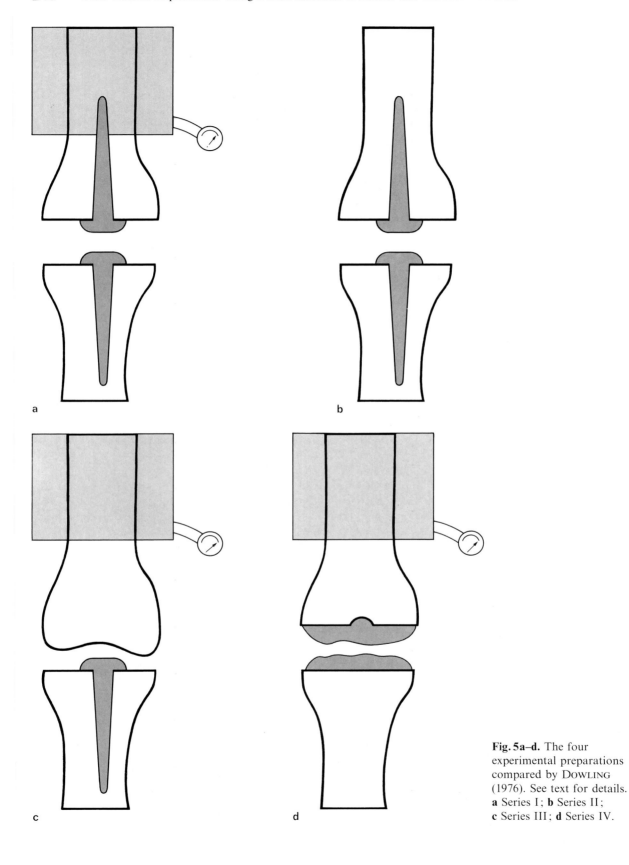

Fig. 5a–d. The four experimental preparations compared by DOWLING (1976). See text for details. **a** Series I; **b** Series II; **c** Series III; **d** Series IV.

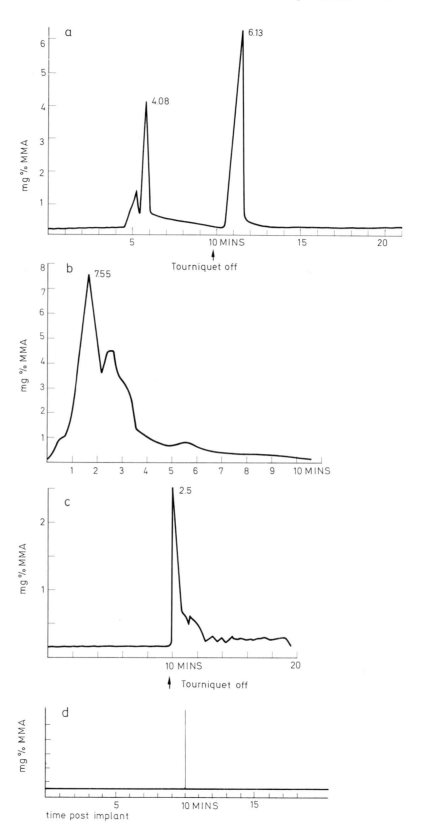

Fig. 6a–d. Monomer blood levels obtained by DOWLING (1976) in series I–IV, respectively. See text for details. *Arrow* indicates removal of tourniquet

ume of monomer migration considering the logarithmic decay.

The amount of monomer detected in some total knee replacement experiments was 20 times the maximum monomer level detected by MCLOUGHLIN et al. (1973) in experimental hip replacement.

Results of experiments in which a tourniquet was used (Series I) indicated a biphasic monomer migration from simulated total knee replacement (Fig. 6). The first phase, probably from the femoral component, enters the circulation 2–6 min after implantation and in profile has a more gradual decay than during the second phase of migration.

First-phase migration could not be reproduced when only the tibial side of a total knee replacement was introduced (series III). It is likely, therefore, that monomer diffuses through the intramedullary cavity and endosteal circulation to the systemic venous system. This route of migration would be uncompressed by a tourniquet. The degree of monomer migration is variable, which is in keeping with clinical experience showing that toxicity and hypotension are not constant features.

The second phase of monomer migration is seen on release of the tourniquet. This always showed a short, sharp rise in monomer level, which is readily explained by the return of circulation to the limb, causing a bolus of monomer to enter the circulation. The higher the level of monomer detected, the more clear-cut the profile of migration.

The findings with respect to "onlay" bone cement are in keeping with clinical experience (WPACOS, 1974) indicating that total knee replacements without intramedullary stems are not associated with acute toxic reactions. No MMA monomer was detected at any stage during these experiments (Series IV).

The high peak level of MMA monomer detected in the inferior vena cava both during exsanguination and on release of the tourniquet does not necessarily signify a very high dose of monomer infusion. The short period during which monomer was detected implies a fast infusion of amounts of monomer similar to that detected during simulated hip arthroplasty.

Patello-femoral Joint

None of the prostheses in this group has a specifically designed surface for the patella, but all allow the patella to come into contact with the anterior surface of the femoral prosthesis during flexion.

The articular surface of the patella is trimmed of osteophytes. More recently ATTENBOROUGH has replaced the patellar surface with a polyethylene surface in selected cases.

The nature of the clinical problems associated with the patella will be considered later. Here it may be said that an obvious problem is encountered by a designer if he wishes both to retain the effective function of the collateral ligaments and at the same time place the patello-femoral surface flush with the anterior femoral surface. If a femoral component is inserted so that it lies flush with the anterior aspect of the femur and the tension of the collateral ligaments is adjusted so that they are taut with the knee extended, no control over the ligaments is possible as the knee is flexed. If, however, the femoral component is placed in relation to the posterior aspect of the condyles, ligament tension can be retained throughout the arc of flexion–extension but the anterior flange of the femoral prosthesis may then lie well in front of the anterior surface of the femur. To retain ligament tension throughout the arc of motion whilst at the same time permitting accurate anterior placement of the femoral component would therefore require a large selection of femoral components to be available for any one case. With any form of complex design this becomes impracticable.

Clinical Results

It is impossible to compare the results obtained with the different prostheses directly and to draw conclusions. Consequently the current results obtained with each type in the hands of the designer will be summarised and some of the particular problems will be analysed.

The principle factor preventing a direct comparison of the results is the wide variation in the pathological conditions requiring replacement in the different series. Most of the patients in these four series had moderately or severely damaged knees, but Table 1 summarises the aetiological conditions in each series. The assessment of function following knee arthroplasty is a complicated procedure. In the author's (SHEEHAN) series, involvement of the contralateral knee, one or both hips, or the feet was frequently present.

Pain, function, and movement have all been differently graded by different designers. The greatest

Table 1. Duration of follow-up and aetiology in the four series

| | Number in series | Maximum follow-up (months) | Aetiology (%) | |
			OA	RA
Sheehan	131	67	19	81
GSB	117	45	56	44
Attenborough	166	45	45	55
Spherocentric	25	23	26	64

Table 2. The incidence of moderate or severe pain in the four series

| | Moderate to severe pain | |
	Before operation	After operation
Sheehan	81%	3%
GSB	95%	13%
Attenborough	Majority	20%
Spherocentric	Grading not applicable	

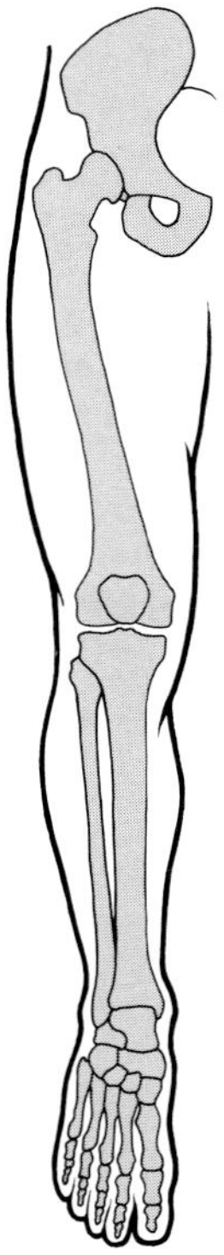

Table 3. The average arc of movement in the four series

	Before operation	After operation
Sheehan	77	91
GSB	66	108
Attenborough	Not recorded	80°+(in over 80%)
Spherocentric	74°	92°

Table 4. Re-operations for patello-femoral symptoms in the four series

Prosthesis used	No. of re-operations
Sheehan	1
GSB	—
Attenborough	10
Spherocentric	1

37 involved + 42 replaced = 60%

47 involved + 34 replaced = 62%

85 involved = 65%

Fig. 7. The incidence of involvement of the joints in the contralateral limb associated with Sheehan arthroplasty

discrepancy is found in the method of recording function. Thus, no attempt at a comparison of this parameter will now be made. A comparison of pre- and post-operative pain and movement is made in Tables 2 and 3, however.

Patello-femoral Symptoms

Re-operation for patello-femoral symptoms has been necessary to a greater or lesser extent with all designs (Table 4). ATTENBOROUGH (1973, 1974)

has had a high incidence of symptoms (necessitating secondary surgery in ten patients) and he now routinely resurfaces the patella with an HDP surface. The patellar symptoms in his series increased with time and accounted for a falling off in the number of good results at 2 years as against the 1-year follow-up.

GSCHWEND (1974) and GSCHWEND et al. (1973) state that patellar pain is not an infrequent finding and that it is attributable less to the destructive changes in the articular surface of the patella than to an uncorrected subluxation. He hopes to be ables to dispense with artificial replacement of the patella in the majority of patients.

In the spherocentric series, approximately 15% of patients have mild to moderate patello-femoral symptoms in the initial post-operative period.

However, these symptoms have resolved spontaneously within the first 6–9 post-operative months and only one patient has so far required revision surgery.

In his own series, the present author had an incidence of 13% of patients with retro-patellar symptoms. One patient required patellectomy but in none of the remaining cases were symptoms severe enough to interfere to any significant extent with function. Where patellar symptoms have occurred, they have improved with time in the majority of patients and an early decision with regard to the need for secondary surgery is not encouraged.

The long-term mechanical stability of patellar replacements is as yet unknown and most designers are reluctant to introduce a further variable into the technique and design at present.

Further Remarks on Individual Series (Tables 5–11)

Sheehan

The grading for function pre- and post-operatively is based solely upon the ability to walk (SHEEHAN, 1978).

Table 5. Ability to walk after Sheehan arthroplasty

	Before operation	After operation
Unable	10	3
Indoors only	33	10
100–200 yards	49	11
440–880 yards	33	34
Normal	0	73

Table 6. Ability to walk after GSB arthroplasty

	No. of patients	Up to 100 m	1 km	>1 km
a) Patients with RA (48)				
Unilateral	35	6	19	10
Bilateral	13	2	7	4
b) Patients with OA (45)				
Unilateral	32	1	11	20
Bilateral	13	0	4	9

Table 7. Pain after spherocentric arthroplasty

Grading
0. None
1. Minimum: does not limit activity
2. Mild: occasionally limits activity
3. Moderate: often limits many activities
4. Severe: constant, disabling and intolerable

Results (average grade)

Before operation	After operation
3.76	0.56

Table 8. Function after spherocentric arthroplasty

Grading
0. Non-walker: in chair or bed all the time
1. Severe restriction: walks only short distance with support, needs help to stand
2. Moderate restriction: definitely limited as to distance walked and terrain walked on. Uses cane, crutches, brace, or walker most of the time
3. Mild restriction: somewhat limited as to distance walked and terrain walked on; seldom uses cane or crutches
4. Walks normally: aware of no limitation

Results (average grade)

Before operation	After operation
1.36	2.98

Table 9. Mechanical complications

Prosthesis	Nature of complication	No. affected
Sheehan	Detachment of tibial plastic in original design	4
	Failure of tibial stud	2
GSB	Failure of tibial component in original design	1
	Loosening: certain	1
	possible	2
Attenborough	Failure of tibial plastic	2
	Loose tibial component	1
Spherocentric	—	—

Table 10. Mortality

Prosthesis	Operative	Post-operative	
		Fat embolism	Pulmonary embolism
Sheehan	1	—	—
GSB	—	1	2
Attenborough	—	—	2
Spherocentric	—	—	—

Table 11. Successful arthrodesis for infection

Prosthesis	No.
Sheehan	1
GSB	3
Attenborough	4
Spherocentric	—

Two patients developed failure of the tibial stud after the insertion of Sheehan prostheses, one at 7 months and the second at 24 months. Both had complete ruptures of the medial collateral ligament due to gross long-standing valgus deformities. This is now considered a contra-indication for this arthroplasty. In four further patients the HDP tibial component became detached from its metal socket. This design was changed in January 1974 and no further case of detachment has since occurred. One patient had a patellectomy for impingement of the patella against the prosthesis.

There has been no case of prosthetic loosening to date and no settling of either component has been detected.

Lucent lines surrounding the cement of both components were detected in two patients — one with bilateral arthroplasties. A further two cases have a lucent line around either the femoral or the tibial component.

Gschwend

GSCHWEND graded function separately for patients with RA and with OA and distinguished between unilateral and bilateral replacements.

Prosthetic failure occurred in one case of an earlier design in which the connecting bridge between the femur and the tibia was thinner than in the current model. It has not occurred with the current design.

Loosening occurred in one case where a hinge joint had previously been implanted.

In a further two cases a radiolucent line of 4 mm is present suggesting loosening. GSCHWEND feels that radiolucent lines of up to 2 or 3 mm round the stem of the prosthesis have no importance as long as they are not found around the articulating part of the prosthesis itself, i.e., at the cement–cancellous bone interface.

Three knees became infected: all had successful arthrodeses with 16–18 hole AO plates.

Attenborough

No detailed breakdown of pre- and post-operative function is available for the Attenborough prosthesis. However, pre-operatively 20% of the patients were unable to walk and a further 38% could only walk indoors, while 12% could walk between a quarter of and half a mile. Post-operatively over 70% could walk a quarter of a mile and in 30%–40% of cases activities were essentially unlimited.

Four patients underwent removal of the prosthesis and arthrodesis of the knee for infection. Three patients now have sound arthrodeses and one has a fibrous ankylosis.

In two patients the tibial component has loosened due to a large amount of residual cement in the back of the knee, causing a sudden block to flexion. In one of these the tibial component broke at the lower end of the stabilising rod. One further patient who was left with a 10° varus deformity had a similar type of fracture of the tibial component.

Ten patients have had secondary operations for patello-femoral pain. In these cases an HDP prosthesis has been implanted on the articular surface of the patella. This is now a routine feature of the Attenborough procedure at the initial operation.

Spherocentric

Only average pre- and post-operative figures for pain and function have been quoted for the spherocentric prosthesis, so that no direct comparison with other prostheses is possible.

The total experience at the University of Michigan is now 140 cases (personal communication,

1978). No mechanical failures have been reported. There have been two re-operations for infection; in both these cases the implant was removed and an arthrodesis attempted. One is a recent case and still undergoing treatment. In the second infected case the infection has been controlled but fusion has not occurred.

A further patient with recurrent haemarthrosis has had a synovectomy and patello-femoral replacement with the Bechtol prosthesis.

Summary

This brief review of the design considerations and early clinical results of semi-stabilised prostheses is an attempt to summarise the present state of the art. These implants combine the qualities of the physiological arc of movement and permit varying degrees of axial rotation (except for the GSB). At the same time they provide inherent stability. In all cases, insertion demands the removal of the cruciate ligaments. Dependence on the collateral ligaments is not essential, but most designers agree that utilisation of these ligaments under adequate tension minimises the stress on the prosthesis and diminishes the risk of loosening. In no instance are these implants designed to replace the monarticular diseased knee in an otherwise healthy young individual.

Results to date indicate a high percentage of satisfactory results. Patellar problems still require further investigation and clarification. With the exception of the Attenborough prosthesis, the re-operation rate for these residual symptoms has been minimal, and the overall impression is that they improve with the passage of time. Time alone will prove whether the current phase of replacing the patellar surface with a convex button will give as good a long-term result as a hemi-arthroplasty of the patella or, if troublesome symptoms persist, a patellectomy.

The ideal design and length for an intramedullary stem is still uncertain. The incidence of stress fractures of the lower femur associated with short stems will be of particular interest in the future. In the present series it is of interest to note that the two cases of stress fracture of the femur and a further two cases of femoral shaft fractures were all associated with short stems.

The increased levels of monomer entering the circulation and the possibility of fat embolism demand that research into both these fields is carried out as a matter of urgency. In the meantime special precautions should minimise these problems.

The ease of insertion and accuracy of alignment of intramedullary stems outweigh their disadvantages. The low incidence of mechanical loosening in these series suggests that many of the problems associated with the rigid hinged prostheses have been eliminated.

A much improved understanding of the muscle vectors about the knee, soft-tissue release procedures, and patellar alignment, as well as the correction of associated foot and hip deformities, augurs for a greater success rate with knee prostheses in the future. Many more years of close observation, collaborative clinical trials, and extensive mechanical analyses are required before the best characteristics of each individual prosthesis are proven. Every designer of a knee implant at present agrees that a great deal remains unknown and unsolved. The clarification and ultimate solution of these remaining problems provide the challenge for the future.

References

ATTENBOROUGH, C.G.: Total knee replacement. In: Proceedings of the international congress on the knee joint. Rotterdam: Excerpta Medica 1973

ATTENBOROUGH, C.G.: Total knee replacement, using a stabilised gliding prosthesis. Proceedings — total knee replacement, p. 92. London: Institution of Mechanical Engineers 1974

AUFRANCE, O.E.: Hinged vitallium prosthesis for knee (Discussion). J. Bone Joint Surg. (Am.) **45**, 1641 (1963)

DOWLING, F.: The Effects of exsanguinating torniquet on the migration of methylmethacrylate monomer in simulated knee arthroplasty. M. Ch. Thesis U.C.D. 1976

GSCHWEND, N.: Total knee replacement using GSB knee. In: total knee replacement, p. 30. London: Institution of Mechanical Engineers 1974

GSCHWEND, N., SCHEIER, H., BAHLER, A.: The GSB knee prosthesis. Proceedings of international congress on the knee joint. Rotterdam: Excerpta Medica 1973

GUNSTON, F.H.: Polycentric knee arthroplasty. J. Bone Joint Surg. (Br.) **53**, 272 (1968)

HOMSY, C.A., TULLOS, H.S., ANDERSON, M.S., FERRANTI, M.D.: Paper presented at orthopaedic research society meeting, New York 1969

HOMSY, C.A., TULLOS, H.S., ANDERSON, M.S., DIFFERRANTE, N.N., KING, J.W.: Some physiological aspects of prosthesis stabilisation with acrylic polymer. Clin. Orthop. **83**, 317 (1972)

KAUFER, H.: Personal communication 1977

MATTHEWS, L.S., SONSTEGARD, D.A., KAUFER, H.: The spherocentric knee. Clin. Orthop. **94**, 234 (1973)

MCLAUGHLIN, R.E., DI FAZIO, C.A., HAKALA, M., ABBOTT, B., MCPHAIL, J.A., MOCK, W.P., SWEET, D.E.: Blood clearance and acute pulmonary toxicity of methylmethacrylate in dogs after simulated arthroplasty and intravenous injections. J. Bone Joint Surg. (Am.) **55**, 1621 (1973)

MORRISON, J.B.: Bio-engineering analysis of force actions transmitted by the knee joint. Biomed. Eng. **4**, 164 (1969)

SEEDHOM, B.B., LONGTON, E.B., DOWSON, D., WRIGHT, V.: Proceedings — The leeds knee and total knee replacement, p.108. London: Institution of Mechanical Engineers 1974

SHEEHAN, J.: Arthroplasty of the knee. Proceedings of the International congress on the knee joint. Rotterdam: Excerpta Medica 1973

SHEEHAN, J.: Proceedings – Total knee replacement, p. 80. London: Institution of Mechanical Engineers 1974

SHEEHAN, J.: Arthroplasty of the knee. J. Bone Joint Surg. (Br.) **60**, 333–338 (1978)

SONSTEGARD, D.A., KAUFER, H., MATTHEWS, L.S.: The spherocentric knee. J. Bone Joint Surg. (Am.) **59**, 602 (1977)

WPACOS (Working party on acrylic cement in orthopaedic surgery): Final report to department of health and social security. London: DHSS 1974

YOUNG, H.: Use of a hinged vitallium prosthesis for arthroplasty of the knee. J. Bone Joint Surg. (Am.) **45**, 1627 (1963)

Chapter 13

Tibio-femoral Replacement Using Two Un-linked Components and Cruciate Resection
(The ICLH and Total Condylar Prostheses)

M.A.R. FREEMAN
The London Hospital, London E1 2AD Great Britain

J. INSALL
The Hospital for Special Surgery, 535 E 70St., New York, NY 10021 USA

This Chapter is in two parts. One, written by FREE-MAN, is concerned with ICLH arthroplasty. The other, written by INSALL, is concerned with the Total Condylar arthroplasty. This material has been combined to form one Chapter, rather than separated into two, because the views of the authors upon most of the topics relevant to replacement of the knee are closely similar, and because both procedures make use of an unlinked two component tibio-femoral prosthesis and cruciate section.

Since cruciate section characterises both the procedures described in this Chapter, it is appropriate at the outset to summarise our view of its advantages. These have been discussed by FREE-MAN et al. (1977 b) and are as follows:

1) Deformities of any magnitude can be corrected. The removal of scarred, adherent cruciate ligaments is an essential element in the soft-tissue release of a fixed valgus or varus deformity, whilst clearance of the intercondylar area of the knee provides full exposure of the posterior capsule and hence facilitates its release for the correction of a flexion deformity. In a knee with a severe fixed deformity in any direction, the intercondylar eminence of the tibia usually abuts against the roof of the intercondylar notch of the femur, so that correction of the deformity is facilitated by the removal of the eminence.

2) One function of the cruciate ligaments (especially the posterior) is to make the femur move backwards across the tibial plateaus as the knee flexes (KAPANDJI, 1970). If the cruciate ligaments are retained, the tibial prosthesis must therefore have a flat, not a dished, upper surface. If a dished tibial component is used, the femoral component will impinge against its posterior lip as the knee flexes: in this event, either the knee will "open like a book" or the tibial component will be depressed posteriorly and elevated anteriorly so

that it loosens. If a flat tibial component is used, its area of contact with the femoral component will be small, and as a consequence, the stresses on the polyethylene must be high. If the cruciate ligaments are removed, a dish-shaped tibial component can be used to reduce the stress on the polyethylene, since the femoral component will no longer move posteriorly as the knee flexes.

3) If the femur is replaced with a bicondylar femoral component, the surgeon can ensure that no cement is left in the posterior compartment of the knee, since after the insertion of both components he has easy access to the back of the joint through the empty intercondylar space.

4) The compressive strength of the replaced tibia can be increased to a value 10–13 times the body weight by resting the component on all aspects of the tibial cortex and/or by using a short intramedullary flange (BARGREN et al., 1978).

5) In pre-operatively stiff knees the range of flexion frequently cannot be increased until scarred and adherent cruciate ligaments have been released.

6) It is technically easier to cut straight across the top of the tibia than to cut around the intercondylar eminence.

7) Finally, our experience with tibial fixation (referred to below) has demonstrated a very considerable advantage that follows from the fact that if the cruciate ligaments, especially the anterior, are resected, the tibia can be subluxed so far forward in the flexed knee as to bring its posterior border in front of the femur. In this way, full uninterrupted surgical access is provided to the sectioned surface of the tibia. This in turn enables the tibial bone surface to be carefully prepared and inspected. The tibial component can then be attached securely to the proximal tibia by driving it vertically downwards into the bone with an appropriate fixation device on its undersurface. It also allows the tibial component to be trimmed so that it makes accurate contact with the whole of the top of the sectioned tibia without overhanging to produce an unacceptable subcutaneous prominence. In this way secure tibial fixation can be obtained with a prosthesis sufficiently strong in compression to resist the forces applied in normal locomotion.

ICLH (Freeman–Swanson) Arthroplasty

Initial Design Considerations

In early 1968 the arthritic knee was treated at The London Hospital by osteotomy, by MacIntosh hemi-arthroplasty, by arthrodesis, by synovectomy (in the case of the early rheumatoid knee), and very occasionally by hinge arthroplasty. The Hospital's experience with the first two of these procedures has been reported elsewhere (ANGEL et al., 1974; FREEMAN et al., 1974). In summary it can be said that the results obtained with all of them were, in different ways, not fully satisfactory. In particular, there was dissatisfaction with the methods of surgical management available to us (arthrodesis and hinge replacement) for the severely damaged arthritic knee. In view of this and of the success then being obtained with the Charnley replacement for the hip, it was decided to investigate the possibility of replacing the knee — or strictly in the first instance the tibio-femoral joint — with cruciate resection and a prosthesis consisting of a femoral and tibial component bonded to the skeleton with polymethyl methacrylate. It was hoped to design a device that could be placed upon conventional arthrodesis surfaces so as to avoid the difficulties of surgical retrieval associated with the failure of some hinge prostheses and to use it for the treatment of the severely damaged knee.

In 1969 and 1970, research along these lines was conducted in the Biomechanics Unit in the Department of Mechanical Engineering at Imperial College. A study was first carried out of the wear properties of existing devices such as the Walldius hinge. This work, (HEATH et al., 1971; SWANSON

et al., 1973) confirmed our clinical impression that cobalt-chromium alloy bearing against itself was an unsatisfactory combination of materials, since it led to the generation of unacceptably high quantities of metal (especially of cobalt) in the solution bathing the prosthesis in vitro and to the production of minute particles of wear debris, which were shown to be carcinogenic in the rat. Subsequent studies demonstrated that the soluble metals released from such prostheses in the laboratory were present in the tissues clinically and that they could sensitise the patient and lead to loosening of the prosthesis (EVANS et al., 1974). For this reason and because of the satisfactory behaviour of polyethylene at the hip, it was decided to design a prosthesis for the replacement of the tibio-femoral joint in which polyethylene was used for one component. Since polyethylene had functioned satisfactorily as the concave component of the hip, it was decided to use it for the tibial component of the knee, since obviously this component can more readily be made concave than can the femoral component.

The decision to use polyethylene as the concave component rather than the convex one has since been vindicated following the failure of devices for the replacement of the hip and ankle in which polyethylene has been used for the convex component (REVELL et al., 1978). Convex polyethylene wears more rapidly than does concave, and thus liberates greater quantities of wear debris into the surrounding tissues. This debris in turn excites a macrophage and giant cell response leading to the production of sheets of such cells which invade the bone–cement interface, cause resorption of the bony anchors to which the cement is attached, and thus lead to loosening of the implant (REVELL et al., 1978).

Having decided that polyethylene should be used in the tibial component, we sought to limit the contact stresses upon the polyethylene articular surface to a level at or below the one already demonstrated to be tolerable in the Charnley prosthesis for the hip. Given a knowledge of the loads acting through the normal tibio-femoral joint from the work of MORRISON (1970), which were subsequently shown to be of the same magnitude in the ICLH knee (PAUL and FREEMAN, 1977, unpublished data), this led to a design having a nominal contact area of 560 mm^2 and hence a nominal contact stress during walking of up to about 4.3 MN/m^2 (as against 5.4 MN/m^2 for the Charnley hip prosthesis). This contact area was achieved by fashioning the tibial component as a trough with an articular surface having a medio-lateral width of 64 mm and a radius of 24 mm, and subtending an arc of 30°. The femoral component was 19 mm narrower at its articular surface than at the tibial surface, and had one radius of curvature (the same as that of the tibial component) so that full area contact could be achieved with the polyethylene throughout the range of movement. The design of a femoral component with a single radius was the first of a number of departures made from the normal anatomy, but not in fact from the normal function of the knee since the tibia normally rotates around what is essentially a single axis (see Chaps. 1 and 2).

In the author's view, one of the possible disadvantages of hinge arthroplasty is the tendency for the prosthesis to loosen in use over the years. This tendency may be attributable to the fact that the bearing of a hinge prosthesis permits no rotational nor abduction–adduction movement. Thus, during use, those forces that tend to produce these displacements are transmitted entirely to the bond between the implant and the skeleton. Although extremely strong bonds can be constructed to meet these forces by the use of long cemented intramedullary stems, the magnitude of the forces themselves, the fact that they are repeatedly applied, and their tendency to generate tensile and shear stresses in the bond all militate against long-term successful anchorage. In an attempt to circumvent this problem, the trough of the ICLH tibial component was designed to be shallow enough to allow the femoral component to slip against, and thus to rotate within, the tibial component at relatively low turning moments. In such a prosthesis rotation inevitably results in the femoral component "climbing" out of the trough, a displacement that in the ICLH prosthesis was accentuated by the provision of sloping surfaces on the tibial component extending anteriorly and posteriorly away from the actual articular area. Thus rotation of the femoral component on the tibial was prevented to some extent by the inherent stability of the roller-in-trough design, but mainly by the fact that as the femoral component rotated on the tibial it climbed, a movement opposed by tension in the soft tissues and the compressive forces acting on the joint generated by the weight of the body and by muscle actions. It was hoped that this design would limit the torsional moments on the bone–prosthesis bond sufficiently to prevent loosening whilst providing sufficient torsional stability for

normal everyday activity. Subsequent laboratory (BARGREN et al., 1978) and clinical experience has confirmed this expectation.

It was hoped that loosening in the face of abduction–adduction moments could be prevented by providing no mechanical link between the two components, so that the femoral component could simply rock on the tibial component in abduction or adduction, without tending to displace either component on its bony bed. To prevent unacceptable instability in use, this meant that the prosthesis had to be inserted in such a way that the collateral ligaments were tight, and that, speaking pathologically, mechanically adequate collateral ligaments had to be present. In an attempt to reduce dependence upon the collateral ligaments, the components were made wide, so as to enhance the extent to which compressive forces acting across the joint stabilised the prosthesis.

These considerations, taken together, defined many of the dimensions of the prosthesis. In the first instance, its overall size was made such that it could be implanted into even the smallest knee. This meant that the prosthesis, especially the tibial component, was very much smaller than the cross-sectional area of the normal tibia in knees of moderate and large size, but this disadvantage was accepted in the interests of manufacturing simplicity. Experience has now shown, however, that a small tibial component in a large knee tends to sink into the tibia (see below), and hence that this decision was unwise. In contrast, the size of the femoral component has proved adequate because in general the bone of the femur is stronger than that of the tibia (COLLEY et al., 1978). The surfaces of the femoral component applied to the bone were designed to allow the component to be fitted onto three straight cuts made essentially at right angles to each other in the lower end of the femur. This design provided inherent stability for the femoral component on the femur and facilitated surgical preparation of the bone. The interface between the bone and the tibial component was at first prepared to be flat, and staples were used to support the bone–cement bond. Very early in our clinical experience, however, this method of fixation was changed to that of a dovetailed stud. The considerations leading to the initial design are discussed in detail elsewhere (FREEMAN et al., 1973a and b; SWANSON and FREEMAN, 1974). With regard to the patello-femoral joint, the initial intention was to carry out a patellectomy at the same time as tibio-femoral replacement, and therefore no great attention was paid to the design of the patellar surface of the femoral component. This surface was made short so that the prosthesis could be fitted to any femur, regardless of the antero-posterior size of the condyles, by "burying" the anterior flange of the prosthesis in the bone of large knees and leaving it slightly proud of the bone in small knees. Our early clinical experience of simultaneous patellectomy and tibio-femoral replacement was disastrous, however: failure of skin healing combined with a failure of healing of the reconstructed extensor mechanism was a not-infrequent complication and led to exposure of the prosthesis, secondary infection, and loss of the implant. For this reason it was soon decided to retain the patella, and therefore the patellar surface of the femoral component was partially redesigned, leaving the anterior flange short but rounding out its contours.

An early question that had to be faced was whether or not to retain the cruciate ligaments. It will be remembered that the ICLH prosthesis was introduced at The London Hospital to manage the severely damaged knee. Any deformity in such a knee can be corrected by arthrodesis or hinge arthroplasty, because both these procedures permit transection of the whole width of the proximal tibia and distal femur and thus allow the femur and tibia to be re-aligned. Put another way: it appeared that the correction of a severe deformity required the resection of the cruciate ligaments and of the intercondylar eminence of the tibia. For this and (in the light of subsequent experience) for other reasons listed above, it was therefore decided to develop a surgical procedure that would include the sacrifice of the cruciate ligaments and to design a prosthesis that would restore their function. Since, for reasons given above, it had already been decided to design the prosthesis as a femoral roller in a tibial trough, the provision of antero-posterior stability of the tibia on the femur in flexion could easily be provided by ensuring that anterior or posterior movement of the tibia was prevented by contact between the posterior or anterior lip of the tibial trough and the femoral roller. This in turn implied that the prosthesis would have to be implanted in flexion, in such a way that the gap between the two components was substantially less than the depth of the trough: were this not to be the case, the trough would be free to slide antero-posteriorly beneath the femoral roller without contact between the two components. Since we wished to allow a little passive

rotational movement in the flexed knee, the aim of the operation became to insert the prosthesis in flexion in such a way that a small gap (about 1–2 mm) existed between the two components (thus permitting some movement) but that larger gaps were avoided (thus providing stability). Clearly this degree of accuracy of implantation could not be guaranteed by "by eye" techniques of insertion, and therefore special instruments were designed to regulate the size of the gap created by bony resection in the flexed knee.

Early Clinical Experience

The first prosthesis for the replacement of the knee designed at Imperial College was implanted at The London Hospital (hence the initials ICLH) in 1970. This prosthesis was at first known as the Freeman–Swanson prosthesis. Early changes included the redesign of the patellar surface of the femoral component, a general rounding out of the corners of this component, and a redesign of the method of attachment of the tibial component to the tibia. These changes led to the prosthesis shown in Fig. 1, which was in use at The London Hospital late in 1971.

The design of the prosthesis at Imperial College over the period 1969–1970 was paralleled by the evolution in theory and in the cadaver of an operative procedure for its insertion. It was clear at the outset that the insertion of this prosthesis could not be accomplished with sufficient accuracy by

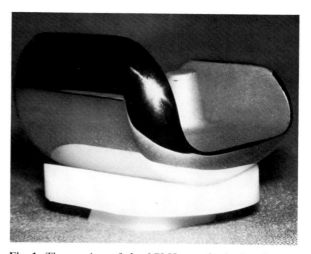

Fig. 1. The version of the ICLH prosthesis that formed the basis of a multicentre clinical trial between 1971 and 1974

Table 1. The evolution of ICLH arthroplasty of the knee

	1969	1970	1971	1972	1973	1974	1975	1976	1977
Femoral prosthesis	Monocondylar, with sharp edges: drawn	Implanted	Edges rounded	—	High anterior flange: drawn	High anterior flange: implanted	Bicondylar: implanted	Bicondylar high anterior flange routine (end 1976)	—
Tibial prosthesis	Small area, fixed with staples: drawn	Implanted	Cemented stud fixation	—	—	Large area: drawn	Large area: implanted	—	Two-peg (cementless fixation optional)
Patellar prosthesis	—	—	—	—	Drawn	Implanted	—	—	Single peg (cementless fixation optional)
Instruments	Unreliable, numerous, and complicated in design	Used	Simplified; still unreliable	—	—	Spacer handle angled. Extension bar and Tenser introduced	—	Consolidated into a set	All steps instrumented

eye. The original intention was to correct angular deformity in the extended knee (to an axis in slight varus relative to the normal) by resecting the femur and tibia at right angles to their long axes and placing the prosthesis on these surfaces. To provide abduction and adduction stability it was intended that the separation of the resected bony surfaces of the distal femur and proximal tibia should be precisely equal to the thickness of the prosthesis in extension so that when the prosthesis was inserted into the gap between the resected bone ends, the ligaments would be rendered taught. Appropriate, but in practice not fully satisfactory, instruments were designed to achieve these objectives.

By 1972 the initial operative procedure and prosthesis had been evolved and stabilized at The London Hospital and the results to that date were communicated to the British Orthopaedic Association (FREEMAN and SWANSON, 1972). Following this communication a multicentre trial was initiated at a number of hospitals in the United Kingdom and Sweden. The trial made use of standardised documentation and computer techniques for the analysis of the data obtained both pre-operatively and at annual intervals post-operatively. These techniques of follow-up have been described elsewhere (FREEMAN et al., 1977d and e; see also Chap. 3).

The evolution of ICLH arthroplasty of the knee before and after 1972 is summarised in Table 1.

Clinical Results Obtained with ICLH Arthroplasty in a Multicentre Clinical Trial up to 1974

The knees operated upon at The London Hospital in 1970 and early in 1971 were few in number and were replaced according to a technique and with a prosthesis that were changed significantly in 1971. The results obtained in this period were reported in 1973 (FREEMAN et al., 1973a and b). At the time they were encouraging, and today some of these knees are still functioning satisfactorily (others have failed or the patients have died). From this very limited experience it may be concluded that if the ICLH prosthesis is correctly inserted, function can be maintained for 8 years.

In 1971 a multicentre trial of the ICLH procedure was initiated and therefore for the next 3 years the implant and operative technique were not changed – even though a number of defects became evident. The results obtained in this period have been reported with regard to (1) the maintenance of function over 2–4 years (BARGREN et al., 1976) and over 3–5 years (FREEMAN, 1977) post-operatively; (2) the usefulness of the procedure in the management of the severely damaged knee (FREEMAN et al., 1977c); (3) the results in RA as against OA (FREEMAN et al., 1977a); and (4) the quality of the results compared with those obtained by osteotomy (FREEMAN et al., 1977a). Although these publications describe knees operated upon up to 1974, they were not published until late 1976 or early 1977, since the intervening years were required for an acceptable post-operative follow-up period to elapse.

Maintenance of Function in the Long Term

BARGREN et al. (1976) studied 209 knees 2–4 years post-operatively. This analysis was subsequently carried 1 year further (i.e., 3–5 years post-operatively) by FREEMAN (1977).

The results up to 4 years are shown in Table 2. At 5 years the results were essentially unchanged, and they are shown in histogram form in Fig. 2. A radiograph of a knee replaced in this period is shown in Fig. 3. Both Table 2 and Fig. 2 refer to a scoring system that is based on function rather than structure and takes account of pain, the ability to walk, and the range of movement (FREEMAN

Table 2. The overall assessment of function 1–4 years after operations in the period 1971–1973

Year of operation	Place of operation	Mean overall functional score at				
		Pre-operative	1 year	2 years	3 years	4 years
1971	London Hospital	35	70	65	95	80
1972	London Hospital	30	80	85	80	—
1973	London Hospital	35	85	85	—	—
1972	Other hospitals	30	85	85	90	—
1973	Other hospitals	30	90	90	—	—

et al., 1977d and e). The details of this system are set out in Chap. 3, Fig. 16.

From Table 2 it can be seen that over the period of follow-up the mean score remained essentially unchanged, implying that the functional state of these knees was maintained over this period.

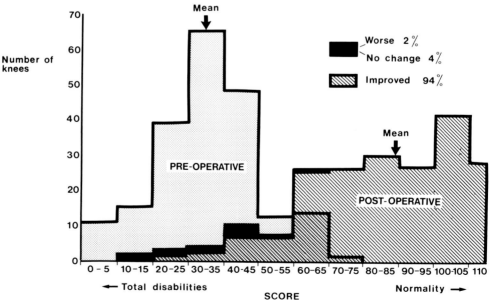

FUNCTION 3–5 YEARS AFTER OPERATION

Fig. 2. A histogram to show pre- (▒) versus post-operative function (▨; ■) 3–5 years after replacement with the prosthesis shown in Fig. 1. The construction of the scores is shown in Chap. 3, Fig. 16. *Arrows* indicate mean scores. ▨, improved (94%); ■, worse (2%) or no change (4%)

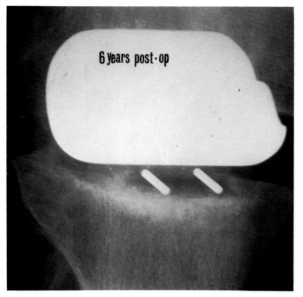

Fig. 3. A radiograph of an ICLH prosthesis inserted in 1972. The patient has RA, and the other knee is arthrodesed. This knee has remained free of pain, permits walking for of 30 min, and has an arc of movement of 90°. Functional score: $50+20+30+10=110$ (see Chap. 3)

Table 3. Correction of severe deformity in 71 severely damaged knees

Nature of deformity before operation	Range of malalignment or flexion deformity before operation (degrees)	Number of knees corrected and stable	Number of knees corrected but unstable	Number uncorrected
Valgus-fixed and/or instability	25–70	23	3	1
Varus-fixed and/or instability	25–30	5	1	0
Combined valgus and varus instability	20 valgus + 30 varus	1	0	0
Combined valgus and fixed flexion	25–40 valgus + 30–70 flexion	5	1	0
Fixed flexion	30–70	30	0	1

Nature of the "Average" Result Obtained

Assuming that no complication developed (see below), the average functional result was a score in the range 85–95 (Fig. 2). This is not a symptomless knee but does represent a very marked functional gain from a pre-operative score of 30–35.

Possibility of Managing the Severely Damaged Knee by this Technique

This question was studied in 71 consecutive knees having pre-operative deformities of at least 25° of valgus, 20° of varus, and/or 30° of fixed flexion, by FREEMAN et al. (1977c).

The structural results obtained are set out in Table 3 and the functional results in Fig. 4.

It will be seen that very severe deformities (e.g., up to 70° of valgus or fixed flexion) could be corrected with this technique, but that satisfactory alignment and stability were not always achieved. This problem is discussed below. Functionally the results were similar to those in the unselected knees followed-up for 5 years, with a post-operative mean score for the group of 85.

Results in RA as against OA

FREEMAN et al. (1977a) analysed the results in RA as against OA, and the results of this analysis are set out in Table 4.

It will be seen that pain relief was similar in the two diseases (90%–93% not requiring analgesics), that the ability to walk post-operatively was rather better in OA than in RA (because other joints interfered with walking in RA), and that the final arc of movement was better in RA than OA (because the knees were stiffer pre-operatively in OA). Overall, the results were similar.

It may be concluded that this procedure, like replacement of the hip, can be used to reconstruct the joint regardless of the initial pathology.

Results Compared with Those of Osteotomy

The results obtained with replacement were also compared with those obtained with osteotomy by FREEMAN et al. (1977a). The results are set out in Tables 5 and 6. Regarding both structure and function the results of replacement were better than those of osteotomy in all groups except varus

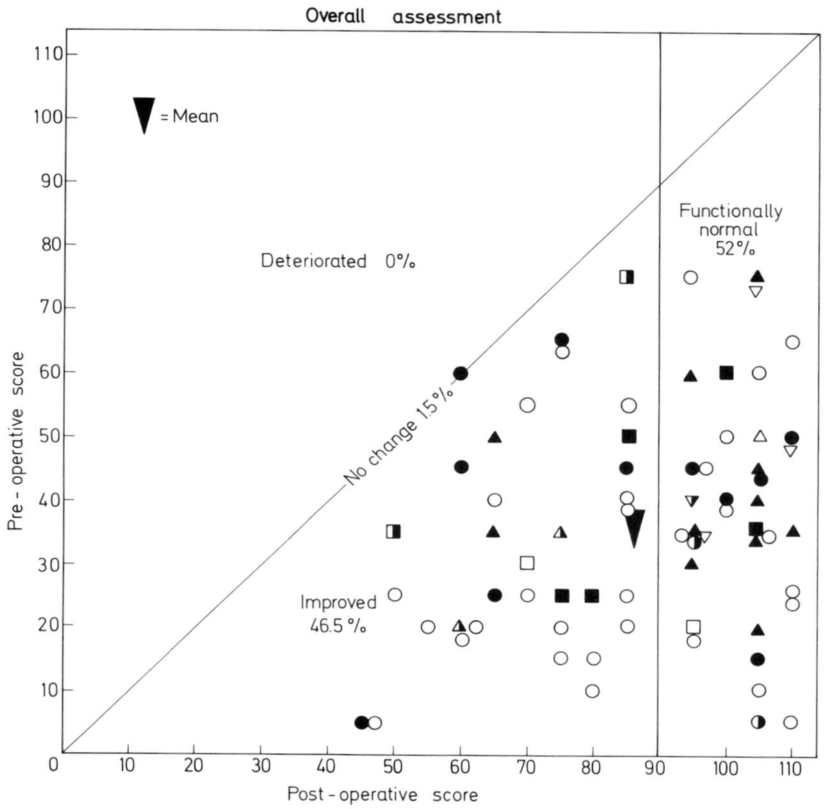

Fig. 4. A diagram to show pre-versus post-operative function in 70 severely damaged knees. (Reproduced from the Journal of Bone and Joint Surgery by kind permission of the Editor). The construction of the scores is shown in Chap. 3, Fig. 11. Each symbol represents one knee. The state of the joint before operation is given on the vertical axis, the state after operation on the horizontal axis. Valgus: instability ▲; fixed ●; fixed and instability ■; Varus: instability ▲; fixed ◐; fixed and instability ◨; Valgus instability and varus instability ▼; Fixed flexion and valgus: instability □; fixed ▽; fixed and instability △; fixed flexion ○

Overall assessment

Table 4. The functional results in RA vs OA[a]

	Pre-operative condition	Result	RA	OA
Pain	Absent or not requiring analgesia		90	93
	Requiring analgesia	Improved	10	3–5
		Unchanged	0	0
		Worse	0	3.5
Walking	Outdoors		85	90
	Indoors or unable	Improved	7.5	0
		Unchanged	5	5
		Worse	2.5	5
Movement	80° plus		67	58
	0°–79°	Improved	4	11
		Unchanged	10	11
		Worse	19	19
Overall score			85	85

[a] All figures are percentages except the overall score, the derivation of which is discussed in the text.

Table 5. The correction of deformity by osteotomy vs ICLH total knee replacement. (Degrees)

		RA		OA	
		Osteotomy	TKR	Osteotomy	TKR
Varus	Pre-op. mean	–	–	10	11
	Post-op. mean	–	–	6	1
Valgus	Pre-op. mean	11	25	20	32
	Post-op. mean	3	5	7	3
Flexion	Pre-op. mean	14	28	9	26
	Post-op. mean	16	5	3	3
Overall	Pre-op. mean	17	27	17	25
	Post-op. mean	12	5	6	2

OA knees, in which the final results were similar. However, the varus OA knees treated by replacement were initially worse than those treated by osteotomy, so that their gain was greater. Therefore a second comparison was made of a small group of pre-operatively comparable OA varus

Table 6. Overall functional scores

Diag-nosis	Pre-operative deformity	Operation	Number of knees	Average overall score		Improvement
				Pre-operative	Post-operative	
OA	Varus	Osteotomy	11	43	81	38
		TKR	6	29	89	60
	Valgus	Osteotomy	7	50	70	20
		TKR	8	37	85	48
	Fixed Flexion	Osteotomy	3	50	72	22
		TKR	12	27	84	57
RA	Valgus	Osteotomy	5	33	64	31
		TKR	21	31	86	55
	Fixed flexion	Osteotomy	8	36	30	−6
		TKR	18	33	88	55

knees: in this group the replaced joints were finally better than those treated by osteotomy.

From this study it may be concluded that ICLH replacement as practised up to 1974 gave better results than did osteotomy (in the case of this comparison, usually a combined tibio-femoral osteotomy) for severe arthritis of the knee; a finding similar to that universally made at the hip. The implications of this finding for the indications for replacement are considered below.

Summary of the Results Obtained up to 1974

The results obtained in this period, as outlined above, were encouraging: they showed that satisfactory function better than that given by osteotomy could be achieved and maintained for up to 5 years, regardless of the initial pathology and the severity of the pre-operative deformity. On the other hand a number of technical deficiencies became manifest, which will now be considered.

Modifications Introduced in 1975 and 1976

It was felt that the results obtained up to the end of 1974 were sufficiently encouraging to justify continued use of the prosthesis but that the complications discussed below necessitated various modi-

fications. These were introduced at The London Hospital (but not elsewhere) over the period 1975–1976, and where they required the manufacture of new instruments or implants, this was done at Imperial College. Unfortunately, there were no facilities for casting cobalt-chromium alloy at Imperial College, and as a consequence we were unable to obtain unrestricted supplies of a suitably modified femoral component until 1977. The development of this implant therefore lagged behind that of the tibial and patellar components and of the instruments.

Femoral Component

In profile the distal and posterior aspects of the femoral component have not been changed. Anteriorly the component has been lengthened to provide a metal surface with a single radius of curvature against which the patella articulates throughout its excursion. Two sizes of this implant (varying in their antero-posterior dimension) are available. Posteriorly the original monocondylar roller has been relieved centrally to provide access, through the intercondylar notch, to the posterior compartment of the knee. This prosthesis is shown in Fig. 5a.

Tibial Component

This still has the same general shape as that used up to 1974, but an implant large enough in area to rest upon the whole of the top of the tibia is now always used. In practice this means that a component of the original, small size is only used in 5%–10% of replacement procedures. An implant that is larger in area is used in the remainder.

A new method of fixation, which does not require cement if the bone is of adequate quality, has been in use since January 1977. Two specially designed ultra-high-molecular-weight polyethylene pegs, integral with the prosthesis itself, are driven into the bone. Their design is such that they provide an immediate interlock with living bone and each has a withdrawal strength approximately equal to that of an AO cancellous bone screw. To date neither loosening nor sinkage has occurred with this implant and pain relief is the same as that achieved with the cemented version. The appearance of the prosthesis and a post-operative radiograph are shown in Fig. 5(a–e).

Patellar Component

The patellar component is countersunk into the patella and can be fixed with or without cement in the same way as the tibial component. It provides area contact against the femoral component because it is concave, not convex (Fig. 5a). These two factors minimise wear (REVELL et al., 1978).

Instruments

Although the principles of the operative procedure have remained unchanged, the steps and their associated instruments have been refined so that the technique is now predictable and does not depend on guesswork. As a consequence, surgeons trained and in training at The London Hospital can now produce reproducible and satisfactory results.

One entirely new instrument has been introduced, the Tenser (Fig. 6). The use of this instrument is essential if anatomical valgus–varus alignment and stability in extension are to be achieved reliably. The operation should not be attempted without it. Two other new instruments are required to fit the tibial and femoral components accurately to the bones.

Finally, all the instruments were redesigned in 1976 (even where their original purpose and dimensions were unchanged) to make them easier to use and to make them into an integrated set (as distinct from a series of separate appliances). This set is now available on a special tray, which is housed in an autoclavable box (Fig. 7). In this way the maintainance of the full set is ensured and their use during an operation is simplified.

The radiographic appearance of a knee replaced with this prosthesis and instruments is shown in Fig. 5.

Prosthetic Complications Encountered in the Period 1970–1974: Nature and Remedies

The general and prosthetic complications encountered in knees examined 2–4 years after operation have been listed by BARGREN et al. (1976), those in severely damaged knees by FREEMAN et al. (1977c), and those in knees replaced after osteotomy by FREEMAN et al. (1977a). These studies and the author's personal experience demonstrated that the prosthetic complications usually fell into one of the following categories:

1) Patellar pain and subluxation
2) Tibial loosening and sinkage
3) Damage to the articular surface of the tibial component, and
4) Failure to restore normal tibio-femoral alignment and to stabilise the tibio-femoral joint.

The incidence, causes and remedies for these complications were described by FREEMAN et al. (1978).

Patellar Pain and Subluxation

Patellar pain occurred in 42% of knees and was of significance in about 15% (FREEMAN et al., 1978). It was due chiefly to the fact that the patella had to move from an exposed area of the femur onto the metal of the femoral component during flexion. No part of this surface was smooth and the prosthetic surface was sharply curved. By using a femoral component whose anterior flange replaces the whole of the patellar surface of the femur with a gently curved metal surface and by shaping the back of the patella to fit the prosthesis, the incidence of patellar pain has been reduced to 12%, with only one knee, in which the patella was not centrally aligned at operation, affected by significant pain.

Replacing the surface of the patella itself with polyethylene further reduces — indeed eliminates — patellar discomfort, but exposes the patient to other possible complications, such as loosening and the necessity for further surgery in the event of spontaneous patellar fracture (HAMMER and FREEMAN, 1978). These two alternative techniques for the management of the patella (i.e., reshaping versus replacement) are at present being compared at The London Hospital.

Patellar subluxation has always been lateral and has been due to a failure to correct tibial external rotation and/or to carry out a release of the lateral patellar retinaculum sufficient to ensure that the patella tracked in the midline of the knee at the time of surgery. If the patella is left laterally subluxed (as it frequently is pre-operatively in a valgus knee), the tibial abduction and external rotation produced by the quadriceps muscle will eventually sublux the tibio-femoral joint. Our experience has been that even with a patellar surface on the femur that is flat from side to side late lateral subluxation of the patella does not occur, provided that the patello-femoral joint is properly aligned in flexion and extension initially.

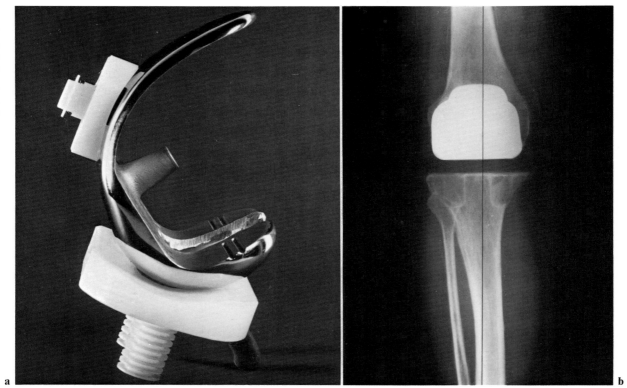

Fig. 5

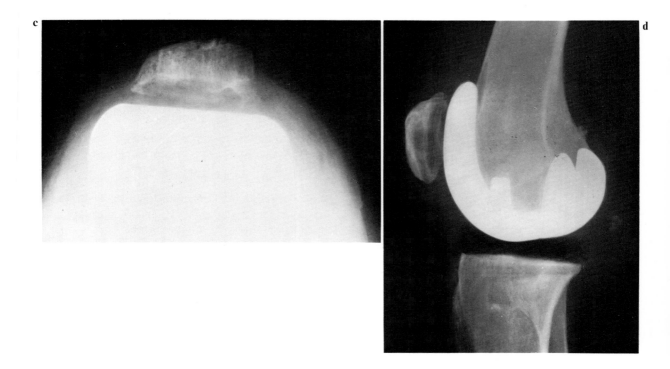

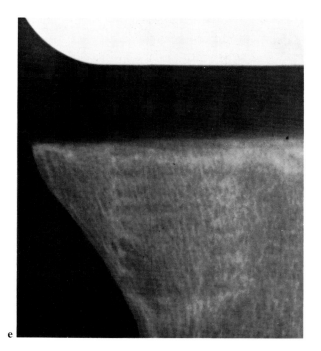

e

Fig. 5. a The current version of the ICLH prosthesis. The use of cement for the tibial and patellar components is optional and depends upon the quality of the bone. This technique and replacement of the patella are undergoing clinical evaluation. **b** Antero-posterior radiograph of a knee replaced with the prosthesis shown in Fig. 5a. The line drawn on this radiograph runs from the centre of the hip proximally to the centre of the ankle distally. The centre of the knee must lie on this line and the prosthesis must be perpendicular to it. **c** A skyline radiograph of the knee shown in Fig. 5b. The correct alignment of the patello-femoral joint, with the patella running in the anterior midline of the prosthesis, is as important as the correct alignment of the tibio-femoral joint. **d** Lateral radiograph of the same knee, showing the absence of cement in the posterior compartment of the joint. **e** A radiograph to show the peg in the tibia securing fixation without cement. Note the presence of bone (shown by the transverse line of radiodensity) in the flanges of the prosthesis. This bone is present immediately after the prosthesis has been implanted, since the flanges flex to interdigitate with the bone. This radiograph was taken 18 months after insertion of the prosthesis

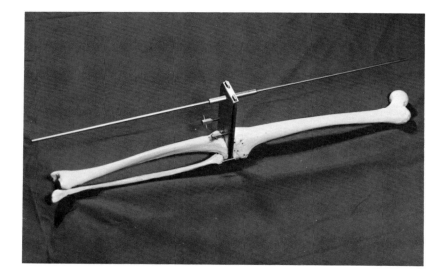

Fig. 6. The Tenser, an instrument used to align and stabilize the knee in extension. The blades are separated in the medial and lateral compartments of the knee until the soft tissues are tight and the ends of the bar lie over the hip and ankle

The advantage of the flat shape used in the ICLH femoral prosthesis is that it enables a polyethylene surface to be designed for the patella that is concave and contacts metal over an area, not a line. Both these factors can be expected to reduce polyethylene wear (REVELL et al., 1978).

Tibial Loosening and Sinkage

Tibial loosening and sinkage were nearly always associated with each other and it was usually im-

possible to determine which was cause and which effect.

The occasional loosening in the absence of sinkage was due to one of three technical errors: failure to engage the stud on the original tibial component in its recess in the top of the tibia (because of the poor exposure of the top of the tibia in the original technique), failure to detect and eradicate defects in the proximal tibia such as a rheumatoid cyst (for the same reason), or failure to place the tibial component on healthy bone after tibial os-

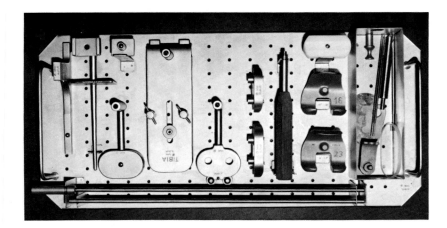

Fig. 7. The instruments used for ICLH arthroplasty in 1977

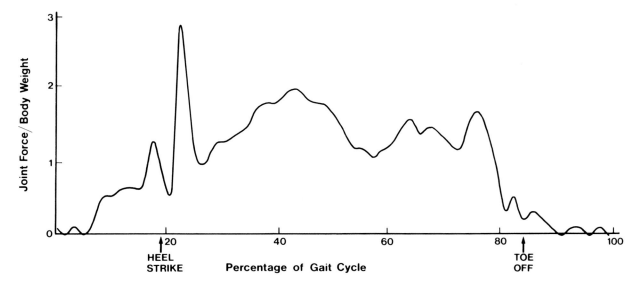

Fig. 8. The load applied to an ICLH prosthesis during level walking. Subject: RA, female, right knee (both knees replaced). *Arrows* indicate heel strike (*left*) and toe off (*right*)

teotomy (FREEMAN et al., 1977a). To some extent the prevention of these errors is a matter of experience, but their avoidance is made easier if (1) the soft tissues are sufficiently released to allow the tibia to be fully subluxed in front of the femur in the flexed knee and (2) the tibial component is implanted first. If these two things are done (as in the present operative technique), sufficient access is obtained to the tibia to ensure that unhealthy tissue is seen and removed and that the prosthesis is accurately placed.

Sinkage, usually leading to loosening, occurred in 12.5% of knees replaced up to 1975 (FREEMAN, et al., 1978). It was due to the fact that the tibial component was deliberately made small in area

so that it could be implanted into even the smallest knee. As a consequence in most knees the component rested on cortical bone only posteriorly. BARGREN et al. (1978) have now shown in the laboratory that the resulting preparation is dangerously weak in compression.

MORRISON (1970) has shown that in the normal knee axial compressive loads of up to 3 times the body weight are transmitted during normal level walking. In three knees in two patients recent studies have shown that loads of a similar magnitude are transmitted after the replacement of the knee with the ICLH prosthesis (PAUL and FREEMAN, 1977, unpublished data; Fig. 8). It is a generally accepted rule of thumb in engineering that if a component is to be cyclically loaded (i.e., if the possibility of fatigue failure arises) and if a life of the order of 10^7 cycles or longer is desired, the strength of the component should be approximately 3 times the strength that would be sufficient for static loading. On this basis, since the knee is cyclically loaded, so that the possibility of fatigue failure does indeed arise, the replaced joint should be capable of withstanding a load of about 9 times the body weight. Thus for the average patient with a body weight of 700 newtons, a strength of about 6 300 newtons should be provided by the replaced tibia. BARGREN et al. (1978) showed that if the proximal tibia were replaced by an implant covering the whole of the transected surface of the bone, the strength of the resulting preparation was about twice this. In contrast, they found that a tibia of average size replaced with the small-area ICLH prosthesis has a strength only just equal to that required to prevent fatigue failure, an observation that conforms with the observation that sinkage of this prosthesis occurred clinically in patients of average or large build.

In the light of these findings, for the past 3 years we have always used a tibial component large enough to cover the whole of the transected tibia. This has meant that we have used the new, large-area component about 10 times as often as the original, small one and that we have had to develop an instrument to trim excess polyethylene from the large prosthesis for those knees for which one component was too small and the other too large.

Since using a prosthesis of adequate size and implanting it first after fully exposing the proximal tibia (i.e. in the years 1975–1978), we have seen neither loosening nor sinkage (FREEMAN et al., 1978).

Surface Damage to the Tibial Component

Surface damage to the polyethylene tibial component was produced by loose fragments of acrylic cement derived from excess acrylic inadvertently left posterior to one or both of the components. With the original ICLH technique, in which a monocondylar femoral component was inserted first and the tibial component second, it was impossible to prevent or even to detect this error at the time of surgery, since cement was carried backwards across the top of the tibia as the tibial component was inserted. Once both components were in place, the posterior compartment of the knee was invisible and inaccessible. A most impor-

tant element in the solution to this problem was proposed by INSALL (J. INSALL, personal communication 1975), who inserted the tibial component first (after which cement posterior to it was fully cleared) and a bicondylar, as against a monocondylar, femoral component was inserted second. The femoral cement was placed on the component, not on the bone. When this is done excess femoral cement flows into the midline space in the knee, where it can be removed easily, not posteriorly, where (certainly with a monocondylar component) it is inaccessible. To date only one knee inserted by this technique has had to be revised (1 year after insertion): the surface of the polyethylene was polished in appearance and showed none of the pitting previously observed. Fixation of the tibial component without cement further reduces the chance of excess acrylic being left in the knee.

A possible objection to the use of a bicondylar femoral component is the fact that a smaller area of the femur is available for load carriage. COLLEY et al. (1978) have shown however, that the use of a bicondylar, as against a monocondylar component, does not in fact weaken the knee in compression.

Failure to Stabilise and Align the Tibio-femoral Joint

Valgus/varus instability and malalignment occurred in 32% of knees operated upon by the original technique (FREEMAN et al., 1978). This complication stemmed partly from (1) a failure to appreciate that fixed valgus and varus deformities could, and should, be corrected by a soft-tissue release procedure before the bone is cut to receive the prosthesis and (2) the fact that in the original technique the collateral ligaments were tensed by traction applied by an assistant. The latter step was unreliable. The use of the Tenser (an instrument now used in ICLH arthroplasty) has eliminated the need for manual traction and has enabled the surgeon precisely to control both collateral ligament tension and the extent to which the soft tissues need to be released before the bone is divided to receive the prosthesis. As a consequence, between the introduction of this instrument at The London Hospital and 1977, only 6% of knees were imperfectly aligned and stabilised, the greatest malalignments being 5° varus and 15° valgus (FREEMAN et al., 1978).

Rotational instability in extension is controlled by the shape of the prosthesis. It occurred rarely and only in knees in which the prosthesis had been inserted after the removal of excessive bone: this results in instability in valgus and varus as well as in rotation. This error has been eliminated by the use of the Tenser.

The restoration of the correct tibio-femoral rotational alignment, particularly the correction of fixed external rotation of the tibia, is as important as the correction of tibial valgus or varus. Its achievement sometimes requires an appropriate soft-tissue release. Its adequacy can be checked by the instruments currently available. (In a severely damaged rheumatoid leg, full correction of a fixed external rotation at the knee may generate problems at the foot — a topic outside the scope of this Chapter.)

Side-to-side instability (translocation) was seen in knees in which the prosthesis had not been inserted horizontally, in which the patella had been left to lie laterally subluxed, or in which all the soft tissues were too lax. The first of these technical errors has been eliminated by redesigning the Spacer (one of the ICLH instruments) so that it acts as a set square for the tibia. The other two defects have already been referred to.

Instability in flexion — especially antero-posterior instability — was seen when too much bone was removed either from the tibia or from the posterior femoral condyles, so that the two components of the prosthesis were widely separable. Such instability resulted in subluxation but never in dislocation. Today, if the Guide (another ICLH instrument) and Spacer are correctly used, this error does not occur.

In summary, instability and malalignment occurred before soft-tissue release procedures and the new set of instruments were introduced. Since their introduction these complications have been virtually eliminated.

Operative Procedure

Space does not permit a full description of the operative technique, but since the quality of the results is very heavily dependent upon the arthroplasty technique, and not just upon the design of the prosthesis, the general principles will be summarised.

It is absolutely fundamental to an understanding of this procedure that it be thought of not simply as a "replacement" of the knee, but as a *reconstruction* of the knee. This distinction emphasises the fact that the procedure involves surgical reconstruction of the soft tissues and, secondly, replacement of the damaged joint surfaces. The prosthesis is of relevance only to the second step. Neither step can be carried out accurately by eye, and thus it is essential to use special instruments by which the alignment of the knee can be regulated and by which the plane and position of the bone sections can be determined before they are made, and checked after they have been carried out.

The principles of the procedure are as follows:

1) Fixed deformities (of the tibio-femoral and patello-femoral joints) are corrected by soft-tissue release, so that the anatomical axis of the limb (i.e. a straight alignment of the hip, knee and ankle) is restored.

2) The bone is cut in such a way as to place the prosthesis perpendicular to the anatomical axis and to create a gap between the bone ends that is exactly equal to the thickness of the prosthesis, both in flexion and in extension with the soft tissues tight. This step ensures the short- and long-term stability of the replaced knee. Put another way, the ligaments must finally be rendered tight and of equal length. Only if this is done will the knee be stable and in anatomical alignment.

Since soft-tissue release procedures allow the bone ends to move apart, the release procedures *must* be carried out first and the bone sections second. If these steps are carried out in the reverse order, too great a gap will eventually be created between the bone ends and the knee will then be unstable in flexion, in extension, or in both.

Technically these two principles are achieved in two basic steps.

1) The knee is flexed to 90°, the cruciate ligaments are resected, and capsular adhesions are released. The femur and tibia are separated as far as possible and a special instrument is used to position cuts in the posterior femoral condyles and in the proximal tibia. The tibia is sectioned (1) at a level such that the gap between it and the sectioned posterior femoral condyles fractionally exceeds the thickness of the prosthesis in flexion and (2) at right angles to its long axis. The femoral section is placed in the coronal plane of the bone.

2) The knee is extended and soft-tissue contractures, if present, are released (see below) until the knee lies in normal alignment with equal soft-tissue tensions medially and laterally. With the soft tissues tensed, the femur is sectioned parallel to the sectioned tibia and at a proximal/distal level such that the gap between this section and that of the tibia equals the thickness of the prosthesis. In the view of the present author (MARF), the Tenser is essential if these steps are to be carried out reliably.

The soft-tissue release procedures that may be required to eliminate fixed deformity are as follows: On the lateral side (to eliminate fixed valgus), (1) the division above the knee of the ilio-tibial tract and of the tendonous portion of the biceps, (2) the division of adhesions between the posterior and lateral aspects of the lateral femoral condyle and the capsule, (3) if necessary, the subperiosteal elevation of the femoral attachment of the lateral collateral ligament. Medially (to eliminate fixed varus), (1) tibial and femoral osteophytes, which tend to "tent" and hence effectively to shorten the medial collateral ligament, are removed, (2) adhesions between the collateral ligament and capsule and the medial femoral condyle are divided medially and posteriorly, and (3) the collateral ligament is elevated if necessary from its tibial or femoral attachments. Posteriorly (to eliminate fixed flexion), (1) adhesions between the posterior capsule and the femoral condyles are divided and (2), if necessary, the posterior capsule is elevated from the femur. It will be appreciated that these procedures are carried out only if fixed deformity is present. Even in the absence of fixed deformity, however, the cruciate ligaments are always removed (for reasons considered above) and the soft tissues attached to the rim of the tibial condyles are divided in the course of removing the proximal tibia. Both these steps are in effect soft-tissue release procedures and are often sufficient by themselves to correct mild fixed deformity. Finally, a release of the lateral patellar retinaculum may be required to correct fixed lateral subluxation of the patella and of the popliteus tendon to correct fixed lateral subluxation of the tibia.

Fixed external rotation of the tibia is the most difficult malalignment to correct. Its reversal usually requires a lateral release, a lateral patellar retinacular release, and the elevation of the soft tissues from the whole circumference of the proximal tibia.

Although they are not strictly essential steps in the reconstruction of the knee by this technique, two manoeuvres become possible if, and only if, the steps already listed are carried out. These are, firstly, that full, uninterrupted access can be obtained to the top of the tibia by levering the bone forwards in the fully flexed knee. This makes it easy to remove all soft-tissue remnants from the cut surface of the bone, to release the soft tissues attached to the back of the tibia (if necessary), to fit the tibial component to the tibia so that it rests on all tibial cortices, to insert the tibial component directly downwards onto its prepared bed (thus enabling secure fixation to be achieved), and to remove all posterior cement. Secondly, when a bicondylar femoral component is used in combination with cruciate resection all excess posterior femoral cement can be removed through the empty intercondylar notch.

If these steps are followed, at the completion of the operation the knee will:

1) lie in full extension and normal valgus, i.e., the centres of the hip, knee and ankle will be in a straight line;

2) be stable in extension and at 90° of flexion;

3) contain a horizontally placed prosthesis;

4) have a patella moving in the midline of the joint; and

5) have no excess cement protruding beyond the prosthesis.

If the post-operative situation departs from these five features in any way, the outcome is uncertain.

Clinical Results

The results of the procedure in its present form can now (1978) be summarised as follows.

Structurally, any knee, regardless of its initial state, can be stabilised and correctly aligned.

Functionally, the patient's pre-operative tibio-femoral pain is abolished but some patellar pain may persist, especially on stairs, unless the patella is replaced. Walking on level ground and standing should not be limited by the knee. Patients should be discouraged from walking over very uneven ground, running, and any kind of sport, since these activites expose the knee to unpredictably high stresses. The range of movement should never be less than 0°–90° (to achieve which a manipulation under anaesthesia may be necessary at 3 weeks).

The exposure of the knee now employed appears to have virtually eliminated failures of wound healing, and no other complication represents a frequent, material problem.

These results might be improved upon by three modifications to the technique, which are under investigation at the time of writing: the regular use of patellar replacement (which awaits a final evaluation of the present alternative technique of limited resection), the effect upon the range of movement of the removal of polyethylene from the postero-superior corner of the tibial prosthesis, and the provision of greater side-to-side stability in the tibio-femoral and/or patello-femoral joints (a feature that might be valuable in knees with severe pre-operative lateral tibial subluxation).

Indications

In the light of the above, ICLH arthroplasty is now used at The London Hospital for the primary treatment of any severely damaged arthritic or osteoarthrosic knee regardless of the pre-operative malalignment or instability.

The procedure should not be used in Charcot's arthropathy, in the absence of a functioning extensor mechanism, in the dysplastic knee, nor in arthrosis secondary to Marfan's syndrome. It should be used with caution, if at all, in the face of past sepsis and in arthrosis secondary to injuries involving rupture of the collateral ligaments or posterior capsule.

The procedure may be used after synovectomy, menisectomy, or debridement, after osteotomy (although the viability of the proximal tibia must then be carefully assessed (Freeman et al., 1977a) and after previous arthroplasty (although this may require the use of a special, revision tibial or femoral component). The author (MARF) has not attempted to use this procedure to revise a hinge arthroplasty or an arthrodesis. It may be unwise to attempt to convert an arthrodesis, because the state of the soft tissues cannot be known pre-operatively. In contrast to this reservation with regard to arthrodesis, a spontaneous ankylosis can be mobilised, because normal soft tissues are present.

These indications leave unsettled the management of the less severely damaged knee: should such a joint be treated by synovectomy in RA and by unicompartmental arthroplasty or by osteotomy in OA, or should it be treated not at all or by total replacement?

The present author (MARF) takes the view that no form of surgical procedure should be undertaken for the rheumatoid knee unless the patient's immediate disability will be sufficiently reduced by surgery to justify the risks and unpleasantness of the operative procedure itself and of its subsequent possible complications. If a procedure existed which had a reliable, worthwhile prophylactic effect, and if knees could be identified that were certain to deteriorate to the point of causing crippling disability unless treated by such a procedure, a case could be made out for exposing patients to the risks of surgery for the sake of future rather than of immediate gain. In a Chapter devoted to a particular form of arthroplasty it is impossible, for reasons of space, to review the literature relevant to the following view, but in the present author's opinion, (1) the future of any particular knee cannot be predicted with complete confidence (so that the prophylactic effect to be obtained from any procedure cannot be determined), and (2) synovectomy has little if any part to play in the inflammatory arthropathies, provided that full modern conservative treatment regimes are available. Thus in RA the author believes that if the disability is such as to require any form of surgical treatment, the joint should be totally replaced.

In early OA the place of osteotomy and of unicompartmental replacement are unsettled: tibial osteotomy appears particularly attractive when the defect is confined to the medial tibial condyle causing minor varus malalignment; unicompartmental replacement may be indicated when degenerative changes are confined to one compartment, especially to the lateral causing valgus malalignment since osteotomy then appears to be less successful. In practice very early OA produces such minor disability that surgery can be postponed — in the elderly sometimes indefinitely — whilst once the disease has advanced to involve more than one compartment total replacement seems the most attractive procedure if the patient is over 60. This appears to leave a relatively limited place for osteotomy and unicompartmental replacement: the former should be considered for varus, mobile knees in patients under 60, whilst the latter should perhaps be considered especially for knees with degenerative changes confined to the lateral compartment.

If these views be accepted, the question remains: at what level of pre-operative disability will the symptomatic gain produced by surgery balance the risks? As far as ICLH arthroplasty is concerned a patient can be told that post-operatively he will have a stable, well-aligned knee with a range of movement from 0°–90° on which he can walk on level ground without significant pain. Once the outcome of the procedure can be reliably predicted in this way, patients can make their own decision: if their disability is only at or below this level, arthroplasty will be rejected; if their disability is greater, it will be considered.

Total Condylar Arthroplasty

Indications

Total knee replacment is required when there is (1) disabling pain, instability, or deformity of the knee joint of a degree that justifies the possibility of failure and subsequent arthrodesis and (2) when there is no satisfactory surgical alternative. The patient's age, occupation, and level of activity are secondary but important issues.

The indications for replacement of the knee in RA are not the same as in OA.

Rheumatoid Arthritis

It is generally agreed that no satisfactory alternative to joint replacement exists. Synovectomy is now seldom used, because although there may be lessening of pain, progression of the arthritis is not affected. Partial replacements of the MacIntosh or McKeever type do not provide the degree of pain relief or level of functional excellence that can be obtained with a cemented prosthesis, and moreover, failure because of infection is likely to lead to arthrodesis whether the implant is partial or complete. Primary arthrodesis should not be done in RA because other joints are often involved. Because of these considerations, in RA joint replacement is acceptable even in youth.

Osteoarthritis

Multiple joint involvement is less common and when disability due to the knee pain is relieved, the patient is likely to engage in activities normal for others of the same age group. In the elderly (over 65) this activity is unlikely to cause prosthetic failure and knee arthroplasty is usually preferred.

A difficulty thus arises in younger patients, as an otherwise healthy and active person may impose

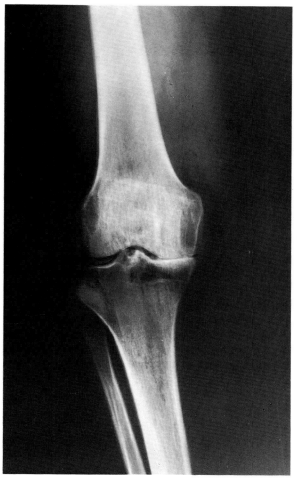

Fig. 9. A radiograph of a knee with medial-compartment OA. There is 5° varus angulation and the knee is stable. High tibial osteotomy gives a predictable result and should be chosen in younger patients

severe stress on a prosthesis, particularly in sports such as golf, tennis, or even ski-ing (these activities may very well be possible after successful knee replacement). Fortunately, tibial osteotomy provides a satisfactory alternative for such patients, because in the earlier stages degenerative arthritis of the knee is a focal, compartmental disease affecting the medial articulation over the lateral in a ratio of about 4 to 1 (Fig. 9). Asymmetrical degeneration leads to secondary angulation (varus or valgus) and only later to instability when the ligament on the convex side of the deformity becomes stretched by the stresses of walking (producing the characteristic "thrust").

Not all deformities are improved equally after tibial osteotomy. When valgus deformity is corrected in this manner obliquity of the joint axis results (COVENTRY, 1965; SHOJI and INSALL, 1973), which leads in time to medial subluxation of the femur and later still to varus angulation. Femoral osteotomy may be considered instead, but our experience suggests that this type of osteotomy is no better (BROWN and INSALL, 1977). On the other hand, the pain associated with varus angulation is often dramatically improved by tibial osteotomy (Fig. 9). This is particularly true if the angular deformity is small (i.e., less than 10°). The results of tibial osteotomy are affected by instability, which in turn is closely related to the degree of angular deformity (INSALL et al., 1974) and knees with less than 10° of angulation (measured on a weight-bearing radiograph) are almost invariably stable. In contrast, knees with over 15° of angulation show subluxation and instability of a degree that will cause tibial osteotomy to fail, so that only knees with between 10° and 15° of deformity require clinical assessment of stability. Additional contra-indications to tibial osteotomy are (1) severe degeneration of the patello-femoral articulation and (2) significant flexion contracture (over 20°).

Even when the selection for osteotomy is correct, the operation will fail unless the post-operative alignment is precise. The author is convinced that the effect of osteotomy is purely mechanical and does not depend on any vascular or "biophysiological" response. BAUER et al. (1969) have shown that when the *post-operative* correction is between 5° and 15° of valgus (for medial OA with varus angulation) the result of the operation is predictably good, but when the alignment falls outside these limits the pain is not relieved. Most of the poor results from tibial osteotomy can be explained by either incorrect initial selection or failure to obtain the critical post-operative alignment that is required. In our own experience the most common technical failure in this respect is undercorrection of the deformity. Overcorrection is unlikely to occur except in unstable knees, which should not have been selected for osteotomy in the first place.

It is necessary therefore to consider both the type and extent of angular deformity as well as age, occupation, and activity before choosing between tibial osteotomy and knee replacement.

Results Obtained with Other Procedures

When knee replacement is selected the surgeon is faced with a second decision — what kind of knee replacement? Some favour a *graduated system* of prostheses depending on type and extent of deformity, while others recommend a single prosthesis for use in all knees. It is worthwhile to consider the development of knee arthroplasty at The Hospital for Special Surgery, because our experience may be unique in the variety of prostheses that have been used in one hospital.

The initial approach was the graduated system concept and began with the development of the uni- and duocondylar prostheses, which were first implanted in patients in 1971. Both prostheses are anatomical replacements for either one or both compartments of the femoro-tibial joint. The femoral component (Vitallium) was designed to replace the *weight-bearing* portion of the femoral condyles as closely as possible, and the dimensions and curvatures were determined from a study of a large number of cadaver knees. The component was initially made in only one size, but later modifications included several sizes. The tibial component(s) (HDP) were separate and also intended to mimic the normal anatomy, being flat in the sagittal and curved concavely in the coronal plane. In the duocondylar prosthesis the two femoral runners were connected by an anterior bar; the unitcondylar was a single unit of similar shape. There was no provision for replacement of the patellofemoral joint with either prosthesis.

The nature of the design limited the application. The *unicondylar* prosthesis is used only in *OA* when there is correctable varus or valgus deformity, no flexion contracture, and an acceptable range of motion (about 90°), as it is not possible to increase motion using this prosthesis. The *duocondylar* implant (Fig. 10) allows limited correction of varus or valgus angulation (up to about 15°). Preservation of the cruciate ligaments is essential, as the prosthesis offers no antero-posterior stability, but slight laxity of one or other collateral ligament can be tolerated because intercondylar stability and resistance to translocation is provided by the median curvature of the tibial components. The duocondylar prosthesis is most suitable for rheumatoid panarthritis with mild to moderate deformity when the bone stock is sufficient to anchor the separate tibial components. The prosthesis is less suitable in OA, as fixed angular deformity is much more frequent.

Because of the limitations of the uni- and duocondylar prostheses, the geometric and Guépar prostheses were used for more severe deformities in both OA and RA.

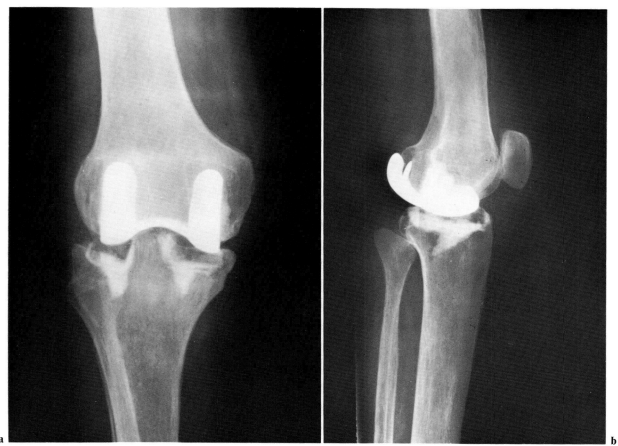

a   b

Fig. 10a and b. An antero-posterior (**a**) and a lateral (**b**) radiograph of a duocondylar prosthesis. This is not strictly a "total" replacement as the patello-femoral articulation is not included. This is a drawback as the patella is some-times painful. Separate tibial components are difficult to align and tibial fixation is insecure because the components rest on cancellous bone. Impingement can occur when the intercondylar bone is not removed

The results of knee arthroplasty with these four prostheses between 1971 and 1973 were reported in 1976 (INSALL et al., 1976a) (Fig. 14, p. 279). A knee rating was used that totalled 100 points, allotting 30 points for pain, 22 points for function (walking, stair climbing, and transfer), 18 points for motion, and 10 points each for muscle strength, flexion deformity, and instability. Subtractions were made for walking aids, extension lag, and residual deformity. In this way average *pre-operative* and *post-operative* ratings were obtained, together with a *point spread* (the difference between the two ratings), and a *percentage improvement*, which related the point spread to the pre-operative rating.

The knees were subdivided into four groups on the basis of the ratings. We designated as *excellent* those knees with a rating of 85 or more. The knees so rated approached the normal and the knee was obviously much improved to both the patient and the examiner. The knees with ratings of 70–84 were considered to have a *good* result. Such knees had obviously been improved by the arthroplasty, but the result was not as good as in the previous group. We designated as *fair* those knees rated 60–69. This group comprised mainly knees in which the result of the arthroplasty was deficient in some way (persistent pain, moderate instability, or unsatisfactory motion), but also included some in which the rating of the arthroplasty was downgraded by the patient's general condition (such as multiple joint involvement in RA). We rated as *failures* those knees that had a post-operative score of less than 60. These knees were evidently unsatisfactory and below the rating achieved by knee fusion. This classification included knees in which the prosthesis had been removed or replaced and knees in which the improvement, if any, did not seem to justify the risk of arthroplasty.

In the entire group of 178 arthroplasties, the results were considered excellent in 47 (26%), good in 66 (37%) fair in 37 (21%), and poor in 28 (16%). There was no significant difference between the results obtained with each of the four prostheses studied. However, because it is easier to improve a "bad knee" than a relatively good one, the percentage improvement was much greater with the Guépar than the unicondylar prosthesis (120% as against 45%).

Three specific problem areas emerged from this study: patellar pain, component loosening, and surgical technique.

Patellar Pain

None of the prostheses makes adequate provision for patello-femoral function, although the Guépar, because of its femoral flange, does make some. Therefore, none of the models used was a total knee replacement in the strict sense. One-third of the entire group had pain related to the patella, and in half of these this was a serious complaint. Patellectomy does not offer a solution to the problem of patello-femoral arthritis. Thirty-eight patellectomies were performed in the group as a whole (three of them were done at a later date than the arthroplasty because of persistent pain). Only five knees with patellectomy had an excellent rating. Six were classified as failures and the others had intermediate ratings. The complaint of pain was as frequent in these patients after patellectomy as in patients in whom patellectomy had not been performed. In addition, patients who had undergone patellectomy suffered from inadequacy of the extensor mechanism. In the GUÉPAR group of 45 knees, pain on patellar compression was found in 22 on follow-up, and patellar erosion was observed in 5. Subluxation of the patella frequently occurred with the Guépar prosthesis, in spite of wide lateral release of the patella retinaculum at the time of arthroplasty. However, this was often not apparent to the patient and may be considered an incidental finding. Subluxation did not necessarily correlate with complaints of post-operative pain.

Component Loosening

A radiolucent line surrounding the prosthetic components was observed with great frequency. With the condylar replacements it was usually seen around the tibial components and was present in 70% of knees with the unicondylar, 50% with the duocondylar, and 80% with the geometric prosthesis. A radiolucent line was observed around the femoral component in 45% of the patients with a Guépar prosthesis. The radiolucency was slightly more frequent in osteoarthritic than in rheumatoid patients; it was observed in all knees treated for OA with the geometric prosthesis. Radiolucent lines are by no means always symptomatic, but when complete, progressive, and associated with pain on weight-bearing they may be considered to indicate failure of fixation. An additional problem is that radiolucency is position-dependent, as can be demonstrated under fluoroscopy where minor degrees of rotation can conceal even a pronounced radiolucent line.

Proven loosening depends on the evidence of an obvious change of position on the radiograph or at re-operation. By this definition the frequency of loosening with the unicondylar and geometric prostheses is 10%, and the frequency with the duocondylar prosthesis is 7%. Femoral component loosening, on the other hand, is very unusual.

It now seems clear that tibial loosening represents a failure in design. The flat cancellous surface of the upper tibia is not a suitable bed for a flat prosthetic component, because of poor resistance to shear stresses; nor is the bone of sufficient strength to resist sinkage even if excavations are made to accommodate fins on the prosthesis. We now believe that *cortical* fixation is essential.

Interpretation of radiolucency around the stems of the Guépar prosthesis is different. In these instances radiolucency always indicates stem loosening, which can be demonstrated by fluoroscopy. Secure cortical fixation such as that obtained by intramedullary cemented stems will not resist indefinitely the severe and repetitive torsional stresses imposed by a constrained prosthesis.

Surgical Technique

The three condylar prostheses are all difficult to insert and align. The necessary retention of the cruciate ligaments dictated by the design of these prostheses made access to the upper tibia awkward, and malalignment of the tibial components was frequently seen (usually this was a varus obliquity of the component). Such malalignment undoubtedly contributed to the incidence of loosening. The shape of the femoral component of all three prostheses also made it difficult to place and align. (This is particularly true of the uni- and duocondylar prostheses, as the deep surface is curved). These prostheses restore alignment and provide stability by a "spacing" effect. It is assumed that the ligamentous structures of the knee are intact and unaltered, having laxity only because of bone erosion, so that when put on stretch by tight insertion of the prosthesis normal length will be restored and the knee will become stable. This concept is often erroneous.

Pathology of Arthritis

In OA the primary lesion is loss of articular carti-lage and later bone erosion. This is nearly always asymmetrical, involving the medial femoro-tibial compartment four times as frequently as the lateral and thereby causing varus or valgus angulation, respectively. By the time knee replacement is neces-sary, almost invariably adaptive changes have taken place in the collateral ligaments. The stress of walking on an angulated limb stretches the liga-ment on the convex side of the deformity (the lateral ligament in the case of a varus angulation and the medial ligament when the deformity is one of valgus). This can be observed clinically by the manisfestation of a "thrust" in the stance phase of walking. *Instability* therefore has two causes: (1) asymmetrical bone loss and (2) *stretch-ing* of one collateral ligament. The other character-istic of an osteoarthritic knee is *deformity*, and this also has two causes: (1) asymmetrical bone loss and (2) *contracture* of the collateral ligament on the concave side of the angulation so that the deformity becomes, in part, fixed or passively un-correctable. In the rheumatoid knee the nature of the disease process is a panarthritis involving all compartments of the knee from the onset, so that the knee is rendered *symmetrically unstable* by the loss of articular cartilage and bone from both fe-moro-tibial compartments. Late in the disease an-gular deformity often develops, so that as in OA secondary adaptive changes take place in the liga-mentous structures. In our experience varus and valgus angulation occur with roughly equal fre-quency: the direction of angulation seems to be determined by chance as it is not uncommon to see a patient with a varus angulation of one knee and a valgus of the other, giving a "wind-swept" appearance. (This is decidedly uncommon in OA).

There are other relevant characteristics of RA.
1) *Valgus angulation is often accompanied by lateral subluxation of the tibia* (translocation) and a fixed external rotation contracture. The author does not know why this is unique to RA, but it is not seen in the osteoarthritic valgus knee.

2) For reasons that are also unclear, *erosion of the femoral condyles* is most pronounced poste-riorly, resulting in a reduction of antero-posterior distance and giving the lower femur viewed from the side a rounded appearance ("drumstick" or "chicken leg" femur). This peculiarity makes the rheumatoid knee more unstable in flexion than in extension.

Flexion deformity or contracture is seen in both OA and RA, although the more extreme degrees are nearly always found in the latter and are often associated with a "chicken leg" femur, producing a knee that is unstable in flexion yet cannot be extended because of contracture of the posterior capsule.

It should be emphasised that no form of arthritis causes lysis or disappearance of ligaments, and even in the most unstable knee the collateral liga-ments are never "absent", (unless, of course, they have been surgically divided).

Relevance of the Pathology to Replacement of the Knee

Instability does not present a problem when *sym-metrical* (although it must be remembered that the instability may be more severe in flexion than in extension). Stability is obtained by the spacing ef-fect of the prosthesis, which makes the ligaments tight.

Asymmetric instability, especially when asso-ciated with fixed deformity, presents a more diffi-cult problem. Alignment of the knee can be re-stored by wedge resection of bone, but if the pros-thesis is then used as a spacer only one collateral ligament can be made taut and in fact, existing laxity of the other will be worse. For this situation there are several solutions:

1) *Prolonged immobilisation* may be prescribed to allow the loose ligament to "tighten". In my experience this may occur at times, but is unpre-dictable and the immobilisation required has the further disadvantage of causing loss of motion (so defeating one of the objectives of knee arthro-plasty).

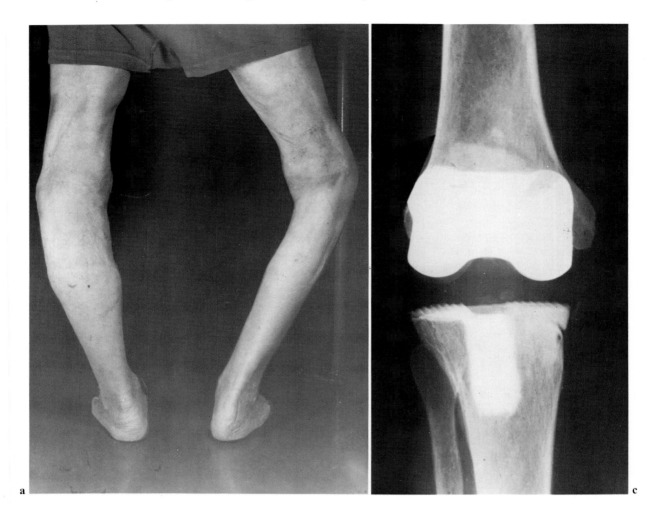

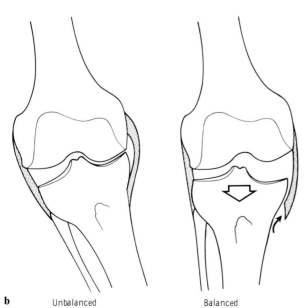

b Unbalanced   Balanced

Fig. 11. a A posterior view of a patient with severe OA of the right knee and a varus angulation of 50°. The TCP can be used provided the ligaments are "balanced" by medial release. **b** Correction (*right*) of varus deformity (*left*) by release of the medial collateral ligament, periosteum, and pes anserinus as a "sleeve" which slides proximally as the deformity is corrected. In smaller deformities than this, the distal portion of the superficial medial collateral ligament is not detached. **c** A radiograph of the same knee 4 years after operation. The knee is stable and the result is rated as excellent

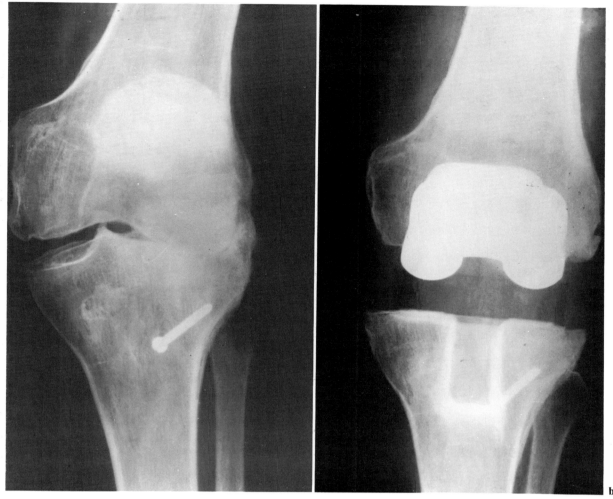

a   b

Fig. 12a and b. Valgus is corrected by a release from the femur. **a** 30° valgus deformity (the screw is from previous reconstructive surgery); **b** same knee after correction and insertion of the TCP Mark II. The Mark II is recommended because extensive lateral release can make stability in flexion difficult to obtain

2) *Surgical tightening* by advancement or reefing of the loose ligament has also been attempted, with equally unpredictable results and with the same disadvantage that prolonged immobilisation is required.

3) *A constrained prosthesis* in which prosthetic design provides the necessary stability may be selected. The stabilocondylar prosthesis allows some degree of triaxial motion and is an example of this type. However, experience suggests that *any* constraint in the design increases loosening and may increase infection.

4) *Asymmetrical instability may be converted to symmetrical instability* by surgical release of the shorter or contracted ligament. This method is the preferred and most successful technique and allows a semi-constrained prosthesis to be used for almost all deformities. In the case of a varus angulation (Fig. 11), a *medial release* is accomplished by elevating from the tibia a "sleeve" consisting of the periosteum, pes anserine insertion, and distal insertion of the superficial medial ligament. Resection of medial osteophytes and division of the semimembranous insertion and posterior capsule complete the release. For anatomical reasons, *lateral release* is done from the femur, dividing the ilio-tibial band and lateral intermuscular septum a hand's breadth above the joint and subsequently releasing the lateral capsule, lateral ligament, and popliteus tendon (Fig. 12). Posterior

capsule release from the lateral femoral condyle is usually required. My experience supports FREE-MAN's contention that peroneal nerve palsy can be prevented by prior isolation of the peroneal nerve to prevent compression by the overlying fascia.

Design Rationale of the Total Condylar Prosthesis (TCP)

The prosthesis designed in 1972 by INSALL, RANA-WAT, and WALKER (Fig. 13) was first implanted in a patient in 1973, and represents The Hospital for Special Surgery's solution to the problems previously encountered with other types of knee replacement. The basic configuration is semi-constrained in that the components conform with each other in extension but allow rotary and gliding motions in flexion. The tibial component has a cupped articulation with a prominent intercondylar eminence to prevent translocation: the femoral component has two separate runners joined anteriorly to form a patellar flange. The femoral runners are of decreasing radius to allow the desired rotary and gliding laxity in flexion. For reasons given previously by FREEMAN, a design of this type requires cruciate ligament excision. In addition, we felt that secure tibial fixation could only be provided by a short, central, intramedullary peg, which necessitated removal of the tibial spines and cruciate attachments to obtain fixation on the posterior cortex of the upper tibia. The prosthesis was designed for a dome-shaped, polyethylene patella component (AGLIETTI et al., 1975). A dome was chosen so that any rotary malalignment incurred during insertion would not cause binding in the femoral groove.

Technical Considerations

There is no doubt that the results of knee arthroplasty depend as much on precise and accurate surgical technique as on prosthetic design itself. While the short-term result of a malaligned prosthesis may be satisfactory, over a longer period malposition causes excessive strain on the components, predisposing to cold flow, excessive wear, loosening, and subluxation. The fit between prosthesis and bone must also be precise so that only a small amount of cement is exposed: third-body abrasion from entrapped cement particles is the most frequent cause of excessive wear (BULLOUGH

et al., 1976). Accurate fit and alignment cannot be achieved "by eye": reliable, and comprehensive instrumentation must be used. A deformed knee is "balanced" as previously discussed by converting asymmetrical to symmetrical instability by means of ligament releases *before* the bone cuts are made. The technique (derived from FREEMAN) uses three instruments to accomplish the three basic steps of the operation. The first (tibial cutter) is in the shape of a cross from which protrudes a stem that is inserted into the intramedullary canal of the femur: the knee is then positioned at 90°. A separate aligning rod is passed into the shaft of the tibia and the cross is aligned with this. The objective is to obtain a right angle resection of the upper tibia. (When laxity in flexion is present, the knee must be distracted before making this cut). The second (femoral shaper) is for cutting the anterior and posterior surfaces of the femur through appropriately placed slots set in a block. With the aid of the handles the knee is distracted and the instrument positioned parallel to the cut surface of the tibia (ligamentous length must previously have been balanced). The third (tibial puller) is for resecting the distal femur after the ligaments have been pulled taut in extension.

Thus, gaps are created in both flexion and extension that will accommodate the thickness of the prosthesis, and if each step is correctly performed the ligaments will be taut in both positions (although not necessarily throughout the full arc of motion).

The patella surface is removed to provide a flat bed and an anchoring hole made centrally for the patella dome.

Clinical Experience

Over 600 Total Condylar Prostheses of the type shown in Fig. 13 have been inserted at The Hospital for Special Surgery since 1973. The first consecutive 223 arthroplasties (in 186 patients) have been examined in detail and were recently reported (SCOTT et al., 1977; INSALL et al., 1979). The preoperative diagnosis was OA in 128, RA in 78, revision of another prosthesis in 9, osteonecrosis in 5, and post-traumatic arthritis in 3 cases. A patellar replacement was used in 188 knees and the patella was not replaced in the remaining 35 knees. The maximum varus deformity corrected was 55° and the maximum valgus 35° (assessed on standing pre-operative radiographs). The maximum flexion contracture was 60°.

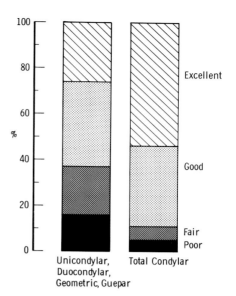

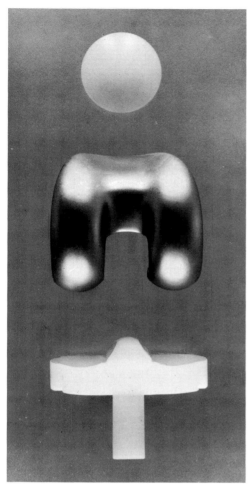

Fig. 13. The Total Condylar Prosthesis

Fig. 14. Results obtained at The Hospital for Special Surgery with the unicondylar, duocondylar, geometric, and Guépar prostheses (left) and the Total Condylar Prosthesis. ▨ , excellent; ▦ , good; ▨ , fair; ■ , poor

Results

The average pre-operative score was 43 and the average post-operative score 82. The results were better in OA (scores 42 and 84) than in RA (scores 43 and 80).

One hundred and twenty knees (54%) were excellent; 81 knees (35%) good; 13 knees (6%) fair; and 9 knees (5%) poor (Fig. 14). In OA the result was excellent in 58%, good in 37%, fair in 2%, and poor in 5%. In RA the result was excellent in 48%, good in 26%, fair in 11%, and poor in 8%.

The causes of fair and poor results were analysed. In three of the thirteen *fair knees* the result was due to severe generalised RA. In three knees there was a residual flexion contracture and three

knees had a decreased range of motion. One knee had patellar pain, which was relieved by subsequent patellar replacement. One knee was painful for reasons unknown. One knee was unstable and in one case the rating was affected by a fracture of the contralateral femur.

There were 12 *poor results*. Three of these were due to deep infection and in three more the failure was associated with severe RA. In two knees there was a posterior subluxation of the tibia. One knee had a residual flexion contracture and one an extension lag. One knee had a separation of the quadriceps mechanism resulting in muscle weakness. One knee had pain for reasons undetermined.

It was clear from assessing these patients that the general level and predictability of the results approach those of total hip replacement and are particularly impressive when compared with the results obtained in our previous group of arthroplasties, which had been assessed in exactly the same manner (Fig. 14). (Unfortunately, we are not able to compare with other published series because there is as yet no uniform method of assessing and reporting the results of knee joint replacement.)

Normal function by The Hospital for Special Surgery rating definition means unlimited walking, normal stair climbing without holding a rail, and the ability to get out of even a deep chair without using the hands. Twenty-two percent of the TCP arthroplasties were in this category, compared with 9% in the comparison group.

The results in OA were definitely better than those in RA ($P=0.025$), and in patients with unilateral OA the results were best of all (average score $87: P=0.01$). Patients with RA did worse in every category assessed, and not surprisingly, the difference was most noticeable in patients attending the combined arthritis programme who, by selection, were those with very severe, generalised disease. Restricted pre-operative motion (less than $50°$) also contributed to a less satisfactory result ($P=0.01$). The reason for a deficient arthroplasty in such a knee was not always restricted post-operative motion: at times it was due to an extension lag, a flexion contracture, or a quadriceps avulsion incurred during manipulation to improve motion.

The presence of severe deformity or a pre-operative flexion contracture did not make any difference to the end result.

Tibial Fixation

In over 600 arthroplasties no case of tibial loosening has been seen, and moreover radiolucent lines around the component are much less frequent (22% compared with 80% with the geometric prosthesis). The radiolucencies with the TCP were all incomplete (did not extend around the fixation peg) and the vast majority were hairline (1 mm or less). The addition of a peg to the tibial component, therefore, has so far eliminated sinkage and loosening, and it does not seem likely that this will be a future problem. In two instances the prosthesis was removed because of late subluxation, and in both there was extreme difficulty in extracting the plastic (the peg must be cut with a saw and removed separately). The peg also makes easier attachment to the upper tibia easier when there is bone deficiency (e.g., in revision operations) and when there is severe asymmetrical bone erosion.

Patellar Replacement

About 750 patellar implants have been used with the total condylar, modified total condylar, stabilocondylar and duopatellar prostheses. There is no doubt that the addition of a third component for the patella has been extremely successful in improving the quality of the arthroplasty. In 188 arthroplasties with both a patellar flange and a patellar replacement, two knees (1.06%) were affected by severe pain, whereas in 30 knees with a flange but without patellar replacement there were also two knees (6.6%) with severe pain. In the comparison group of 178 arthroplasties in which there was neither flange nor patellar replacement, 28 knees (16%) were severely painful. Thus the addition of a flange to the femoral component does reduce the incidence of patellar pain, but not as effectively as when combined with patellar replacement.

The increased complications when a third component is added must be set against this improvement. These have been very few. In 750 patellar replacements with several different types of prosthesis, there have been two instances of loosening (0.3%). One of these was in a suspected neuropathic joint, is only mildly symptomatic, and has not been treated. The other case was associated with a subluxation of the tibial component and at the time of revision the patella was removed. The other complication has been patellar fracture in two cases (0.3%). One involved the lower pole and occurred spontaneously 3 weeks after operation when the patient was standing. This fracture was treated by immobilisation for 6 weeks; it healed satisfactorily, and has not influenced the result of the arthroplasty. The other fracture, involving the upper pole, occurred 1 year after operation and presented as mild anterior knee pain. The patient was not seen for some weeks after the onset of pain and at that time the fracture had partially healed, so that no treatment at all was given. The arthroplasty now has an excellent rating. In addition to our own cases, we have heard reports from other centres of five more fractures: all have been transverse fractures across the centre of the patella and all have required operative repair or patellectomy. In one of these cases the patella showed evidence of avascular necrosis. This type of fracture has not been seen at The Hospital for Special Surgery and I am inclined to believe that some technical error may be responsible (excessive removal of patellar bone or an excessively large centering hole). Another possibility is that a lateral release was done to centre the patella, which might have caused devascularisation (at The Hospital for Special Surgery a lateral release has seldom been required).

The patellar component (Fig. 15) is now available in five sizes (31–44 mm). The largest possible

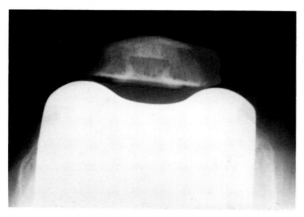

Fig. 15. The patellar implant conforms with the femoral flange. Rotary alignment is not necessary. The addition of the patellar implant definitely improves the "quality" of the arthroplasty and is now included routinely

size should be used to cover the patellar surface fully so that there can be no impingement at the edges although, because the patella is oval, there will then be overhang superiorly and inferiorly: this is of no consequence.

Posterior Subluxation

Although the results obtained with the TCP were very good, one problem exists. In 600 arthroplasties there have been five cases of posterior subluxation. In the same group there are four infections (0.66%), so that posterior subluxation is the most frequent serious complication.

The cause is sometimes technical and therefore avoidable. A mistake that may cause posterior subluxation is an initial loose fit in flexion. This error in a knee that is stable to begin with is completely avoidable with the proper technique. Difficulty may arise, however, when dealing with a severely deformed knee requiring ligament release, for then only one ligament (either the medial or lateral collateral) remains intact, because the other has been released and the cruciates have been excised to achieve correction. In this situation, while it is relatively easy to accomplish stability in extension, it may be very difficult, and sometime impossible, to attain the required stability in flexion. Another contributory factor is patellectomy, which, by removing the normal anterior pull of the patellar tendon in flexion, allows the hamstrings to act unopposed. Of the five cases of subluxation, three occurred in severely deformed knees and the

patella had been previously excised in the other two.

While this complication has been infrequent, it is possible that more cases will be seen. MURRAY, using a knee simulator, has shown a similar dislocation occurring after an estimated 7 years of use, due to plastic deformation.

For these reasons a modification of the TCP has been developed. The intercondylar eminence of the tibial component has been enlarged and reshaped, and the corresponding area between the femoral runners is now covered to form a shallow box. The intercondylar cam of the tibial component articulates within the femoral box, preventing posterior dislocation in flexion as well as hyperextension. The posterior lip of the tibia has also been lowered to obtain greater flexion.

One hundred and ten modified prostheses have been used and I believe that providing anteroposterior stability in the design is an advantage.

References

AGLIETTI, P., INSALL, J., WALKER, P.S., TRENT, P.: A new patella prosthesis. Design and application. Clin. Orthop. **107**, 175 (1975)

ANGEL, J.C., LIYANAGE, S.P., GRIFFITHS, W.E.G.: Double osteotomy for the relief of pain in the arthritis of the knee. Rheumatol. Rehabil. **13**, (3), 109 (1974)

BARGREN, J.H., FREEMAN, M.A.R., SWANSON, S.A.V., TODD, R.C.: ICLH (Freeman/Swanson) Arthroplasty in the treatment of the arthritic knee: A 2 to 4 year review. Clin. Orthop. **120**, 65 (1976)

BARGREN, J.H., DAY, W.H., FREEMAN, M.A.R., SWANSON, S.A.V.: Mechanical tests on the tibial components of non-hinged knee prostheses. J. Bone Joint Surg. (Br.) **60**, 256 (1978)

BAUER, G.C., INSALL, J., KOSHINO, T.: The effect of angular deformity on stability and pain in osteoarthritis of the knee. Arthritis Rheum. **12**, 279 (1969)

BROWN, G., INSALL, J.: Femoral osteotomy for valgus deformity. Unpublished (1977)

BULLOUGH, P.G., INSALL, J., RANAWAT, C.: Wear and tissue reaction in failed knee arthroplasty. J. Bone Joint Surg. (Am.) **58**, 754 (1976)

COLLEY, J., CAMERON, H., FREEMAN, M.A.R., SWANSON, S.A.V.: Loosening of the femoral component in surface replacement of the knee. Arch. Orthop. Traumat. Surg. **92**, 31–34 (1978)

COVENTRY, M.B.: Osteotomy of the upper portion of the tibia for degenerative arthritis of the knee. A preliminary report. J. Bone Joint Surg. (Am.) **47**, 984 (1965)

EVANS, E.M., FREEMAN, M.A.R., MILLER, A.J., VERNON-ROBERTS, B.: Metal sensitivity as a cause of bone necrosis and loosening of the prosthesis in total joint replacement. J. Bone Joint Surg. (Br.) **56**, 626 (1974)

FREEMAN, M.A.R.: A three to five years' follow-up of the Freeman-Swanson replacement arthroplasty of the knee. J. Bone Joint Surg. (Br.) **59**, 119 (1977)

FREEMAN, M.A.R., SWANSON, S.A.V.: Total prosthetic replacement of the knee. J. Bone Joint Surg. (Br.) **54**, 170 (1972)

FREEMAN, M.A.R., SWANSON, S.A.V., TODD, R.C.: Total replacement of the knee using the Freeman-Swanson knee prosthesis. Clin. Orthop. **94**, 153 (1973a)

FREEMAN, M.A.R., SWANSON, S.A.V., TODD, R.C.: Total replacement of the knee: Design considerations and early clinical results. Acta Orthop. Belg. **39**, 181 (1973b)

FREEMAN, M.A.R., ANDERSSON, G.B.J., JESSOP, J., MASON, R.M.: MacIntosh arthroplasty in rheumatoid arthritis. Acta Orthop. Scand. **45**, 245 (1974)

FREEMAN, M.A.R., BARGREN, J., MILLER, I.: A comparison of osteotomy and joint replacement in the surgical treatment of the arthritic knee. Arch. Orthop. Unfallchir. **88**, 7 (1977a)

FREEMAN, M.A.R., INSALL, J.N., BESSER, W., WALKER, P.S., HALLEL, T.: Excision of the cruciate ligaments in total knee replacement. Clin. Orthop. **126**, 209 (1977b)

FREEMAN, M.A.R., SCULCO, T., TODD, R.C.: Replacement of the severely damaged arthritic knee by the ICLH (Freeman/Swanson) arthroplasty. J. Bone Joint Surg. (Br.) **59**, 64 (1977c)

FREEMAN, M.A.R., TODD, R.C., CUNDY, A.D.: The presentation of the results of knee surgery. Clin. Orthop. **128**, 222 (1977d)

FREEMAN, M.A.R., TODD, R.C., CUNDY, A.D.: A technique for recording the results of knee surgery. Clin. Orthop. **128**, 216 (1977e)

FREEMAN, M.A.R., TODD, R.C., BAMERT, P., DAY, W.H.: ICLH arthroplasty of the knee: 1968–1978. J. Bone Joint Surg. (Br.) **60**, 339 (1978)

HAMMER, A., FREEMAN, M.A.R.: Patellar fracture after replacement of the tibio-femoral joint with the ICLH prosthesis. Arch. Orthop. Traumatic Surg. (1978) (in press)

HEATH, J.C., FREEMAN, M.A.R., SWANSON, S.A.V.: Carcinogenic properties of wear particles from prostheses made in cobalt-chronium alloy. Lancet **1971 I**, 7699, 564

INSALL, J., RANAWAT, C.S., AGLIETTI, P., SHINE, J.: A comparison of four models of total knee-replacement prosthesis. J. Bone Joint Surg. (Am.) **58**, 754 (1976a)

INSALL, J., RANAWAT, C.S., SCOTT, W.N., WALKER, P.: Total condylar replacement. Preliminary report. Clin. Orthop. **120**, 149 (1976b)

INSALL, J., SCOTT, W.N., RANAWAT, C.E.: The total condylar knee prosthesis. J. Bone Joint Surg. (Am.) **61**, 173 (1979)

INSALL, J., SHOJI, H., MAYER, V.: High tibial osteotomy. A five year evaluation. J. Bone Joint Surg. (Am.) **56**, 1397 (1974)

KAPANDJI, I.A.: The mechanical role of the cruciate ligaments. In: The physiology of the joints, Vol. II, p. 120. London, Edinburgh: Churchill Livingstone 1970

MORRISON, J.B.: Biomechanics of the knee joint in relation to normal walking. J. Biomech. **3**, 51 (1970)

MURRAY, D.: Unpublished data

REVELL, P.A., WEIGHTMAN, B., FREEMAN, M.A.R., VERNON-ROBERTS, B.: The production and biology of polyethylene wear debris. Arch. Orthop. Traumatic Surg. **91**, 167 (1978)

SCOTT, W.N.: The total condylar prosthesis. Orthop. Trans. **1**, 103 (1977)

SHOJI, H., INSALL, J.: High tibial osteotomy for osteoarthritis of the knee with valgus deformity. J. Bone Joint Surg. (Am.) **55**, 963 (1973)

SWANSON, S.A.V., FREEMAN, M.A.R.: The design of a knee joint implant. Biomed. Eng. **9**, 348 (1974)

SWANSON, S.A.V., FREEMAN, M.A.R., HEATH, J.C.: Laboratory tests on total joint replacement prostheses. J. Bone Joint Surg. (Br.) **55**, 759 (1973)

Advances in Artificial Hip and Knee Joint Technology

Editors: M. Schaldach, D. Hohmann
In collaboration with R. Thull, F. Hein
1976. 525 figures. XII, 525 pages
(Engineering in Medicine, Volume 2)
ISBN 3-540-07728-6

R. Bombelli

Osteoarthritis of the Hip

Pathogenesis and Consequent Therapy

With a Foreword by M. E. Müller
1976. 160 figures (70 in color). X, 136 pages
ISBN 3-540-07842-8

J. Charnley

Low Friction Arthroplasty of the Hip

Theory and Practice

1979. 440 figures, 205 in color, 22 tables.
X, 376 pages
ISBN 3-540-08893-8

Current Concepts of Internal Fixation of Fractures

Editor: H. K. Uhthoff
Associate Editor: E. Stahl
1980. 287 figures, 51 tables. IX, 452 pages
ISBN 3-540-09846-1

H.-R. Henche

Arthroscopy of the Knee Joint

With a Foreword by E. Morscher
Translated from the German by P. A. Casey
1980. 163 figures, most in color, diagrams by
F. Freuler, 1 table. XII, 85 pages
ISBN 3-540-09314-1

Late Reconstructions of Injured Ligaments of the Knee

Editors: K.-P. Schulitz, H. Krahl, W. H. Stein
With contributions by M. E. Blazina,
D. H. O'Donoghue, S. L. James, J. C. Kennedy,
A. Trillat
1978. 42 figures, 21 tables. V, 120 pages
ISBN 3-540-08720-6

R. Liechti

Hip Arthrodesis and Associated Problems

Foreword by M. E. Müller, B. G. Weber
Translated from the German edition "Die Arthro-
dese des Hüftgelenkes und ihre Problematik" by
P. A. Casey
1978. 266 figures, 35 tables. XII, 269 pages
ISBN 3-540-08614-5

Manual of Internal Fixation

Techniques Recommended by the AO Group
By M. E. Müller, M. Allgöwer, R. Schneider,
H. Willenegger
In collaboration with W. Bandi, A. Boitzy,
R. Ganz, U. Heim, S. M. Perren, W. W. Rittmann
T. Rüedi, B. G. Weber, S. Weller
Translated from the German by J. Schatzker
2nd, expanded and revised edition 1979.
345 figures in color, 2 templates for Preoperative
Planning. X, 409 pages
ISBN 3-540-09227-7

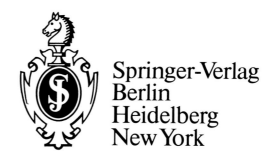

Springer-Verlag
Berlin
Heidelberg
New York

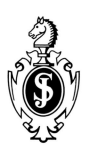